Transvaginal Sonography
A Clinical Atlas

Transvaginal Sonography
A Clinical Atlas

Arthur C. Fleischer, MD
Professor of Radiology and Radiological Sciences
Professor of Obstetrics and Gynecology
Chief, Diagnostic Sonography
Vanderbilt University Medical Center
Nashville, Tennessee

Donna M. Kepple, RT, RDMS
Chief Sonographer
Senior Technical Manager, Ultrasound Section
Vanderbilt University Medical Center
Nashville, Tennessee

With Nine Contributors

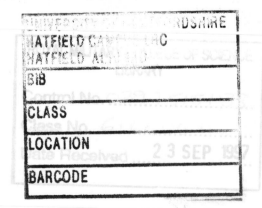

J.B. LIPPINCOTT COMPANY
Philadelphia

Acquisitions Editor: **Lisa McAllister**
Sponsoring Editor: **Emilie Linkins**
Project Editor: **Bridget C. Hannon**
Production Manager: **Caren Erlichman**
Production Coordinator: **MaryClare Malady**
Design Coordinator: **Melissa G. Olson**
Interior Designer: **Holly Reid McLaughlin**
Cover Designer: **Richard Spencer**
Indexer: **Lynne E. Mahan**
Compositor: **Achorn Graphic Services, Inc.**
Printer/Binder: **Quebecor/Kingsport**
Cover Printer: **Lehigh Press**
Color Separator: **Princeton Polychrome Press**

2nd Edition

6   5   4   3   2   1

Library of Congress Cataloging-in-Publication Data

Fleischer, Arthur C.
    Transvaginal sonography : a clinical atlas / Arthur C. Fleischer,
Donna M. Kepple ; with nine contributors. — 2nd ed.
        p.   cm.
    Includes bibliographical references and index.
    ISBN 0-397-51513-8 (alk. paper)
    1. Transvaginal ultrasonography—Atlases. I. Kepple, Donna M.
II. Title.
    [DNLM: 1. Genital Diseases, Female—ultrasonography—atlases.
2. Prenatal Diagnosis, Female—methods—atlases. WP 17 F596t 1995]
RG107.5.T73F56 1995
618'.047543—dc20
DNLM/DLC
for Library of Congress   95-7919
                                                                      CIP

⊗ This paper meets the requirements of ANSI/NISO Z39.48-1992 (permanence of
paper).

The authors and publisher have exerted every effort to ensure that drug selection and
dosage set forth in this text are in accord with current recommendations and practice
at the time of publication. However, in view of ongoing research, changes in
government regulations, and the constant flow of information relating to drug
therapy and drug reactions, the reader is urged to check the package insert for each
drug for any change in indications and dosage and for added warnings and
precautions. This is particularly important when the recommended agent is a new or
infrequently employed drug.

To our clinical and imaging colleagues who, by their thoughtful inquiries, encourage refinement and expanded applications of diagnostic sonography. And to our children Hillary and Jarrod, Braden, Jared and Amy, who will use new technologies to contribute to the future betterment of mankind.

Contributors

Jeanne A. Cullinan, MD
Assistant Professor of Radiology and
  Radiological Sciences
Assistant Professor of Obstetrics and
  Gynecology
Clinical Director of Ultrasound
Vanderbilt University Medical Center
Department of Radiology
Nashville, Tennessee

Arthur C. Fleischer, MD
Professor of Radiology and Radiological
  Sciences
Professor of Obstetrics and Gynecology
Chief, Diagnostic Sonography
Vanderbilt University Medical Center
Nashville, Tennessee

Patricia C. Freeman, RDMS, RDCS
Staff Sonographer
Vanderbilt University Medical Center
Department of Radiology
Nashville, Tennessee

Joyce Kelly, RDMS
Staff Sonographer
Vanderbilt University Medical Center
Department of Radiology
Nashville, Tennessee

Donna M. Kepple, RDMS
Chief Sonographer
Senior Technical Manager
Vanderbilt University Medical Center
Department of Radiology
Nashville, Tennessee

Jodi P. Lerner, MD
Assistant Professor of Clinical Obstetrics and
  Gynecology
Sloane Hospital for Women
College of Physicians and Surgeons
Columbia University
Assistant Professor of Clinical Obstetrics and
  Gynecology
Columbia-Presbyterian Medical Center
New York, New York

Ana Monteagudo, MD
Assistant Professor of Clinical Obstetrics and
  Gynecology
Columbia University
Columbia-Presbyterian Medical Center
New York, New York

Ronald R. Price, PhD
Professor of Radiology
Director, Radiologic Sciences
Vanderbilt University Hospital
Nashville, Tennessee

Martin J. Quinn, MD, MRCOG
Senior Registrar in Obstetrics and
Gynecology
University Hospital of Wales
Cardiff, Wales
United Kingdom

Ilan E. Timor-Tritsch, MD
Professor of Clinical Obstetrics and
Gynecology
Columbia University, College of Physicians
and Surgeons
Director, Obstetric and Gynecologic
Ultrasound
Co-Director, Obstetrical Service
New York, New York

Jaime M. Vasquez, MD
Assistant Professor
Vanderbilt University Hospital
Vanderbilt University Medical Center
Vanderbilt Hospital
Nashville, Tennessee

Preface

The changes in figures and text of this book reflect the new developments and applications of transvaginal sonography (TVS) since the publication of the last edition. Most notably, the higher frequency TVS probes with greater line density have improved sonographic depiction of the endometrium and myometrium and these have become integrated into the clinical evaluation of pre- and post-menopausal patients. More extensive experience has also been gained with transvaginal color Doppler sonography and the expanded chapters on these gynecologic and obstetric applications reflect the current state of the art.

This clinical atlas provides an extensive visual overview of common disorders encountered with transvaginal sonography, with or without color Doppler imaging. It is intended to provide gynecologists, sonographers and sonologists with the latest images and most up-to-date references on the full range of applications of transvaginal, transperineal, and transrectal sonography. This book provides testament to the ever expanding role of transvaginal sonography in gynecology and obstetrics. We hope that you will become as impressed as we are with the improved clinical outcomes provided by the earlier detection and enhanced knowledge of those disease processes depicted by TVS.

A.C.F.
D.M.K.

Preface to the First Edition

Transvaginal sonography (TVS) has greatly enhanced sonographic visualization of pelvic structures. As this clinical atlas demonstrates, major improvements in sonographic diagnosis brought about by TVS have occurred in definitive diagnosis of ectopic pregnancy and evaluation of adnexal masses, as well as detailed depiction of endometrial and myometrial disorders, and early embryonic anatomy.

The purpose of this clinical atlas is to familiarize the reader with the typical sonographic appearances of a variety of disorders. This is done by displaying the native image, without annotations that may distort it, next to a line drawing to draw attention to the areas that need to be noted as well as a line drawing demonstrating the scanning plane in which the image is obtained. When available, the image is compared with the gross pathology, thus enhancing the reader's comprehension of the correlation of the sonographic features with the actual specimen.

The text also includes short chapters on new and specialized applications of TVS such as evaluation of the lower urinary tract and cervix, and the use of transperineal and/or transrectal sonography in a variety of obstetric and gynecologic disorders. The preliminary experience with color Doppler sonography obtained with a transvaginal probe is also discussed.

The reader can refer to this clinical atlas for familiarization with the expected sonographic findings in a particular abnormality. Thus, we hope it is a useful guide for sonographers and sonologists who perform transvaginal sonography.

A.C.F.
D.M.K.

Acknowledgments

The authors would like to acknowledge the contribution of Charles Odwin, RT, RDMS, for his assistance with the line drawings and computed diagrams, John Bobbitt for his photography, Paul Gross, MS, for his artistic drawings and Alice Hammond for her secretarial help with the manuscript. We also thank our contributors Ron Price, PhD, Jeanne Cullinan, MD, Jodi Lerner, MD, Ana Monteagudo, MD, Ilan Timor-Tritsch, MD, Martin Quinn, MBChB, Pat Freeman, RDMS and Joyce Kelly, RDMS, for adding their expertise to this book. Finally, our staff sonographers are thanked for their help in obtaining many of the images. They include Pat Freeman, RDMS, RDCS, Joyce Kelly, RDMS, Kevin Walters, RDMS, Amy Arnold, RT, Cheri Moore, RDMS, Pam Crum, RDMS, RDCS, and Cheryl Norris. We also appreciate the efforts of Emilie Linkins, Lisa McAllister, and Bridget Hannon at J.B. Lippincott for producing a quality text-atlas.

Contents

Transvaginal Sonography

A Clinical Atlas

Transvaginal Sonography: A Clinical Atlas, Second Edition,
edited by Arthur C. Fleischer and Donna M. Kepple.
J.B. Lippincott Company, Philadelphia, © 1995.

CHAPTER **1**

Instrumentation Used in Transvaginal and Transrectal Sonography

Ronald R. Price, PhD
Arthur C. Fleischer, MD

INTRODUCTION

Transvaginal sonography is a recent innovation that requires knowledge of pelvic anatomy, clinical obstetrics and gynecology, and the instrumentation used to obtain diagnostic images. This chapter discusses the instrumentation used in transvaginal and transrectal sonography.

Improvements in sonographic (ultrasound) instrumentation have primarily resulted from more complete integration of high-speed digital electronics. Special-purpose microcomputers are used to steer and dynamically focus array transducers, which allows greater flexibility and control over image formation and which produces images with higher spatial and intensity resolution. Recent developments in real-time color Doppler systems have also been the product of high-speed special-purpose microprocessors.

Selection of a satisfactory ultrasound system

can be puzzling and time consuming. Although there are no definite guidelines, there are general considerations.

This chapter discusses the principles of ultrasound and ultrasound imaging for both transvaginal and transrectal systems, describes the advantages and disadvantages of each, and discusses recent advances in instrumentation design. The features of various transducer-probes relative to their clinical use are also emphasized.

SCANNER CHARACTERISTICS

Real-time instruments rapidly sweep the ultrasound beam through a sector, rectangular or trapezoidal field-of-view by either mechanical or electronic means. Frame rates greater than 15 frames per second are required to produce flicker-free images and to observe moving structures. Because real-time

1

probes are not attached to an articulated scanning arm, the sonographer has great flexibility in selecting the image plane orientation.

Ultrasound scanning systems typically consist of the following:

1. A mechanical or electronic means of moving the ultrasound beam through an image plane
2. An electronic signal processing unit with controls for varying the transducer power output, overall receiver gain, and other operational parameters such as time-gain compensation (TGC)
3. A gray scan display unit equipped with controls for varying the image brightness and contrast
4. A device to permanently record the images (Polaroid, multiimage format camera, paper prints, videotape, or disk).

The console also has a keyboard to superimpose patient identification, examination date, and study information on the recorded image.

TRANSDUCER DESIGNS

Transducers are characterized by their frequency and size or, for arrays, effective aperture and degree of focusing. The typical range of frequency for diagnostic ultrasound imaging is 3.5 to 10.0 MHz. The degree of focusing is either short (1 to 4 cm), medium (4 to 8 cm), or long (6 to 12 cm). Focusing is achieved internally by the crystal shape, externally by an acoustic lens, electronically by selective pulsing of individual elements of an array, or by a combination of these three methods. The length of the zone available for focusing (the Fresnel zone) is governed by the effective transducer aperture and its operating frequency. In selecting a transducer that has the optimum combination of frequency, aperture size, and focal zone for a particular type of examination, the following points should be considered:

1. Increasing transducer frequency generally results in enhanced axial resolution at the expense of reduced tissue penetration. The highest frequency consistent with adequate tissue penetration should be used.
2. For a selected transducer frequency, decreasing the transducer aperture improves lateral resolution in the near field. The length of the Fresnel zone (useful working range of the transducer) is reduced, however, and lateral resolution beyond this zone (the Fraunhaufer

zone) is degraded because of beam divergence. Decreasing the transducer aperture also decreases its sensitivity. Many new array systems provide the capability of dynamic aperture, that is, the effective aperture size can be varied by using smaller or larger subunit transducers, depending on the depth of focus chosen.
3. Larger aperture transducers are more suited to lower frequencies to preserve good lateral resolution at depth, whereas smaller apertures are better suited to higher-frequency transducers to provide improved lateral resolution over the shorter range. The transvaginal probe is limited because of the size of the transducer contact area, or footprint, relative to anatomic constraints.
4. Focused transducers provide improved lateral resolution and sensitivity at the depth of the focal zone, which is limited by the length of the Fresnel zone. The choice of focal zone, therefore, depends on the depth of structures to be resolved.

ALTERNATIVES IN SCANNER DESIGN

The evolution of real-time scanners has led to development of a variety of equipment designs and configurations. In general, no single design provides maximum performance of all imaging parameters; rather, they optimize some imaging parameters at the expense of others. Examples of these are the trade-off of axial resolution obtained from higher frequencies with loss of penetration; good lateral resolution at a specific depth resulting from a large-aperture transducer with decreased lateral resolution at other depths; the convenience of fully electronic scanners against less expensive mechanical scanners; and the large echo-dynamic range of mechanically driven single-element transducers against the more rapid multielement arrays, which may have a more limited echo-dynamic range. Real-time scanners can be grouped according to how they form the beam (focusing) and how the beam is steered (directed) to form the image. In each case (focusing and steering), the task may be accomplished either mechanically or electronically. The use of acoustic lenses is frequently called mechanical focusing. Single-element transducers use mechanical means exclusively for beam focusing, whereas multielement arrays use pulse timing to bring about a convergent beam in the plane of the array and use mechanical means to converge the beam in the "slice-thickness" direction (perpendicular to the array axis). Beam steering can be accomplished either by mechanically moving the transducer (or an acoustic mirror) or by electronic steering by means of pulse-timing sequences in multielement systems. Hybrid systems use a combination of array focusing and mechanical steering.

Advances in real-time ultrasonic imaging are largely the result of more complete integration of high-speed dedicated digital electronics (computers) into the imaging systems. The term "computed sonography" is used to emphasize this increased dependence of the ultrasound image formation on the digital computer.

Single-Element Mechanically Steered Scanners

Most single-element mechanically steered scanners produce a sector (pie-shaped) format image. The sector opening angles may range from 30° to 120°. Most are approximately 90°.

Mechanically steered scanners have two main advantages over electronically steered scanners. First, the use of a single-element transducer requires less sophisticated electronics and generally allows for a more simple transducer head design. Second, there are fewer image artifacts caused by side lobes and grating lobes (unique to electronically steered beams).

There are several disadvantages of mechanically steered arrays. First, the beam focus and beam pattern are fixed for a given transducer. To change the focus, the entire transducer must be changed. Second, the image framing rate depends, in part, on how rapidly the transducer is oscillated. The framing rate is governed by the line density needed to produce an image of diagnostic quality and the depth of the field of view. The velocity of ultrasound in tissue is the ultimate factor governing the oscillation rate of the transducer. The framing rate may become low when large fields of view that require large excursions of the transducer element are chosen. Finally, field-of-view and image frame rates compete in sector format images when the total number of scan lines per image is constant. Thus, large opening angles are needed for large field sizes and small opening angles are required for high resolution, that is, the sector angle must be decreased to achieve higher line density. This problem is not unique to mechanical scanners, however, and is discussed again in relation to electronically steered scanners.

Although there are many variations on the mechanical oscillating transducer design, the most common design is a transducer that oscillates around a single fixed point and yields a sector-shaped image format (Fig. 1-1).

When a single-element wobbler transducer is placed in contact with the skin surface, it is rocked

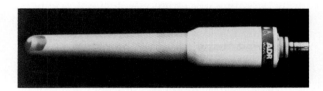

A

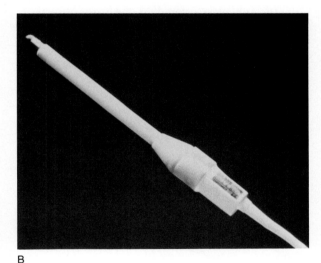

B

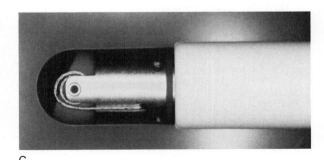

C

FIGURE 1-1
Single-element mechanical sector transvaginal probes. (**A**) Advanced Diagnostic Research/Advanced Technology Laboratories (ADR/ATL) transvaginal probe. (**B**) Diasonics transvaginal probe. (**C**) Close-up view of Diasonics probe showing single-element transducer and its electrical wire.

from side to side in a small arc by means of an electrical motor. Each individual line of the B-mode image is produced and displayed as a radius of a circle with the transducer at the center.

Beam formation in mechanical scanners is achieved through mechanical focusing using either a shaped transducer (internal focus) or an acoustic lens attached to the transducer surface (external focus) (Fig. 1-2). A disadvantage of this design is that the focal zone cannot be conveniently changed during scanning. Electronically focused scanners achieve focusing by delayed pulse sequences, which allow the focal zone to be changed without physically altering the scanner.

Another common design for mechanical scanners is the rotating wheel, which consists of multiple (usually two or three) transducers mounted on a wheel that is rotated by an external motor (Fig. 1-3). The wheel is rotated in the same direction, making the mechanical assembly much simpler. The wheel and transducer are housed in a fluid-filled case with an acoustic window at the lower surface that makes contact with the patient. As the transducers rotate, the output is switched from one transducer to the next in sequence, depending on which transducer has rotated in front of the acoustic

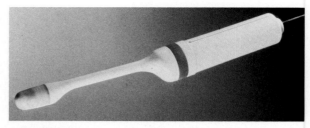

FIGURE 1-3
Dual-element (5.0 and 7.5 MHz) rotating-wheel transvaginal probe (Siemens).

window. This design allows for rapid framing without flicker—typically 30 frames per second. It produces a sector-shaped field of view and allows a wide opening angle of 90° or more. It also allows the incorporation of transducers that have more than one frequency. This allows the use of lower-frequency transducers for the deeper aspects of the field of view and higher-frequency transducers for nearer structures (Fig. 1-4).

Electronically Steered Scanners

Included in the category of electronically steered scanners are linear phased arrays, multielement linear-sequenced arrays, and multielement annular arrays. Through the proper phasing of the transmit/receive timing of the transducer elements used to fabricate the arrays, a composite ultrasonic beam can be created. In this manner, the beam can be focused and steered electronically. Fundamental to electronic focusing is that this element of the array must generate an ultrasonic wave with a definite phase relationship with the waves from the other elements. The ultrasonic waves generated by each element can be superimposed in a precise manner to create the effect of a single wavefront.

Multielement linear-sequenced arrays sequentially pulse subunits of transducers to produce a wavefront that moves normal to the transducer face, yielding a rectangular field, whereas linear phased arrays pulse all of the available transducers for each line and thus must steer as well as focus (Figs. 1-5 and 1-6). A variation on general field geometry is the field shape produced by curvilinear array transducers (Fig. 1-7). Radial or curvilinear arrays operate like conventional linear-sequenced arrays, but instead of being aligned in a straight line, the transducer subelements are aligned along an arc. The arc of the transducer elements may be

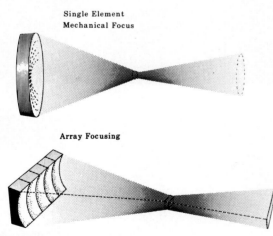

FIGURE 1-2
Single-element scanners require curved transducer crystals or an attached acoustic lens to achieve focusing (*top*). Single-element transducers are thus focused to a specific depth (fixed focus). Array focusing is achieved by altering the times at which each subelement is pulsed, thus allowing multiple focal depths (*bottom*). (Fleischer A, James AE Jr. Diagnostic Sonography: Principles and Clinical Applications. Philadelphia: WB Saunders, 1988.)

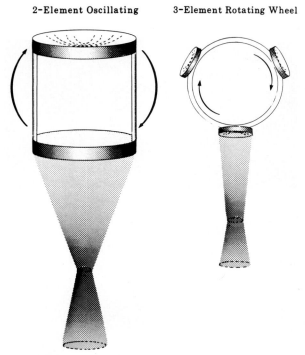

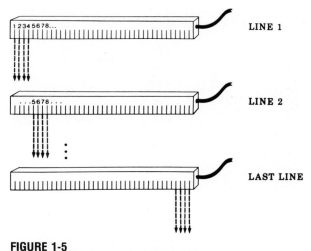

FIGURE 1-5
Linear-sequenced arrays scan the beam by sequentially pulsing transducer subgroups (N-4 illustrated) along the length of the array. Thus, only a small portion of the crystals is used to form any one line. (Fleischer A, James AE Jr. Diagnostic Sonography: Principles and Clinical Applications. Philadelphia: WB Saunders, 1988.)

FIGURE 1-4
Rotating-wheel mechanical scanners with multiple elements provide more rapid frame rates than single-element scanners and may also produce wider fields of view. (Fleischer A, James AE Jr. Diagnostic Sonography: Principles and Clinical Applications. Philadelphia: WB Saunders, 1988.)

these conditions, the field from the N elements are focused at a depth that depends on the magnitude (time interval) of the delays. By changing the delay magnitude, the focal zone can be chosen for a specific depth. The elements may also be sensitive to the returning waves as determined by the same de-

configured to various radii, with the tightest arc giving the highest line density (see Fig. 1-7C). There are several advantages to this design. Better transmission is achieved by launching the ultrasound wave perpendicular to the transducer face as well as to the skin. Beam steering is achieved geometrically rather than by pulse timing, thus eliminating the increased grating lobe artifacts seen in phased arrays at large steering angles and increasing the depth of the field of view, unlike conventional sequenced arrays, which produce rectangular fields of view.

The transducer array is usually composed of many (typically 128 to 256) small piezoelectric crystals (M) arranged in a row (see Fig. 1-5). Because the field from a single small crystal element diverges rapidly, several elements (N) are driven simultaneously and electronic focusing is used. In the subgroup of N crystals, the outer crystals may be pulsed first and the inner crystals delayed. Under

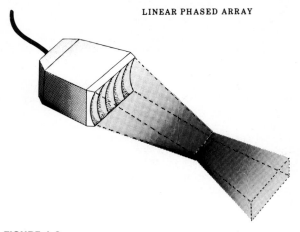

LINEAR PHASED ARRAY

FIGURE 1-6
Linear-sequenced arrays produce rectangular fields of view and use both transmit and receive array focusing.

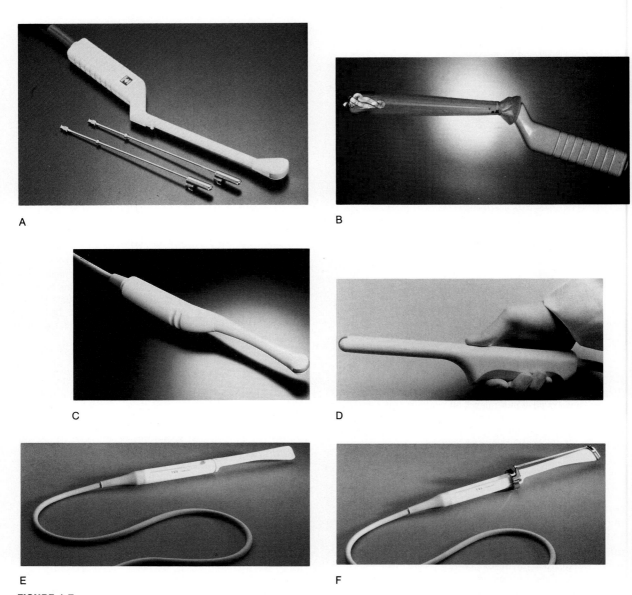

A

B

C

D

E

F

FIGURE 1-7
PHASED CURVILINEAR ARRAYS, are steered to produce a sector-shaped field of view and also use both transmit and receive focusing. (**A**) Curvilinear array (Toshiba America Ultrasound, Inc.) transvaginal probe. The probe has needle guide attachments. (**B**) The same probe with condom covering and gel coating. (**C**) "Tight" curvilinear 6.0-MHz transducer with high line density (Courtesy of Toshiba Ultrasound America, Inc., Tustin, CA). (**D**) ATL curvilinear transvaginal probe, which uses frequencies between 5 and 9 MHz (Courtesy of Advanced Technology Laboratories, Bothell, WA.) (**E**) Acuson transvaginal probe, which allows imaging with three different frequencies. The footprint is "tilted." (Courtesy of Acuson Inc.) (**F**) Same as *E* with needle guide attached (Courtesy of Acuson Inc.).

lay factors used in transmission, resulting in a focusing effect on the returning signals. A single scan line in the real-time image is formed in this manner. The next adjacent scan line is generated using another group of N crystals, formed by shifting the previous N crystals one crystal position along the transducer array. The same transmit/receive pattern is repeated for this set of N crystals, and for all other sets of N crystals along the array in a cyclic manner. Focusing in the plane of the transducer elements improves lateral resolution as well as sensitivity by increasing the amount of energy in the focal zone (constructive interference) (see Fig. 1-6). Focusing in the plane perpendicular to the scan lines determines the slice thickness and is accomplished by the use of mechanically focused elements.

The linear phased array is frequently called the electronic sector scanner because the resulting field is pie-shaped, with the field diverging as the distance from the transducers is increased (Fig. 1-8 and see Fig. 1-7). Creation of the main beam and side lobes is illustrated in Figure 1-9. The outside trans-

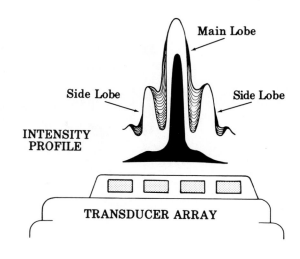

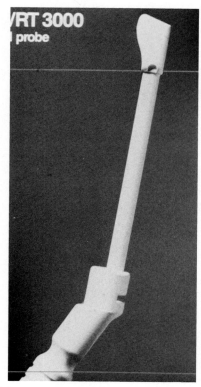

FIGURE 1-8
Phased-array transvaginal probe (General Electric Co.).

ducers are activated first and the inner transducers are delayed, with the central transducer delayed the most to yield a wave axis perpendicular to the plane of the transducer. By varying the order of the delay, the wave can be focused at a specified depth and the wave axis can be scanned through a sector of 60° to 90°. Properly selected delays can produce steering and focusing simultaneously. One distinction between linear-sequenced arrays and linear phased arrays is that, in the phased array, every element is used to form the beam for each line and, in the linear-sequenced array, only a small subset of the transducers is used to create a given line.

The phased annular array scanner is a hybrid system and has characteristics of both mechanical and electronic designs. The transducer is comprised of a series of independent transducers. Each element is shaped like an annular ring and multiple elements are arranged in concentric rings around a central transducer element (Fig. 1-10).

Beam formation and focusing is achieved electronically by proper phasing of the transducer elements. An advantage of this design is that focusing is achieved in two dimensions, similar to a single focused element, but, unlike mechanical focusing, the focal zone can be changed without physically changing the transducer. Conversely, beam steering must be achieved mechanically. Either the beam is swept through a trapezoidal field of view with an oscillating mirror or the transducer is oscillated. As with other mechanically steered scanners, the trans-

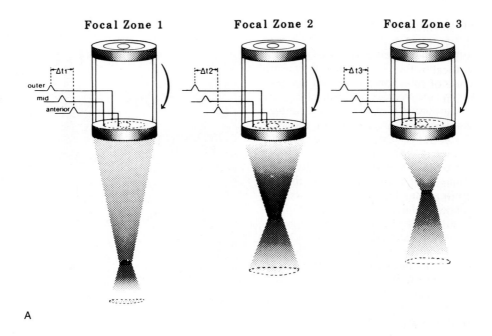

A

B

FIGURE 1-10
Phased annular arrays are capable of dynamic, both transmit (**A**) and receive (**B**) focusing and offer the added advantage that the beam is focused in two dimensions, unlike linear arrays, which are capable of electronic focusing in the plane of the array only. Receive-focus is carried out in real time by means of high-speed digital processors capable of monitoring the response received by each transducer element. By using predetermined time-delay patterns, the system can distinguish echoes that come from different depths by the relative time delays (Δt) observed by the array elements. For linear arrays, focusing in the slice-thickness direction must be accomplished mechanically. Annular arrays also must be steered mechanically. (Fleischer A, James AE Jr. Diagnostic Sonography: Principles and Clinical Applications. Philadelphia: WB Saunders, 1988.)

ducers, mirrors, or both are contained within a fluid-filled housing.

Commercially available annular array scanners offer a variable focal zone option that allows the user to specify one of several focal zones. The systems also operate in a survey–scan mode in which the transducers are cyclically scanned through the focal zones while the operator observes the images. Once a particular depth of interest is specified, the operator selects that focal zone. Some transducers can image at various frequencies. This allows low-frequency imaging for deeper structures and higher-frequency imaging for more superficial ones. The transducer elements can be configured to operate at selectable frequencies. Scanning while the patient is on a pelvic examination table allows the patient's legs to be suspended. The examiner can bring structures of interest closer to the transducer by palpation (Fig. 1-11).

DISPLAY AND STORAGE OF REAL-TIME IMAGES

The number of gray shades displayed in the ultrasound image depends on the characteristics of the scan converter, which translates the pressure change received by the transducer into numbers that are stored in the digital scan converter (Fig. 1-12). In these systems, the analog voltage levels that correspond to the returning echo amplitudes for each line of the image are digitized by an analog-to-digital converter. The generated array of numbers is then stored in a digital memory. The digital memory is divided into a number of picture elements, or pixels. The size of the memory is described by the number of pixel elements, such as 512 × 512. Each pixel represents a region in the body, the size of which is equal to the image field of view divided by the number of pixels. For example, a 25-cm field of view imaged with a 512- × 512-pixel matrix yields pixel sizes of approximately 0.5 × 0.5 mm. The memory can then be interrogated and the image displayed on a video monitor. The brightness of the television signal representing each picture element is controlled by the value stored in the corresponding digital word. The number of shades of gray is determined by the size of the digital word used to store the information for each picture element. The size of the word is measured in terms of the number of bits, frequently referred to as the depth of the memory. Three-bit words provide the capacity for displaying 8 shades of gray, 4 bits provide 16 shades of gray, and 5 bits provide 32 shades of gray. Most digital memories used for real-time scanners are at least 512 × 512 by 6 to 8 bits deep (64 to 256 shades of gray).

The discreteness of both the spatial domain and the gray-scale shades provides an image that is not as smooth as the analog image. The appearance of the image is different, and the margin between picture element pixels is more definite than with analog displays; however, as the number of pixels increases and the size of the pixels becomes smaller, it becomes difficult to distinguish the two types of images. Images are frequently processed by linear interpolation in order to soften the edges of the pixels. Interpolation fills in between picture elements without altering the original image data. The digital system is more stable, however, does not drift, and is less sensitive to heat, which eliminates long start-up time and allows the institution of predigital and postdigital image processing.

The most common methods for permanent archiving of ultrasound images are multiimage format film, paper print, and videotape. Multiformat film imagers are the recording device of choice for not only ultrasound but also computed tomography, scintigraphy, and magnetic resonance imaging (Fig. 1-13A). Due to the transportability of most ultrasound systems, multiformat cameras of compact design are usually chosen. In most applications, the

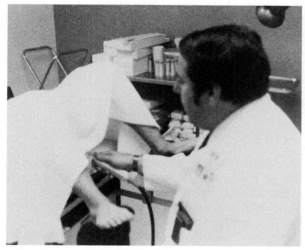

FIGURE 1-11
A pelvic examination table is preferred for transvaginal sonography. Advantages of the table include support of the patient's legs and placement of the patient in a reverse Trendelenburg position, which assists collection of physiologic fluid around the uterus, tubes, and ovaries.

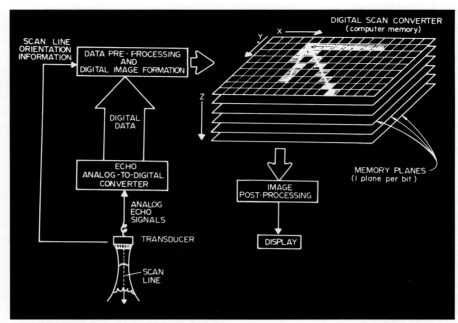

FIGURE 1-12
Block diagram of a digital ultrasound system. Echo signals detected by the transducer are digitized and stored in computer memory (digital scan converter), which is read out to a video monitor. (Fleischer A, James AE Jr. Diagnostic Sonography: Principles and Clinical Applications. Philadelphia: WB Saunders, 1988.)

9-on-1 format on 8- by 10-inch film is adequate for viewing and measurements. If larger recorded images are desired, the 6-on-1 format is also readily available. Paper printers are economical, and can produce a variety of different formats. (see Fig. 1-13*B*). They do not require processing but do not have as great a gray scale latitude as cut film.

The most recent innovation in image display involves storage of many (60 to 80) images on a single disk. These systems allow several scanners to be connected to a single recording device.

Videotape recorders are also popular storage devices because they allow a real-time study to be recorded as it is performed, often with superimposed audio from the operator for further clarification of orientation and other descriptive findings.

Videocassette recorders (VCR) using 0.5-inch VHS standard videotape are relatively inexpensive and store several hours of video on a single tape with acceptable resolution. These units generally include slow and fast motion playback modes, still-frame replay mode, and automatic search capabilities. In most units, when still-frame imaging is used, the number of displayed lines is reduced to approximately one half of the real-time display resolution. Super VHS VCRs improve image resolution by increasing the number of lines in the image but are more expensive than conventional VCRs (see Fig. 1-13*A*).

COMPUTERIZED ULTRASOUND

In addition to the use of digital scan converters, which has become common in current real-time systems, several manufacturers are replacing many of the traditional analog portions of pulsing and receiving hardware with digital components. Digital components provide flexibility through software programmability that analog systems cannot. Only recently have the price and speed of digital systems been such that the replacement of analog circuits could be considered. High-speed parallel processors under program-control driving multielement array transducers have made it possible to dynamically

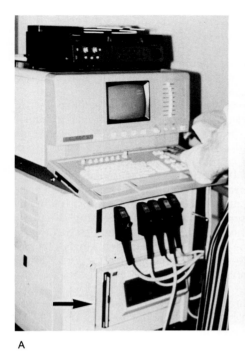 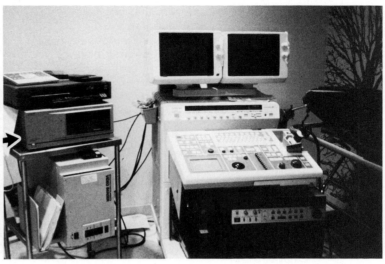

A   B

FIGURE 1-13
Recording devices. (**A**) A multiformat camera (*arrow*) records hard-copy film. A VCR is used for videotaping on top of Acuson 128. (**B**) Color and black-and-white printer attached to Toshiba 270 scanner (*arrow*).

vary pulsing and receiving signal processing steps. Analog circuits must be physically changed each time a change in signal processing is made.

As described previously, a beam can be formed and steered by pulse timing of transducer arrays. The focal depth of the beam depends on the values of the time delays between the pulsing of the outer transducer elements relative to the center elements. Once a beam is launched from the transducer, it cannot be controlled further. In the case of transmit focus, the primary benefit of digital flexibility benefit is that the focal zone can be chosen before each scan without having to physically change the transducers. This is a practical benefit that does not change the resultant image quality compared with analog systems.

The most significant improvement in image quality that results directly from the use of digital systems is the benefit derived from dynamic signal processing on the returning echoes. This is often referred to as "receive focusing" or "dynamic focusing." Although the transmitted beam can have only a single focal zone, it is possible to selectively "lis-ten" to the returning echoes. Returning echoes from different depths arrive at different times, that is, nearby reflections are detected first, followed by reflection from deeper sites. Accepting only those echoes that have the proper pattern of arrival times ensures that the returning signals are in focus for each depth. This is the essence of dynamic focusing. To accomplish dynamic focusing, the system must have almost complete control over the pulsing and receiving of each transducer element, which requires the power of high-speed parallel processing. Conventional multielement scanners sum the received signal with equal weighting from the various elements to produce the echo signal. In the parallel processed systems, the gain of each element is controlled separately. This dynamically variable gain capability is referred to as "dynamic apodization." Dynamic variations in the individual gains can be used to discard echoes from off-axis sites to minimize side lobe and grating lobe artifacts. The same technique can be used to change the size of the aperture during the scan, depending on whether the near or far field is being scanned.

ENDOLUMINAL TRANSDUCER-PROBES

Recent advances in transducer designs have resulted in development of transducers that can be mounted on probes and placed within various lumina of the body. The two major types of endoluminal probes that have gained clinical application include transvaginal transducer-probes for imaging the uterus, early pregnancy, and adnexa and transrectal transducer-probes for imaging the cervix, uterus, and parametrium.

Because of the proximity of the organ of interest to the transducer, both transvaginal and transrectal probes can use transducers with frequencies of 5 or 7.5 MHz. In general, the use of these probes can contribute to increased diagnostic specificity by the improved resolution afforded by the proximity of the transducer to the area of interest and the higher transducer frequencies that can be used.

Transvaginal transducer-probes significantly enhance the sonographic evaluation of the uterus and adnexa. There are numerous different types of commercially available probes (Table 1-1) (Platt, 1987). The major types of transvaginal probes include those that use a single-element mechanical oscillating transducer, those with a curved linear array, those that use an electronically phased steering of multiple transducer elements, and those that use a single-element transducer that rotates (see Figs. 1-1 through 1-9).

Probe focus and other parameters are summarized in Table 1-1. In general, the field of view of most transvaginal probes is approximately 10 cm, with the focal range varying from 2 to 7 cm depending on the type and design of the transducers. The sector of the field of view is typically 90° to 100°, with some rotating wheel designs going as high as 240°. The design of the probe housing ranges from one in which a straight shaft with a transducer is mounted on the end to one in which the transducer's face is inclined relative to the handle.

Needle guides that attach to the shaft are available on several transvaginal transducer-probes; some are flush with the shape of the probe, and others are outrigged (Fig. 1-14). When probes with an outrigged needle guide are used, the operator must be careful no to press on the area of the anterior urethra. The path of the needle can be superimposed on the imaging monitor, thereby providing precise guidance for a variety of interventional procedures such as a follicular or cyst aspiration.

Each transvaginal transducer-probe varies according to the size of the actual contact surface or footprint, the size of the shaft, and the angle of the handle. Handles that assist the operator in determining probe orientation are preferred. Probes with the smallest shaft size may be preferred in virgins or young girls and older women with less distensible vaginas.

Transrectal probes are used extensively for prostate evaluation, but can be used for guidance of cerclage, intrauterine tandem placement, guided dilation and curettage, or intrauterine contraceptive device retrieval (Fig. 1-15A) (Fleischer and coworkers, 1990). These probes usually contain at least one array of transducers. For imaging in the sagittal plane, a series of linear array elements with electronic or phased-array focusing is usually used. For those probes that have two elements, the axial view is usually obtained by a single-element mechanically oscillated transducer, curved linear array, or phased-array transducer array (see Fig. 1-15B).

Transducers that can be placed on an examiner's fingertip are being developed (Fig. 1-16). These also may have biplanar imaging capabilities, with a curvilinear array mounted at the top of the housing and a slightly curved linear array mounted below.

DOPPLER SYSTEMS

Doppler systems have evolved from the relatively simple continuous wave (CW) units, which yielded an audible frequency to the user's earphones, to current pulsed-Doppler systems capable of yielding color-coded flow images in real time. This evolution has been made possible, in large part, by the advent of relatively inexpensive high-speed parallel-processing computers. The basic interaction of the Doppler effect has not changed over the years, but the ability to rapidly process and analyze the returning echo data has improved (Taylor, 1987).

Ultrasound passing through the body is either absorbed (a decrease in beam intensity of about 1 dB/cm/MHz) or reflected. Ultrasound is reflected at each point along the beam where the relative acoustic impedance changes. If this reflecting interface is stationary, the frequency of the reflected wave is identical to the incident beam. If the interface is moving, the reflected echo frequency is shifted up or down (relative to the incident wave) by an amount proportional to the velocity along the beam direction. This shift is called the Doppler shift and is given by the following equation:

TABLE 1-1
Transvaginal Transducer-Probe Characteristics

Manufacturer	Freq (MHz)	Focal Range (mm)	Sector Size	Type	Insertion Length (cm)	"Footprint" Diameter (cm)	Needle Guide	Color Doppler
Acuson	5.0	15–40	90°	Phased-array sector	16.0	0.8	Flush	+
ADR/ATL Ultra-sound	2.5, 5.0, 6.5	15–40	90°	Phased-array sector	16.0	0.8	Flush	+
ADR/ATL Ultra-sound	3.0 5.0	40–60 30–60	90° 90°	Mechanical sector	16.0	1.9–2.5	Flush	+
Ausonics/ Universal	6.0 (5–9)	15–60	150°	Curvilinear convex	2–4	1.9	Flush	+
Ausonics/ Universal	7.5	20–40	90°	Mechanical sector	17.0	1.2–2.5		
Bruel & Kjaer	7.5	10–60	115°	Mechanical sector	7.2	2.1–3.8	Flush	
Bruel & Kjaer	5.0	30–70	112°	Mechanical sector	15.0	1.2–2.6	Outrigged	
Cone Instruments/ Kretz	7.5	20–50	240°	Mechanical sector	14.0	1.6–2.0		
Corometrics Med Systems (Aloka)	5.0 5.0	15–45 15–50	60° 88°	Curvilinear convex	17.9	1.9–2.7		+
Diasonics	7.5	20–40	100°	Mechanical sector	20.2	1.5–1.7	Outrigged	
Elscint	6.5	20–60	30–105°	Mechanical sector	16.1	2.6	Outrigged	
GE Medical Systems	5.0	25–80	90°	Phased-array sector	19.2	1.0–2.5	Flush	
Hewlett-Packard	5.0	20–80	110°	Mechanical sector	16.0	1.4–2.6	Outrigged	
Hewlett-Packard	6.5	15–45	80°	Curvilinear convex	14.0	1.6–2.0	Flush	
International/ ESAOTE Biomedica	5.0, 7.5	15–70	90°	Annular array sector	14.0	1.8–2.2	Flush	
Philips Ultrasound International	5.0 7.5	30–70 20–65	90°	Mechanical sector	15.0	2.3–3.3		
Picker Interna-tional	3.5, 5.0, 7.5	~20–40	~100°	Mechanical sector	~23	2.0		
Pie Medical USA	5.0	Sector: 40–120 Linear: 40–80	Sector: 110° Linear: 5 cm	Mechanical sector or linear	Sector: 15 Linear: 19 20.0	Sector: 3.5 Linear: 1.2–2.2 2.0–2.3		
Siemens Medical Systems	5.0, 6.0, 7.5, Selectable	20–70	220°	Annular array sector	14.0	1.8	Flush	
Shimadzu	5.0	20–120 (auto-focus)	115° or 90°	Curvilinear convex or phased array sector	15.0	0.7		
Toshiba Medical Systems	5.0	50 (auto-focus)	86°	Curvilinear convex	20.0	2.2–2.7	Flush	+
Toshiba Medical Systems	6.0	35	121°	Curvilinear convex	14.5	2.3–2.6	Flush	+

13

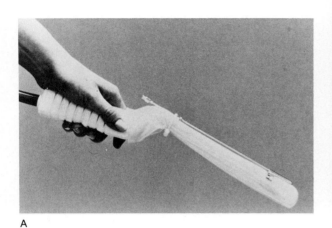

A

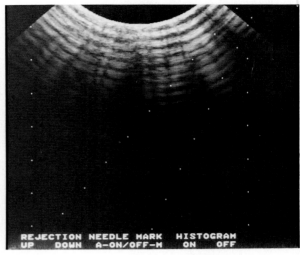

B

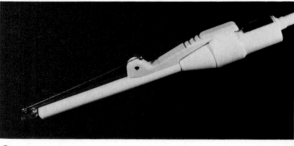

C

FIGURE 1-14.
Needle guides. (**A**) Needle-guide attachment to a curvilinear array transvaginal probe. (**B**) Needle path display on imaging monitor. (**C**) Mechanical sector transvaginal probe with outrigged needle guide. (**D**) Needle path display on imaging monitor.

D

$$\Delta f = \frac{\pm 2V f_0}{c} \cos \theta$$

where Δf = Doppler shift frequency (Hz)
          V = velocity of the moving interface (cm/sec)
          f_0 = frequency of the incident sound (Hz)
          c = velocity of sound in tissue (cm/sec)
          θ = the angle in degrees between the sound beam direction and the direction of the moving interface

The actual received frequency (fr) from the moving interface is:

$$fr = f_0 \pm \Delta f$$

When the impinging ultrasound beam passes through a blood vessel, the ultrasound wave scatters. In this process, small amounts of sound energy are absorbed by each red cell and are reradiated in all directions. If the red blood cell is moving with respect to the source, the backscattered energy returning to the receiving transducer is shifted in fre-

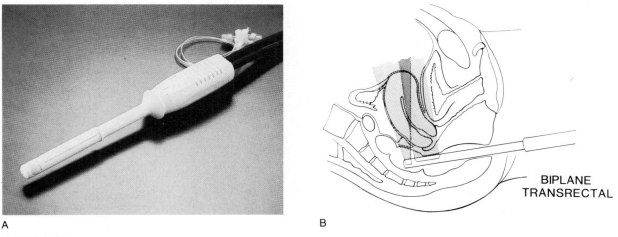

A   B

FIGURE 1-15
Biplane transrectal probe. (**A**) Transrectal probe with biplanar capability has both linear and sector scanners incorporated into a single probe. (**B**) Diagram of field-of-view and scan-plane orientations for the dual transducer transrectal probe.

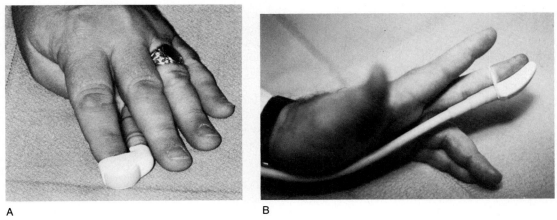

A   B

FIGURE 1-16
Fingertip transducers. (**A**) ''Fingertop'' curvilinear array transducer. (**B**) Longitudinally oriented curved linear array. (Courtesy of Hitachi Corporation.)

quency; the magnitude and direction of this shift is proportional to the velocity of the respective cell. If the ultrasound beam is considered to fill the entire lumen of a blood vessel, then the backscattered signal consists of all the Doppler shifts produced by the red cells moving through the ultrasonic beam. Because there is always a range of velocities, from zero at the vessel wall to a peak value near the center of the vessel lumen, there is always a spectrum of Doppler shift frequencies. The frequency spectrum is derived by applying a mathematical operation (i.e., a Fourier transformation) to the returning echo wave train. This spectrum can become complex with pulsating blood flow and vessel wall motion, especially when blood flow disturbances due to anatomic defects are present. Vessel wall irregularity, ulcerated plaques, narrowed or partially occluded vessels, or other abnormalities such as stenotic heart valves cause velocity variation that can be readily detected by differences in the frequency spectrum of the Doppler signal.

A number of imaging schemes have been devised to give the user some information on the vessel anatomy in addition to blood flow. The simplest of these uses a CW Doppler transducer fixed to a mechanical arm. As the transducer moves over a vessel of interest, an image corresponding to each site of inquiry is produced on a storage oscilloscope. This simple continuous wave (CW) Doppler instrument is deficient in depth resolution.

A practical means to add depth resolution to a Doppler instrument is to pulse the source and add a range gate to the receiver. These pulsed Doppler devices are similar to a pulse-echo instrument in that bursts of ultrasound are emitted at a regular rate into the body tissue. A new pulse is not transmitted until echoes from the previous pulse cease or are significantly diminished. The depth of a pulse can be determined by noting the time of its flight to an interface and of its return. Relatively short bursts of approximately 0.5 to 1.0 μsec can be used to give high axial resolution for detection of the location and separation of interfaces to within 1 mm or less.

The principle of pulsed Doppler is different from that of a pulse-echo instrument. To determine the Doppler spectrum of a reflected wave from many depths simultaneously requires fast parallel processing to calculate the frequency shift of each pixel. Because of the relatively long time needed to perform a Fourier transformation, faster phase-sensitive calculations are often used instead. To display these multidimensional data (i.e., flow magnitude, direction, and location), color-coded images

are often used. In the image, color is used to encode direction, and hue is used to encode relative magnitude. Red is usually assigned to flow toward the transducer; blue is used for flow away from the transducer; lighter hues represent high-frequency shifts in areas of flow with increased velocities. Turbulent flow can be imaged as a mosaic of yellows and greens.

A disadvantage of pulsed Doppler scanners is their inability to accurately determine rapid flow. Consequently, they may present aliased results in which a high-flow location is actually presented as a low-flow location. The maximum flow measured by a pulsed Doppler system is determined by the pulse repetition (PRF) of the system. Specifically, the detected Doppler shift frequency (Δf) cannot be greater than PRF/2. Increasing PRF to allow estimates of rapid flow limits the field of view to superficial structures and adds the potential for range ambiguity errors. Range ambiguity errors occur when echoes from previous lines are received as echoes from the current line (Gill and coworkers, 1989). Flow aliasing can often be recognized and generally does not lead to mistaken diagnoses.

Recently, color Doppler sonography can be displayed as a function of the power spectrum. For this application, the pixel elements are assigned color wherever there is flow. This process is thought to be three to four times more sensitive than conventional color Doppler sonography (Rubin, 1994).

QUALITY CONTROL

The purpose of a quality assurance program is to ensure that the diagnostic quality of all ultrasonic images is maintained at the maximum attainable level. Part of this program must include monitoring procedures that ensure the proper and consistent operation of all equipment. Equipment acceptance tests must be performed on new equipment and repeated whenever major equipment repairs are made. Quality assurance tests should be performed on a routine basis to detect deviations from the baseline acceptance tests. Quality assurance is the joint responsibility of the sonologist, sonographer, and service support personnel.

There are numerous test objects and instruments available for assessing the performance of ultrasonic equipment. Also available are detailed protocols for establishing a quality assurance program. The most versatile and complete test object is probably the American Institute of Ultrasound in Medicine (AIUM) Standard 100 mm Test Object. The standard AIUM test object is filled with a relatively nonattenuating medium. Phantoms with a similar configuration but filled with an attenuating tissue-equivalent material are also commercially available. These tissue-equivalent phantoms provide system beam-parameter measurements in a more clinically pertinent situation (Fig. 1-17). The ability to discern closely spaced wires in the far field corresponds to axial resolution capabilities, whereas the width of the echo returned from centrally placed wires corresponds to lateral resolution properties. The ability to depict variously sized cysts as shown within the soft tissue matrix correlates to the ability to discern cystic structures within organs.

A minimal quality assurance program should include routine monitoring of the performance of the gray scale photography, the image system sensitivity, the axial resolution, and the accuracy and linearity of distance markers. In addition to evaluation of the gray scale system, the AIUM Test Object may be used to assess each of the other system parameters. The minimal quality assurance program provides relative parameter values, which are useful for detecting early changes in image system characteristics. Absolute measurements of system parameters are more difficult and may require additional test objects and equipment.

Of equal importance to the performance testing is documentation of the test results. These recorded data are essential for accurate monitoring of equipment performance and are useful to both the equipment service personnel and the equipment manufacturer. Such documentation may become required by government regulatory and certifying agencies.

The initial camera settings, scan converter output controls, or both largely depend on individual points of reference. Once a baseline is established, a daily evaluation should be made to ensure that the same range of echo amplitudes as previous test exposures can be seen.

Most systems generate a gray scale bar displayed to one side or at the bottom of the image. This bar should be examined daily for consistency of step distribution and display. The comparison can be made either by visual inspection or with the aid of a densitometer, which is more quantitative.

A simple test for system sensitivity stability can be performed with the AIUM phantom. After carefully positioning the transducer directly above the reference wires, which are spaced 2 cm apart, and,

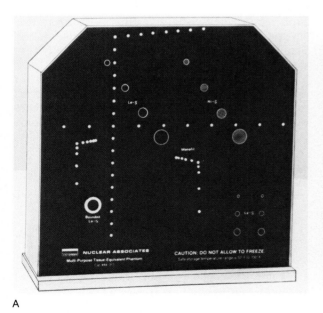

A

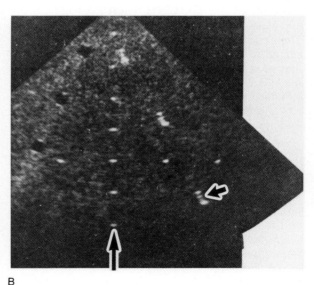

B

FIGURE 1-17
Phantom. (**A**) Photograph of soft tissue cyst phantom. (**B**) Image from phantom illustrating axial resolution as the ability to depict closely spaced wires (*short arrow*), lateral resolution of beam as the size of the center dot (*long arrow*), and cysts within the soft tissue matrix. (Courtesy of Nuclear Associates.)

after ensuring that the transducer face is flat against the phantom surface, the system gain (attenuation or output) settings should be adjusted to display a one-division echo from the most distant wire. The gain setting should not change on subsequent recordings. Similarly, the minimum gain settings required to yield a discernible echo in the B-mode image should not change with time. This method determines the stability of the instrumentation over time.

A single image of the AIUM phantom provides data on axial resolution as well as the accuracy and linearity of the distance markers. Axial resolution is assessed from the minimum resolvable spacing in the set of diagonal wires at the center of the phantom. Within this set, wire spacings range from 1 to 5 mm. Most imaging systems should exhibit the ability to resolve 2-mm wire spacings, and this value should remain constant.

The accuracy and linearity of the system-generated distance markers can be evaluated by measuring the distances of the vertical and horizontal wires from a B-mode image. The distance between the top and bottom wires in the 2-cm spaced groups is actually 10 cm, and this distance, as estimated by the markers, should not differ by more than 2 mm.

BIOEFFECTS CONSIDERATIONS

Theoretic extrapolation from bioeffects that have occurred at intensities and magnitudes higher than that used for diagnostic sonography has suggested that there is a threshold for possible production of bioeffects at 100 mW/cm^2. There has never been a biologically significant adverse bioeffect attributed to diagnostic ultrasound, however (Merritt, 1989).

Manufacturers must report the intensities used for diagnostic imaging, duplex, and color Doppler imaging. Most manufacturers have complied with the Food and Drug Administration recommendation of intensities lower than 94 mW/cm^2. Before purchasing a transvaginal probe, manufacturer data on the intensities used should be reviewed.

Some researchers believe that transvaginal sonography, with the probe nearer to the embryo than in conventional sonographic scanning, delivers more of the incident beam to potentially sensitive tissue. Because higher frequencies and more well-focused beams are used for transvaginal sonography, however, less of the incident beam is actually propagated (Goldstein, 1989).

A case of excessive pressure on a follicle-bearing ovary or hemorrhagic ovarian mass potenti-

ating rupture or torsion has not been reported. A more likely complication, however, is the potential for infection when the probe is not properly prepared with a bacteriostatic medium between studies. We recommend the use of a bacteriostatic spray (Sporocidin) or sanitizing cloth to be applied to the probe after each study (Odwin and coworkers, 1990); however, each manufacturer has specific recommendations for disinfection of its transducers.

PROBE PREPARATION, COVERS, AND GEL

There are several products and methods for disinfection of transvaginal and transrectal probes. The most practical and efficacious one involves spraying the probe with a disinfectant before use. Sporocidin is sufficiently bacteriostatic and virostatic (including being effective against the human immunodeficiency virus) because it kills on contact (Odwin and coworkers, 1990). The use of this spray does not require that the probe sit in disinfectant. Because each probe is made to different specifications, however, each manufacturer recommends a specific method for disinfection (Table 1-2).

Latex condoms can be used as probe covers. To secure the condom with sufficient tension to the probe, it can be twisted over the shaft before it is secured with rubber bands. Most departments use Sani-cloth (Nice-Pak Products, Orangeburg, NY) to disinfect the probe between uses.

There are a variety of acoustic gels used for transvaginal scanning. A sufficient amount of gel needs to be placed both within and around the condom to provide adequate acoustic coupling. Some

TABLE 1-2
TVS Transducer Disinfection Policy

1. Before initiating any TVS examination, the transducer must be disinfected by wiping it clean with a Sani-cloth. This procedure should be followed if transducers are changed during the examination.

2. All TVS transducers must have excess gel removed from the shaft of the transducer before disinfecting the transducer with Metri-spray (gluetaraldehyde). Excess liquid will drain off the transducer and should be placed in an appropriate container by the sink. The transducer should be wiped off with a Sani-cloth before preparing it for the next patient.

3. At the conclusion of each patient's TVS examination, all transducers are wiped off and cleansed to remove any remaining excess gel.

gels may affect sperm motility and should not be used in patients undergoing insemination (Odwin and coworkers, 1990).

SUMMARY

This chapter has discussed and illustrated the pivotal and clinically pertinent principles involved in transvaginal and transrectal sonographic imaging. An understanding of the probe design can optimize transvaginal imaging with these transducer probes.

REFERENCES

Fleischer A, Burnett L, Jones H. Guidance for intraoperative uterine procedures with transrectal sonography. Radiology 1990;176:576.

Gill RW, Kossoff MB, Kossoff G, Griffiths KA. New class of pulsed Doppler US ambiguity at short ranges. Radiology 1989;173:272–275.

Goldstein A. Advances in transducer technology, digital circuitry and software have enhanced ultrasound image quality. Diagnostic Imaging 1989;11.

Merritt C. Ultrasound safety: What are the issues? Radiology 1989;173:304.

Odwin C, Fleischer A, Kepple D, et al. Probe covers and disinfectants for transvaginal transducers. J Diagnostic Medical Sonography 1990;6:130.

Platt LD. New look in ultrasound: The vaginal probe. Contemp Obstet Gynecol 1987;30:99.

Rubin JM, Bude RO, Carson PL, Bree RL, Adler RS. Power Doppler US: A potentially useful alternative to mean frequency-based color Doppler US. Radiology 1994;190:853.

Taylor KJW. Going to the depths with duplex Doppler. Diagnostic Imaging 1987;9:106.

Transvaginal Sonography: A Clinical Atlas, Second Edition,
edited by Arthur C. Fleischer and Donna M. Kepple.
J.B. Lippincott Company, Philadelphia, © 1995.

CHAPTER **2**

Normal Pelvic Anatomy and Scanning Techniques

Arthur C. Fleischer, MD
Donna M. Kepple, RDMS

INTRODUCTION

Transvaginal sonography (TVS) provides better resolution of the uterus and ovaries than conventional transabdominal sonography (TAS). Although the proximity of the transducer-probe to the pelvic organs allows more detailed depiction with TVS than with TAS, the limited field of view and unusual scanning planes depicted with TVS make it more difficult for the sonographer to become oriented to the images (Fig. 2-1).

As the sonographer develops a systematic approach for examining the uterus and adnexal structures, the examination becomes easier to perform. Usually, we first depict the uterus in long axis in a sagittal plane, then we delineate the adnexa in a semicoronal or semiaxial plane. The last images are obtained of the cervix and cul-de-sac as the transducer is withdrawn from the vaginal fornices.

This chapter describes the sonographic appearances of the uterus, ovary, and other adnexal and pelvic structures, with emphasis on how they are best depicted during a TVS examination.

SCANNING TECHNIQUE AND INSTRUMENTATION

The three scanning maneuvers used in TVS include:

1. Vaginal insertion of the probe with side-to-side movement within the upper vagina for oblique sagittal imaging (Fig. 2-2*A*).
2. Transverse orientation of the probe for imaging of the adnexa and uterus in various degrees of semiaxial to semicoronal planes (see Fig. 2-2*B*). This is the best orientation for examining the adnexa in most patients.
3. Variation of the depth of probe insertion for optimal imaging of the fundus and corpus; imaging of the cervix is optimized by gradual withdrawal of the probe into the midvagina (see Fig. 2-2*C*).

Other maneuvers, such as placing the patient in a decubitus position to bring a floating yolk sac/embryo closer to the probe, can be used in selected cases (see Fig. 2-2*D*).

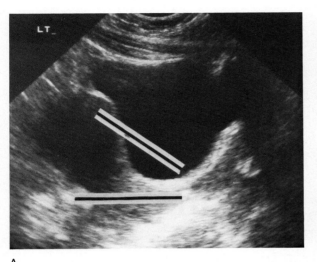
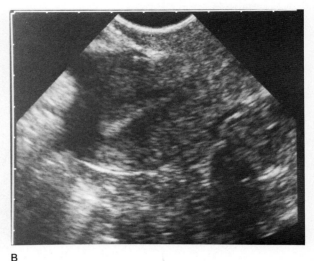

A   B

FIGURE 2-1
Comparison of transabdominal and transvaginal pelvic sonography. (**A**) Sector seen in TVS superimposed on a transabdominal pelvic sonogram. (**B**) Transvaginal image showing field of view depicted in *A*.

Unlike TAS, bladder distension is not required for TVS. Overdistension can hinder TVS by placing the desired field of view outside of the optimal focal range of the transducer. In patients with a severely anteflexed uterus, minimal distension straightens the uterus relative to the imaging plane.

As with conventional sonographic equipment, the operator should select the highest frequency transducer that allows adequate penetration and depiction of an area of interest. Thus, 5.0- and 7.5-MHz transducers are preferred, but these higher frequency transducers limit the field of view to within 6 to 8 cm of the probe.

The major types of transducer-probes used for TVS include those with a single-element oscillating transducer, those with multiple small transducer elements arranged in a curved linear array, and those with multiple small elements steered by an electronically phased array (see Chap. 1). All of these transducer-probes depict the anatomy in a sector format encompassing between 85° and 100°. In our experience, the greatest resolution is achieved with a curved linear array that contains multiple (up to 124) separate transmit/receive elements. Mechanical sector transducers may be subject to minor image distortions at the edges of the field because of the hysteresis (stopping and starting) that occurs with an oscillating transducer. Reverberation artifacts can be created by suboptimal coupling of the surfaces of the condom, probe, or vagina (Fig. 2-3) or by lack of tautness of the condom as it is stretched over the probe. Although degradation of image

quality by side lobe artifacts can occur in the far field in a phased-array transducer, the image in the near field is not degraded significantly. Therefore, phased-array transducers have resolution capabilities similar to sector and curved linear transducers when used in transvaginal examinations.

After the transducer probe is completely covered by a condom and the condom is secured to the shaft of the probe by a rubber band, the probe is inserted within the vagina and manipulated around the cervical lips and into a fornix to depict the structures of interest in the most detail. When the transducer is oriented in the longitudinal, or sagittal, plane, the long axis of the uterus can usually be depicted by slight oblique angulation off midline. The uterus is used as a landmark to depict other adnexal structures. Once the uterus is identified, the probe can be angled to the right or left of midline in the sagittal plane to depict the ovaries. The internal iliac artery and vein appear as tubular structures along the pelvic sidewall. Low-level blood echoes can occasionally be seen streaming within these pulsating vessels. The ovaries typically lie medial to these vessels. Hypoechoic follicles within the ovaries facilitate their identification. After imaging in the sagittal plane, the transducer can be turned 90° counterclockwise to depict these structures in their axial or semicoronal planes. Counterclockwise movement maintains standard right-to-left orientation on the semicoronal scans.

Particularly in larger patients, it is helpful for the sonographer to use one hand to scan while

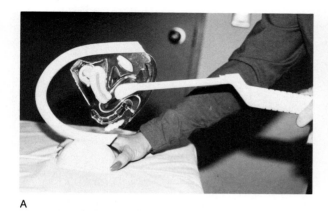

A

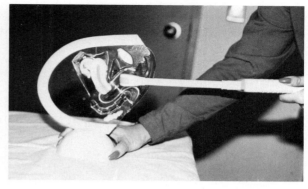

B

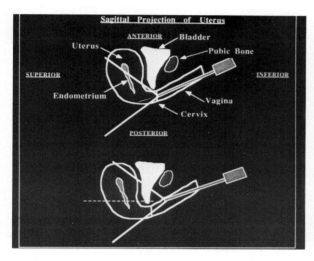

C

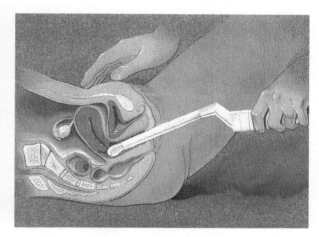

D

FIGURE 2-2
Scanning planes used in TVS. (**A**) Oblique sagittal planes. (**B**) Semicoronal planes. (**C**) Diagrams showing field of view with various degrees of probe insertion. Varying the degree of probe penetration alters the field of view. (Courtesy of Bill Carrano.) (**D**) Diagram showing application of abdominal pressure while transvaginal probe is within the vagina. This maneuver brings the structure of interest closest to the transducer probe. Displacement of the adnexa relative to the uterus is a sign of the presence of pelvic adhesions (sliding organ sign).

using the other to gently palpate the abdomen to move structures such as the ovaries closer to the transducer and to displace bowel.

Placing the patient in a decubitus position occasionally helps to bring the area of interest closer to the transducer. This maneuver is used particularly in early pregnancy examinations when the yolk sac/embryo complex may lie in the far field or on the edge of the sac. Left-lateral decubitus positioning of the patient is preferred.

A pelvic examination table is preferred for TVS, primarily because it supports the patient's legs, enabling her to relax her abdominal, leg, and perineal muscles (Fig. 2-4). If such a table is not available, an inverted bed pan can be placed under the patient's buttocks to elevate the pelvis from the stretcher surface. This allows the examiner to displace the handle of the probe posteriorly to direct the probe and beam anteriorly.

SCANNING PLANES

Transvaginal sonography affords examination of the pelvic organs in three major imaging planes: sagittal, semicoronal, and semiaxial. The sagittal

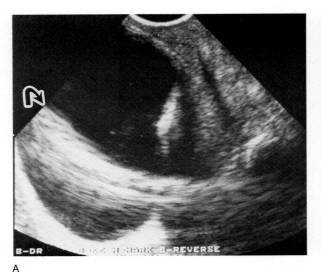

A

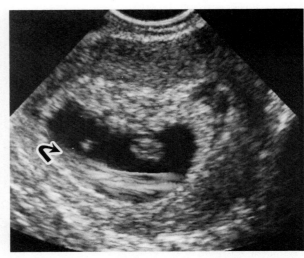

B

FIGURE 2-3
Artifacts. (**A**) Side-lobe artifact (*curved arrow*) projected over the bladder. (**B**) Same artifact displayed
as if within the gestational sac.

plane usually is used initially to identify the uterus in the long axis. Once the uterus is adequately depicted, the transducer probe can be directed into the right or left adnexa where the ovary and iliac vessels are seen. Various degrees of pressure with the probe can be used to move the organs of interest closest to the transducer while displacing bowel. The semicoronal and semiaxial images are then obtained by turning the probe 90° counterclockwise. If the probe is directed in the coronal plane, the image is a semicoronal image. Semiaxial images are obtained when the beam is directed anteriorly. Fi-

nally, a posteriorly directed image of the cul-de-sac is obtained when the probe is withdrawn from the vaginal fornices into the midvagina.

IMAGE DISPLAY

To distinguish a transvaginal from a transabdominal sonogram, "TV" should be displayed at the top left of the viewing screen. For oblique sagittal and semicoronal images, the main bang should be displayed at the top of the screen with the cephalic direction

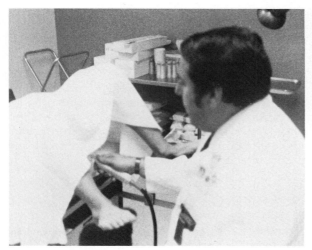

A

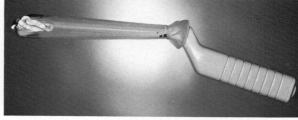

B

FIGURE 2-4
Equipment used for TVS. (**A**) Patient on pelvic examination table in slight reverse Trendelenburg position. This position affords collection of physiologic fluid in the cul-de-sac and allows the patient's legs to be supported. (**B**) Transvaginal transducer probe covered with a condom. A small amount of gel is placed on the condom to facilitate insertion and contact.

displayed at the left of the screen. European operators tend to orient the image with the apex at the bottom of the screen. For semicoronal planes, the patient's right side should be displayed on the left side of the screen. Neither display from the top or the bottom of the screen is anatomically correct, but this method of display correlates with the conventional method established by the American Institute of Ultrasound in Medicine and is used extensively in the United States.

UTERUS

Examination of the uterus begins with its depiction in the long axis. The endometrial interface, which is typically echogenic, is a useful landmark to depict the long axis of the uterus. Once the endometrium is identified, images of the uterus can be obtained in the sagittal, semiaxial, and coronal planes. In the oblique sagittal plane, an anteflexed uterus displays the fundus to the left of the image, and a retroflexed uterus displays the fundus to the right of the image (Fig. 2-5).

It may be difficult to determine the flexion of the uterus on the hard-copy images obtained by TVS alone, except in extreme cases of anteflexion or retroflexion. Uterine flexion can be surmised during the examination, however, by the relative orientation of the transducer probe needed to obtain optimal images of the uterus. For example, retroflexed uteri are best depicted when the probe is in the anterior fornix and angulated in a posterior direction.

The endometrium has a variety of appearances depending on its stage of development (Fleischer and coworkers, 1988). In the proliferative phase, the endometrium measures 4 to 8 mm in anteroposterior (AP) dimension (width). This measurement includes two layers of endometrium. A hypoechoic interface can be seen within the luminal aspects of echogenic layers of endometrium in the periovulatory phase and probably represents an edema in the inner layers of endometrium. In the few days after ovulation, a small amount of secretion into the endometrial lumen can be seen. During the secretory phase, the endometrium typically measures 8 to 14 mm in width and is surrounded by a hypoechoic band representing the inner layer of the myometrium. The endometrium should only be measured in a straight sagittal image; measuring it in a semicoronal image is inaccurate.

An endometrial volume may be calculated by measuring its length by long axis, with AP and transverse dimensions. In the axial plane, the place where the endometrium invaginates into the area

of ostia in the region of the uterine cornu can be used as a landmark.

Because the transducer probe is close to the cervix, the cervix is not as readily depicted as the remainder of the uterus. If the probe is withdrawn into the vagina while the endometrium is visualized, however, images of the cervix can be obtained. The mucus within the endocervical canal usually appears as an echogenic interface. This may become hypoechoic during the periovulatory period because cervical mucus has a higher fluid content.

OVARIES

Ovaries are typically depicted as oblong structures measuring approximately 3 cm in the long axis and 2 cm in AP and transverse dimension (Fig. 2-6). On angled long-axis scans, the ovaries are immediately medial to the pelvic vessels. They are particularly well depicted when they contain a mature follicle that is typically 1.5 to 2.0 cm in diameter. It is not unusual to depict multiple immature or atretic follicles in the 3- to 5-mm range that serve as sonographic markers of the ovary.

The size of an ovary is related to the patient's age and phase of follicular development (Granberg and Wikland, 1987). When the ovary contains a mature follicle, it can become twice as large in volume as one that does not contain mature follicles. The ovaries of postmenopausal women are usually small ($2 \times 2 \times 1$ cm) and featureless (Rodriguez and coworkers, 1988; Fleischer and coworkers, 1990), whereas the normal ovaries of a premenopausal woman can range up to $5 \times 3 \times 2$ cm or 10 cm^3; the normal postmenopausal woman's ovaries should not measure more than 8 cm^3 (Cohen, 1989).

OTHER PELVIC STRUCTURES

Transvaginal sonography can depict several other pelvic structures in addition to the uterus and ovaries. These include bowel loops within the pelvis (Fig. 2-7), iliac vessels, and, occasionally, distended fallopian tubes. Even small amounts of intraperitoneal fluid (1 to 3 mL) can be detected surrounding the uterus or in the cul-de-sac.

As discussed, the major pelvic vessels appear as relatively straight tubular structures that course obliquely on either pelvic sidewall. The internal iliac arteries have a typical width of 5 to 7 mm and tend to pulsate with expansion of both walls, whereas the iliac vein is larger (approximately 1 cm) but does not demonstrate this pulsation. Occasionally, low-

(text continues on page 34)

FIGURE 2-5
Uterus

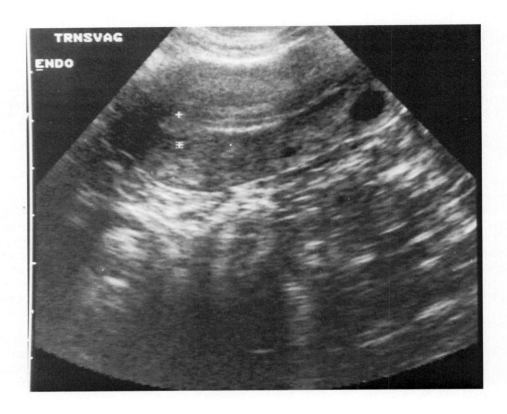

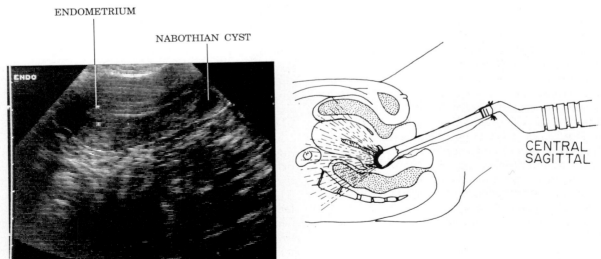

Figure 2-5A. Long axis view of the uterus and endometrium (between cursors) in the secretory phase appearing as echogenic tissue. A Nabothian cyst is also present.

Uterus *(Continued)*

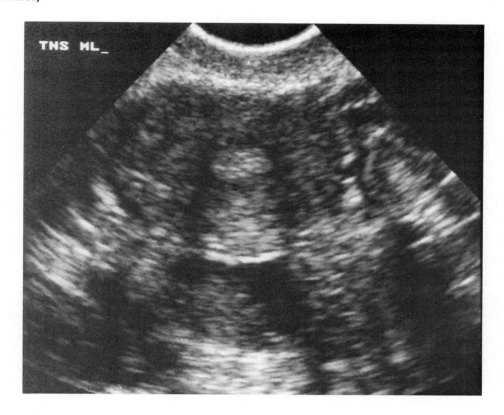

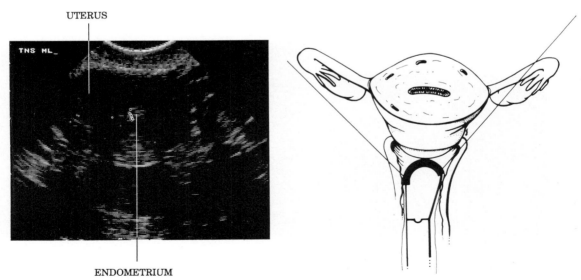

Figure 2-5B. Same as Figure 2-5*A* in semicoronal short axis.

Uterus *(Continued)*

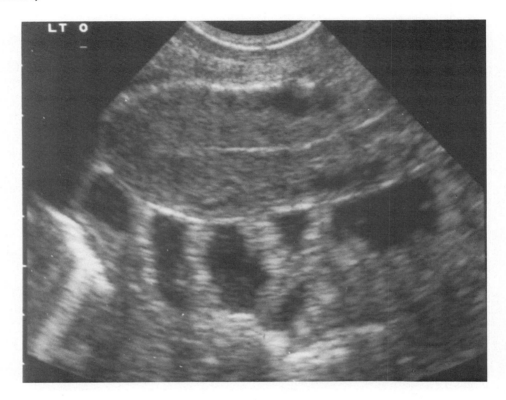

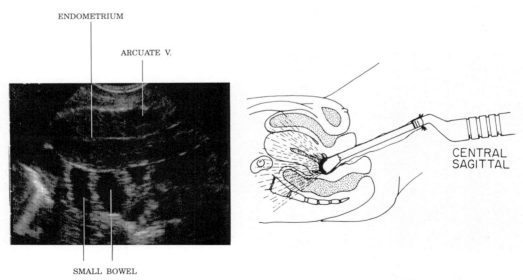

ENDOMETRIUM

ARCUATE V.

SMALL BOWEL

CENTRAL SAGITTAL

Figure 2-5C. Sagittal image showing penetrating vessels within the outer myometrium at the level of the internal cervical os.

FIGURE 2-6
Ovaries and Fallopian Tubes

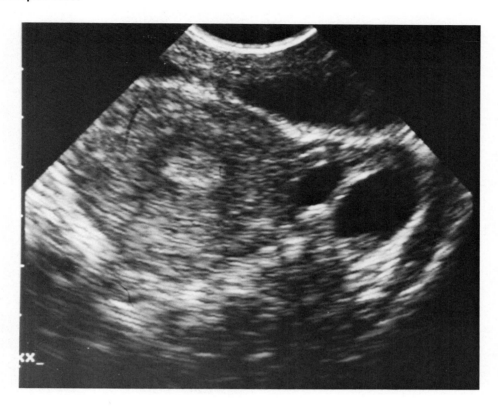

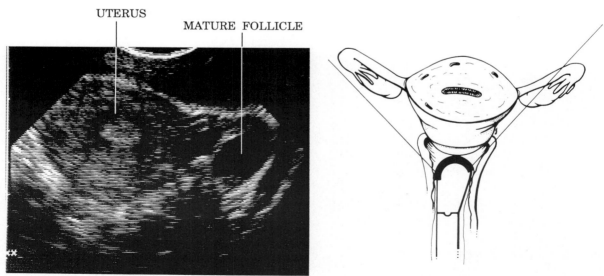

Figure 2-6A. Left ovary containing a mature follicle. The proximal portion of the left tube is also seen.

Ovaries and Fallopian Tubes *(Continued)*

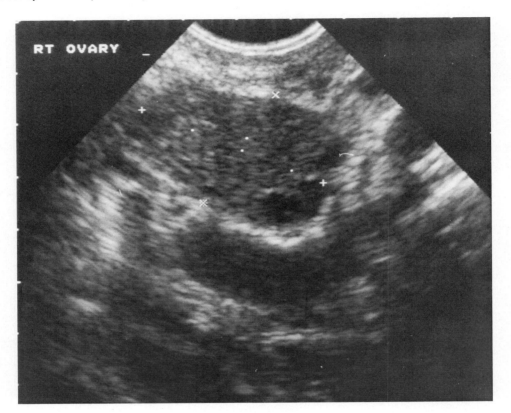

INVOLUTED CORPUS LUTEUM

Figure 2-6B. Right ovary containing an involuted corpus luteum.

Ovaries and Fallopian Tubes *(Continued)*

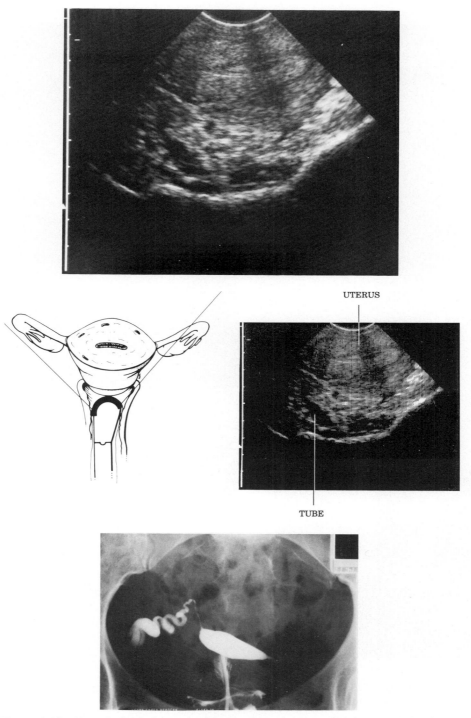

UTERUS

TUBE

Figure 2-6C. Normal distal right tube lying in the cul-de-sac. The hysterosalpingogram showed a normally patent tube.

FIGURE 2-7
Bowel

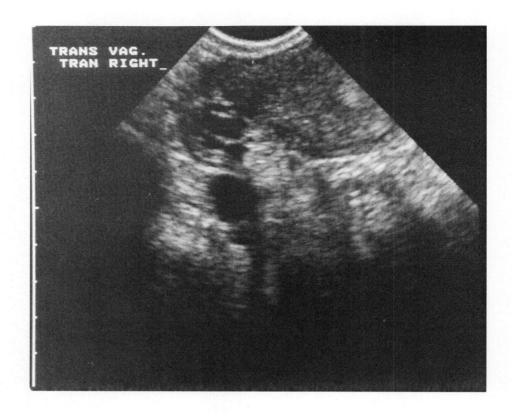

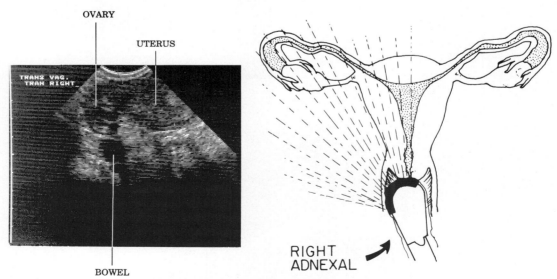

Figure 2-7A. Fluid-filled loop of small bowel adjacent to the right ovary.

Bowel *(Continued)*

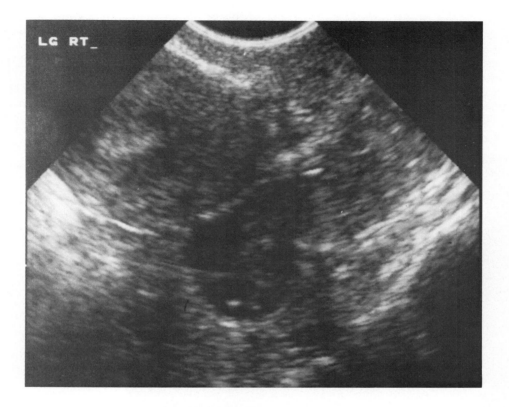

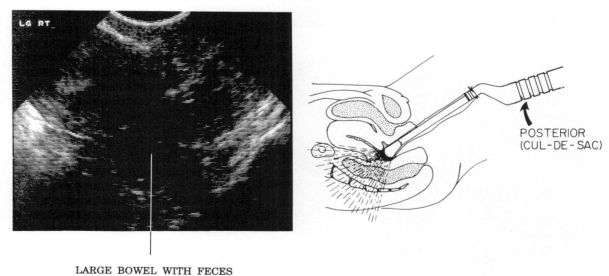

LARGE BOWEL WITH FECES

POSTERIOR
(CUL-DE-SAC)

Figure 2-7B. Large bowel, partially filled with feces, adjacent to the uterus.

level blood echoes are seen streaming within the vein. The transducer can be manipulated or pivoted to demonstrate these vessels in their long axis. Occasionally, a distended distal ureter may have this appearance but not demonstrate pulsations. In most patients, the larger branches of the uterine vessels are demonstrable by TVS as tubular structures coursing in the paracervical area.

The nondistended fallopian tube is difficult to depict on TVS, probably because of its small intra-luminal size and serpiginous course. Occasionally, the origin of the tubes can be identified by locating the invagination of endometrium depicting the area of the tubal ostia and following the invaginated en-dometrium laterally in the axial or coronal plane. The ovarian and infundibulopelvic ligaments usu-ally cannot be depicted.

Sonographic delineation of the fallopian tubes is facilitated by surrounding the tubes with intra-peritoneal fluid that may be present in the cul-de-

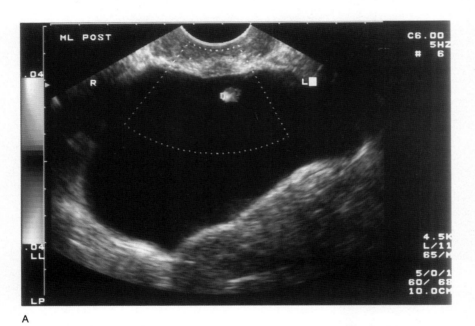

A

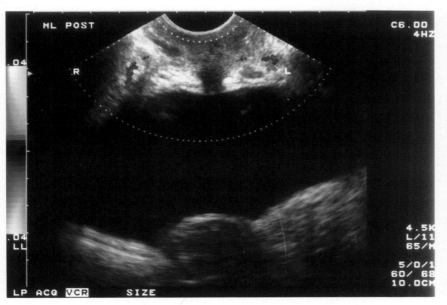

B

FIGURE 2-8
Distal ureters and urethra. (**A**) Transvaginal color Doppler sono-gram showing ureteral jet squirting from left ureteral orifice. (**B**) Trans-vaginal color Doppler sonogram taken in semicoronal phase show-ing long axis of hypoechoic urethra and vesicle vessels at the base of the bladder.

sac (Timor-Tritsch and Rottem, 1987). By placing the patient in a reverse Trendelenburg position, the fluid can be collected around the tube. When surrounded by fluid, the normal tube appears as a 1-cm tubular echogenic structure that usually courses from the lateral aspect of the uterine cornu posterolaterally into the adnexal regions and cul-de-sac. In some patients, flaring of the fimbriated end of the tube can be seen because it approximates its nearby ovary. Transvaginal depiction of the tube is also facilitated when it contains intraluminal fluid.

The urethra is seen as a hypoechoic tubular structure when imaged in the long axis as the transducer is partially withdrawn from the vagina and directed anteriorly. The hypoechoic texture is thought to be the result of a circular orientation of the smooth muscle bundle surrounding the urethra. The distal ureters can be seen at the base of the bladder as they empty into the area of the bladder trigone (Laing and coworkers, 1994). Their location can be confirmed by observing ureteral jets arising from the distal ureteral orifice (Fig. 2-8).

The transvaginal appearance of the round ligaments is somewhat similar to that arising from a nondistended tube, except the course of the round ligaments is straighter and more parallel to the uterine cornu.

Bowel is typically recognized as a fusiform structure frequently containing intraluminal fluid; its configuration changes frequently with peristalsis. If there is fluid within the lumen, periotic intraluminal projections resulting from the valvulae conniventes can be seen from small bowel, as can the haustral indentations that are characteristic of large bowel.

SUMMARY

Transvaginal sonography affords detailed depiction of the uterus and ovaries. It requires systematic evaluation of these pelvic structures for their complete delineation in light of the limited field of view of transvaginal transducer-probes. An understanding of the anatomic relationship of these structures gained from previous experience with TAS, combined with the anticipated findings from previous palpation of these structures during a pelvic examination, is necessary.

REFERENCES

Cohen H. The normal size of the ovary: It's bigger than we think. Radiology 1989;173(suppl):142.

Fleischer AC, Gordon A, McKee M, et al. Transvaginal sonography of postmenopausal ovaries with pathologic correlation. J Ultrasound Med 1990;9:637.

Fleischer AC, Mendelson E, Bohm-Valez M. Sonographic depiction of the endometrium with transabdominal and transvaginal scanning. Semin Ultrasound CT MRI 1988;9:81.

Granberg S, Wikland M. Comparison between endovaginal and transabdominal transducers for measuring ovarian volume. J Ultrasound Med 1987;16:649.

Laing F, Benson C, DiSalvo D. Distal ureteral calculi: Detection with vaginal US. Radiology 1994;192:545.

Rodriguez M, Platt L, Medearis A, Lacarra M, Lobo R. The use of transvaginal sonography for evaluation of postmenopausal ovarian size and morphology. Am J Obstet Gynecol 1988;159:810.

Timor-Tritsch IE, Rottem S. Transvaginal ultrasonographic study of the fallopian tube. Obstet Gynecol 1987;70:424.

Transvaginal Sonography: A Clinical Atlas, Second Edition,
edited by Arthur C. Fleischer and Donna M. Kepple.
J.B. Lippincott Company, Philadelphia, © 1995.

CHAPTER **3**

Differential Diagnosis of Pelvic Masses

Arthur C. Fleischer, MD

INTRODUCTION

Transvaginal sonography (TVS) is particularly useful for evaluation of patients with pelvic masses of 10 cm in diameter or less that lie in the true pelvis. For larger pelvic masses, TVS has only an adjunctive role to transabdominal sonography (TAS). Because TVS can define the size, location, and internal consistency of pelvic masses, it is the imaging modality of choice for most pelvic masses (Coleman and coworkers, 1988; Fleischer and coworkers, 1989; Mendelson and coworkers, 1988; Tessler and coworkers, 1989; Andolf and Jorgensen, 1990; Lande and coworkers, 1988; Vilaro and coworkers, 1987).

The clinically pertinent features of a pelvic mass depicted by TVS include its size and location (e.g., ovarian, uterine), its internal consistency (e.g., totally cystic, low-level echoic, septated, or containing papillary projections, fat, calcifications), and its associated abnormalities (e.g., presence of intraperitoneal fluid).

Rather than classifying masses into cystic, complex, and solid categories as with TAS, TVS affords a more specific differential diagnosis based on more precise delineation, such as the location and internal consistency of the mass. A more specific classi-

fication is afforded by TVS than has been possible with conventional TAS. Table 3-1 is a guide for differential diagnosis of pelvic masses using TVS primarily as an adjunct to TAS.

Specific morphologic features such as wall thickness, septa regularity, and echogenicity have been incorporated into a scoring system that reflects the relative probability that a mass is malignant (Fig. 3-1). Even though these concepts are useful, they may not be necessary to specifically score each mass (Granberg and coworkers, 1989; Sassone and coworkers, 1991).

OVARIAN MASSES

Masses that are confined to the ovary typically demonstrate a rim of ovarian tissue surrounding the abnormal lesion. In some cases, immature follicles appear as hypoechoic structures within the ovarian parenchyma that help identify the tissue surrounding a mass as ovarian.

The ovary is the site of a variety of pelvic masses, ranging from physiologic cysts to malignant ovarian carcinoma (Figs. 3-2 through 3-6). It is the site of not only primary tumors but also meta-

TABLE 3-1
Differential Diagnoses of Pelvic Masses by TVS

Location	Consistency		
	Cystic	*Complex*	*Solid*
Ovarian	Physiologic cysts Neoplastic cysts	Dermoid cysts Neoplastic cysts	Metastases Primary ovarian tumors
		Hemorrhagic cysts Tubo-ovarian abscess	Fibroma
Adnexal extra- ovarian	Paraovarian cysts, hydrosalpinx		Tubal tumor
Uterine			Pedunculated fibroid
Other		Arteriovenous malfor- mation	Bowel tumor, lymph- adenopathy

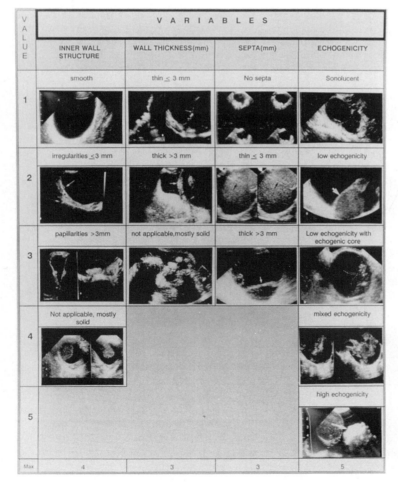

FIGURE 3-1
Scoring system based on inner wall structure, wall thickness, septa, and echogenicity. Each category is scored between 1 and 5. Most benign lesions have a cumulative score of less than 9; most malignant lesions score more than 12. (Sassone A, Timor-Tritsch I, Anfuer A. Transvaginal sonographic characterization of ovarian disease: Evaluation of a new scoring system to predict ovarian malignancy. Obset Gynecol 1991;78:70.)

static lesions from gastrointestinal and breast primary carcinomas. It can also be the site of tumor sequestration in patients with leukemia.

Physiologic cysts are typically larger than 3 cm in diameter and are anechoic, smooth-walled structures. Luteal cysts have a thicker wall than hydropic follicles. Either may contain low-level echoes arising from internal hemorrhage.

Ovarian epithelial tumors tend to demonstrate septa with or without solid areas. Mucinous cystadenomas typically have thin internal septations, whereas serous cystadenomas may be unilocular. Mucinous tumors may contain internal echogenic material arising from the mucin.

Malignant tumors tend to have irregular walls, papillary excrescences, or both. If tumor has spread beyond the capsule, intraperitoneal fluid is usually present as well. Other sonographic features that suggest malignancy include irregularly thick wall or septa and internal solid areas.

Dermoid cysts have a variety of sonographic appearances, ranging from anechoic to solid lesions containing echogenic sebum. The anechoic dermoids tend to be encountered in young girls and have a neuroectoderm lining. Dermoids that contain sebum, hair follicles, or both demonstrate echogenic internal material. In some cases, the sebum collects anteriorly.

Solid tumors of the ovary may represent primary tumors, metastases, or benign lesions such as fibromas. Hemorrhage may appear as a solid area within an ovary, and these ovaries may twist (see Fig. 3-6). Ovarian torsion should be suspected when an enlarged ovary, usually associated with intraperitoneal fluid, is seen in a patient with pelvic pain. Color Doppler sonography may be used to definitively confirm the presence of ovarian torsion by the lack of flow to the ovary (Fleischer and coworkers, 1990). The amount of perfusion is related to the completeness of torsion and its chronicity.

ADNEXAL EXTRAOVARIAN MASSES

Adnexal extraovarian masses arise from adnexal structures outside the ovary. These include masses such as paraovarian cysts and endometriomas, which can typically be identified as separate from the ovary itself (Fig. 3-7).

Endometriomas have a spectrum of sonographic appearances, ranging from anechoic to echogenic, depending on the extent of clot and organization within them. Typically, however, these masses have internal echoes combined with excellent through transmission, indicating that they are predominantly cystic in consistency.

Paraovarian cysts are structures arising from the wolffian duct remnant in the mesovarium. These have similar appearances to peritoneal inclusion cysts, which may arise as a sequela from intraperitoneal surgery. Peritoneal inclusion cysts form from fluid accumulation that is walled off and becomes localized to surrounding serosal structures.

Occasionally, tubal masses appear as extraovarian cystic structures. When a tube becomes maximally distended, it is difficult to distinguish it from an ovarian mass. When it is only moderately distended, however, its continuity with the region of the uterine cornu can be established, thus identifying it as a tubal structure.

Isolated tubal torsion can occur in women who have undergone tubal ligation. The tube can undergo torsion, resulting in a thickened wall (Fig. 3-8).

Solid masses that are extraovarian may, on rare occasions, represent pedunculated fibroids or tubal carcinoma. In pedunculated fibroids, the sonographer can usually maneuver the probe between the mass and the uterus, showing the pedicle of the pedunculated fibroid. Tubal carcinoma is rare, appearing as a solid fusiform mass adjacent to the uterus and ovary.

UTERINE MASSES

The most common uterine mass is the leiomyoma (Fig. 3-9). These masses may simulate the appearance of a pelvic mass if they become subserosal and pedunculated. Usually, however, the intrauterine location of these masses can be established by using the landmarks of the endometrium and applying a small amount of pressure to the uterus to displace the pedicle of a pedunculated fibroid from the uterus proper.

OTHER MASSES

Masses arising from a bowel may, on rare occasions, appear as pelvic structures (Fig. 3-10). Inflamed terminal ileum and bowel tumors appear as fusiform solid structures, usually distinguishable from the uterus and ovary by TVS. Diverticulosis appears as a multilayered fusiform structure with punctate hypoechoic areas arising from the diverticula themselves.

Pelvic vessels may appear as a true mass. Color Doppler sonography can establish the vascular nature of these masses and the presence of arteriovenous fistulas or varices.

SUMMARY

Transvaginal sonography provides important information regarding the size, location, and internal consistency of pelvic masses. Using these parameters and combining the information with clinical data enable TVS to provide a relatively specific diagnosis. More extensive experience and larger studies will assist in evaluating the efficacy of TVS as a means for early detection of ovarian tumors and other pathologic gynecologic disorders.

REFERENCES

Andolf A, Jorgensen C. A prospective comparison of transabdominal and transvaginal ultrasound with surgical findings in gynecologic disease. J Ultrasound Med 1990;9:71.

Coleman BG, Arger PH, Grumbach K, et al. Transvaginal and transabdominal sonography: Prospective comparison. Radiology 1988;168:639.

Fleischer A, Gordon A, Entman S. Transabdominal and transvaginal sonography of pelvic masses. J Ultrasound in Medicine and Biology 1989;15:529.

Fleischer A, Rao B, Kepple D. Transvaginal color Doppler sonography: Preliminary experience. Dynamic Cardiovascular Imaging 1990;3:52.

Granberg S, Wikland M, Janion I. Macroscopic characterization of ovarian tumors and the relation to the histologic diagnosis: Criteria to be used for ultrasound evaluation. Gynecol Oncol 1989;35:139.

Lande IM, Hill JC, Cosco FE, Kator NN. Adnexal and cul-de-sac abnormalities: Transvaginal sonography. Radiology 1988;166:325.

Mendelson EB, Bohm-Velez M, Joseph N, Neiman HL. Gynecologic imaging: Comparison of transabdominal and transvaginal sonography. Radiology 1988;66:321.

Sassone A, Timor-Tritsch I, Anfuer A. Transvaginal sonographic characterization of ovarian disease: Evaluation of a new scoring system to predict ovarian malignancy. Obstet Gynecol 1991;78:70.

Tessler F, Perrella R, Fleischer A, Grant E. Endovaginal sonography of dilated fallopian tubes. AJR 1989;153:523.

Vilaro MM, Rifkin MD, Pennell RG, et al. Endovaginal ultrasound: A technique for evaluation of nonfollicular pelvic masses. J Ultrasound Med 1987;6:697.

FIGURE 3-2
Cystic Ovarian Masses

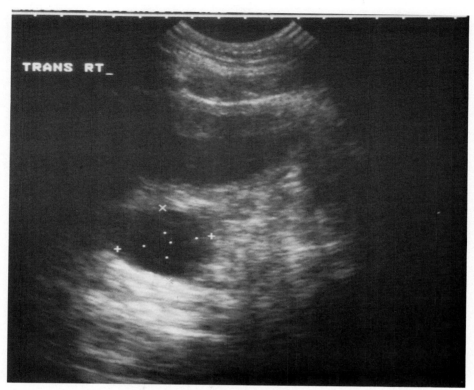

Figure 3-2A. TAS showing an anechoic right adnexal mass (between cursors).

Cystic Ovarian Masses *(Continued)*

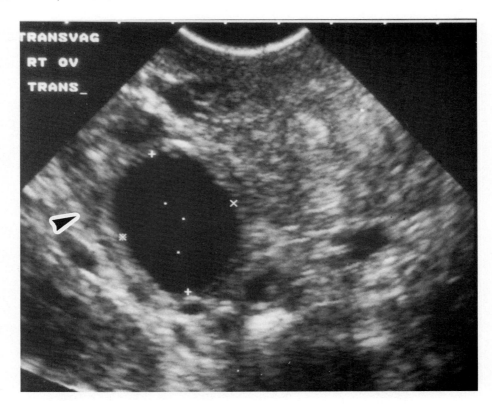

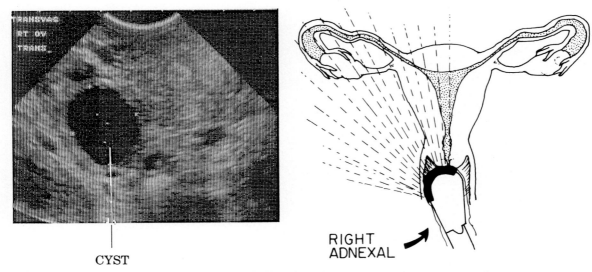

CYST

RIGHT
ADNEXAL

Figure 3-2B. TVS of same patient as in Figure 3-2A demonstrating the cyst (between cursors) within the compressed residual ovarian tissue (*arrow*).

Cystic Ovarian Masses *(Continued)*

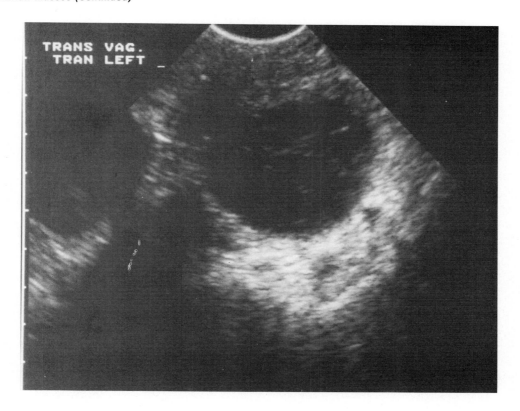

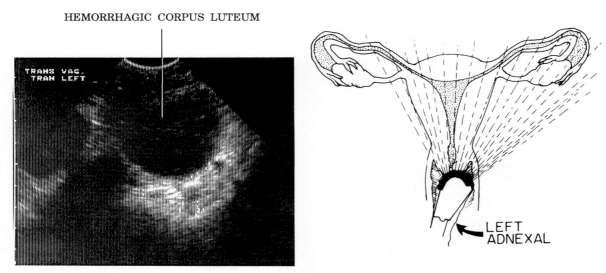

Figure 3-2C. TVS of a hemorrhagic corpus luteum containing multiple thin synchae.

FIGURE 3-3
Septated Ovarian Masses

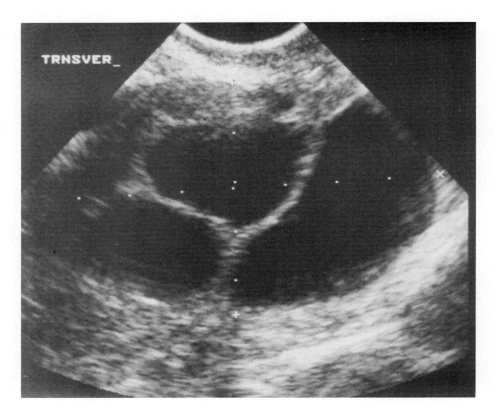

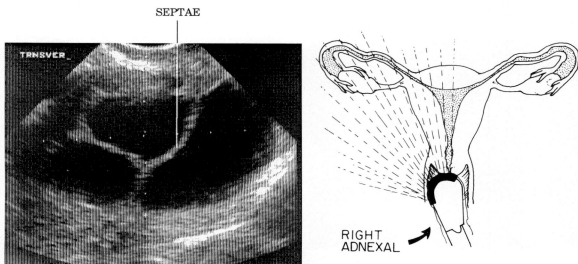

Figure 3-3A. TVS of mucinous cystadenoma (between cursors) with multiple septae.

Septated Ovarian Masses *(Continued)*

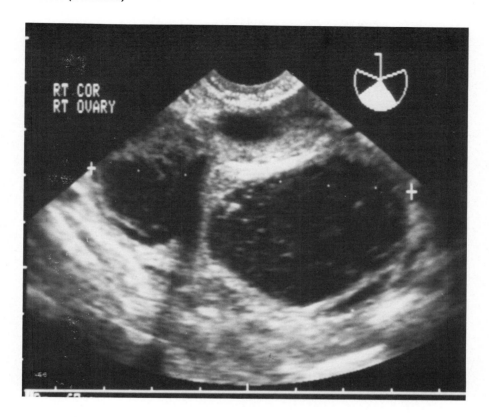

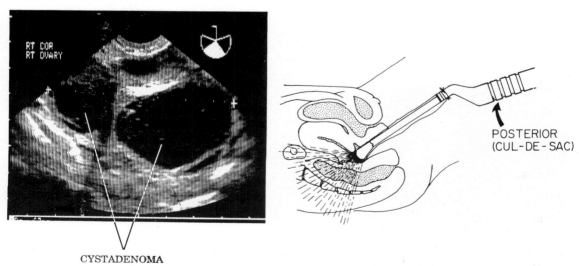

CYSTADENOMA

Figure 3-3B. TVS of bilateral cystadenomas (between cursors) with numerous septae.

Septated Ovarian Masses *(Continued)*

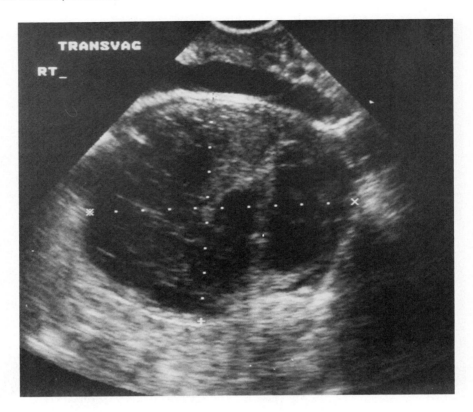

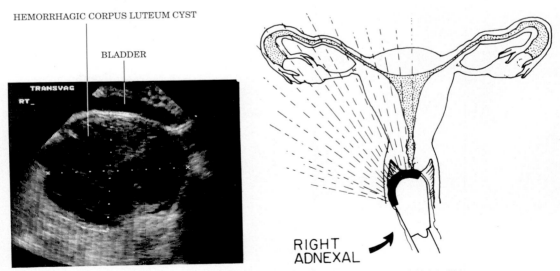

Figure 3-3C. TVS of an 8- by 12-cm complex mass containing septae and solid material. This was a hemorrhagic ovarian cyst.

FIGURE 3-4
Cystic Ovarian Mass Containing Solid Elements

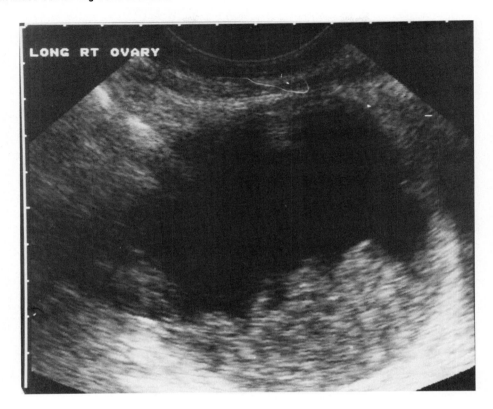

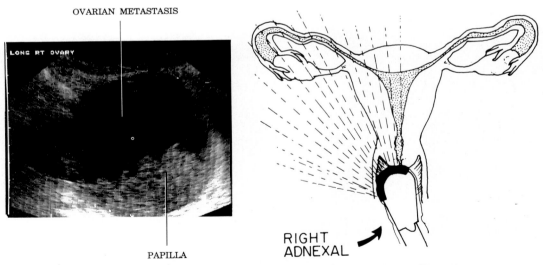

Figure 3-4A. TVS of metastases from gastrointestinal primary lesion containing papillary excrescences.

Cystic Ovarian Mass Containing Solid Elements *(Continued)*

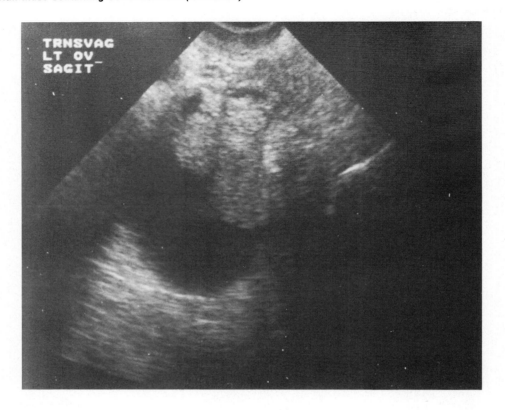

SOLID AREA

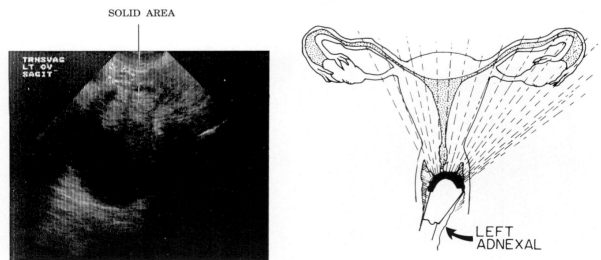

LEFT
ADNEXAL

Figure 3-4B. TVS of an endometrioid carcinoma containing an irregular solid area.

Cystic Ovarian Mass Containing Solid Elements *(Continued)*

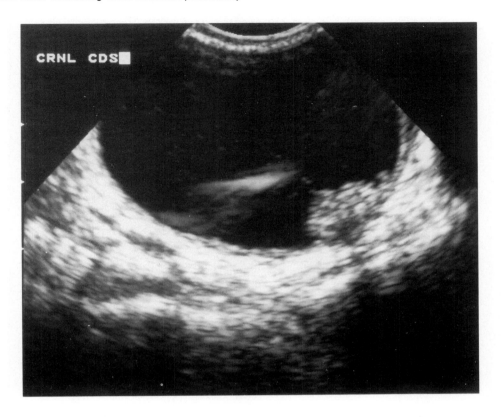

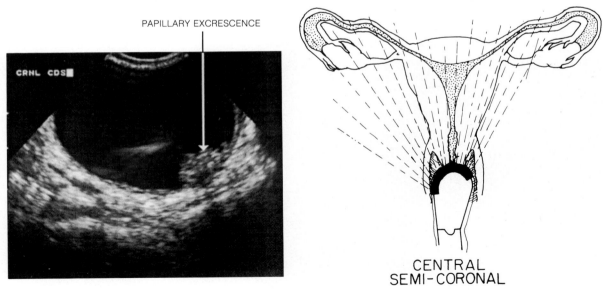

Figure 3-4C. Papillary excrescence within a papillary serous cystadenocarcinoma. This finding is highly indicative of malignancy.

Cystic Ovarian Mass Containing Solid Elements *(Continued)*

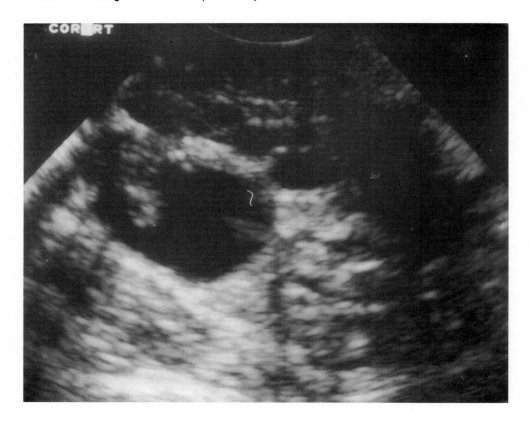

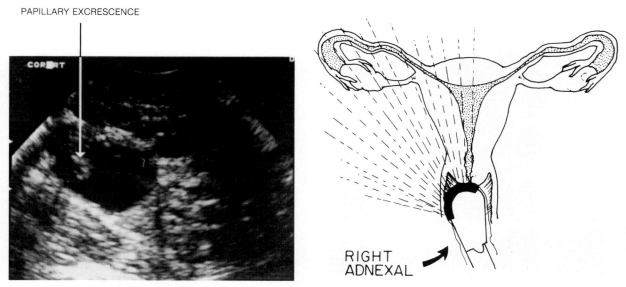

Figure 3-4D. Papillary excrescence within a cystadenofibroma.

FIGURE 3-5
Complex Adnexal Masses

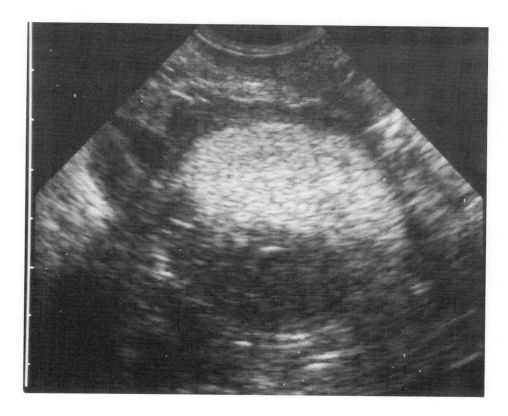

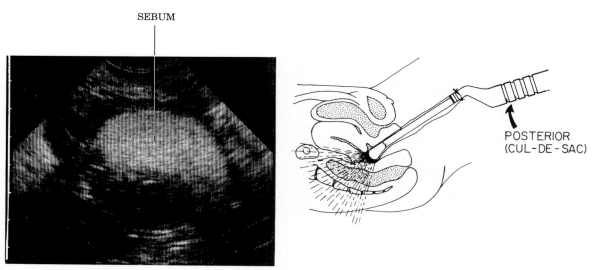

Figure 3-5A. TVS of a dermoid cyst containing a layer of sebum.

Complex Adnexal Masses *(Continued)*

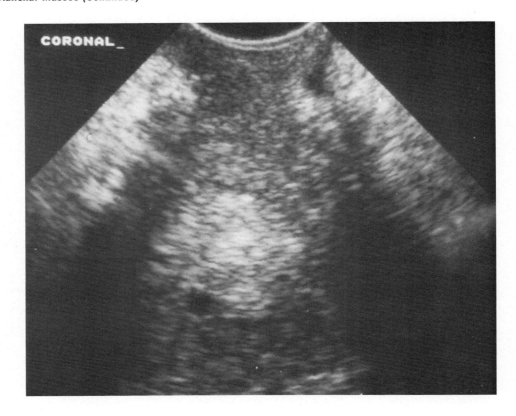

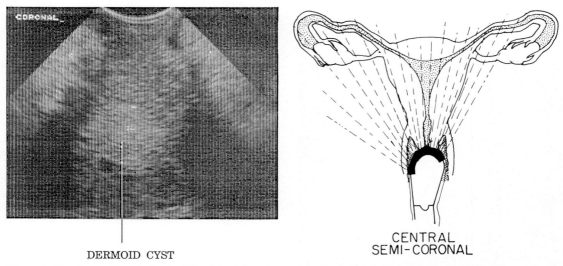

DERMOID CYST

CENTRAL
SEMI-CORONAL

Figure 3-5B. Dermoid cyst that is difficult to delineate due to echogenic interfaces created by hair and fat.

Complex Adnexal Masses *(Continued)*

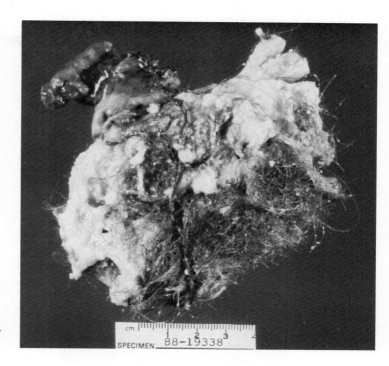

Figure 3-5C. Sectioned dermoid cyst that appeared on TVS in Figure 3-5*B.*

FIGURE 3-6
Solid Ovarian Masses

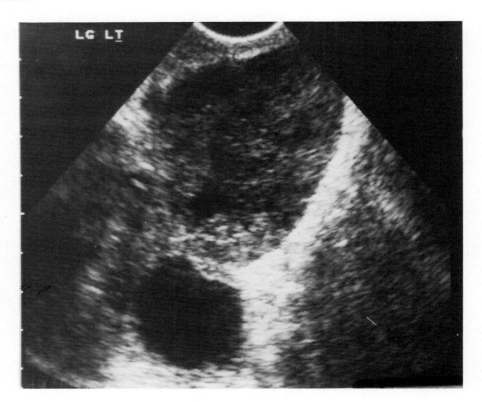

ENDOMETRIOMA

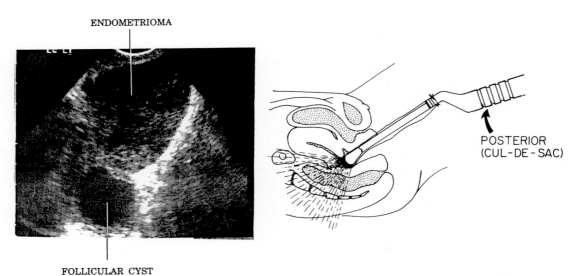

FOLLICULAR CYST

Figure 3-6A. TVS of an endometrioma adjacent to a follicle-containing right ovary. The endometrioma appears solid due to the organized clot it contains.

Solid Ovarian Masses *(Continued)*

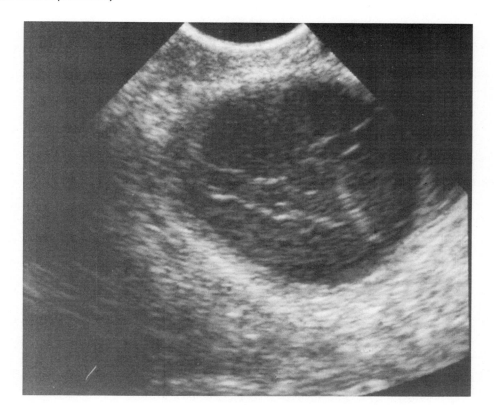

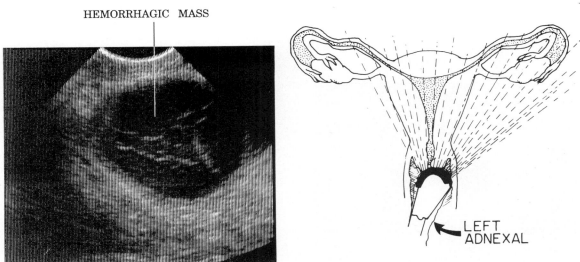

Figure 3-6B. TVS of a solid ovarian mass containing fibrous strands. The mass is the result of extensive hemorrhage within the left ovary.

FIGURE 3-7
Adnexal Extraovarian Masses

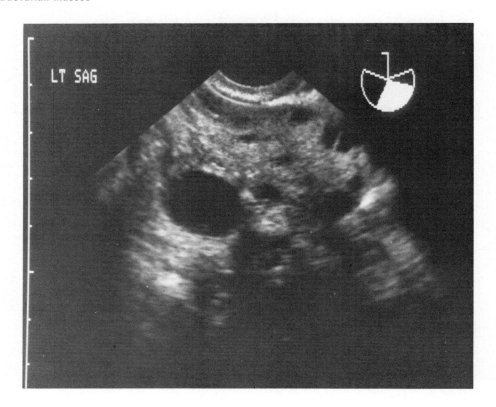

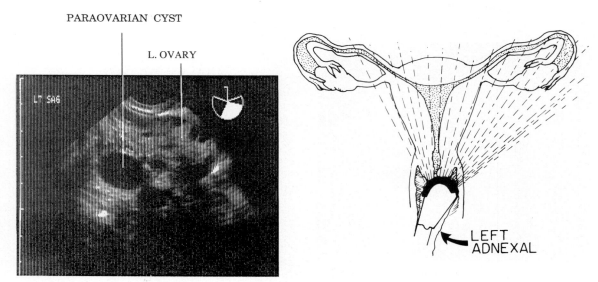

Figure 3-7A.   TVS of a paraovarian cyst that is separate from the ovary.

Adnexal Extraovarian Masses *(Continued)*

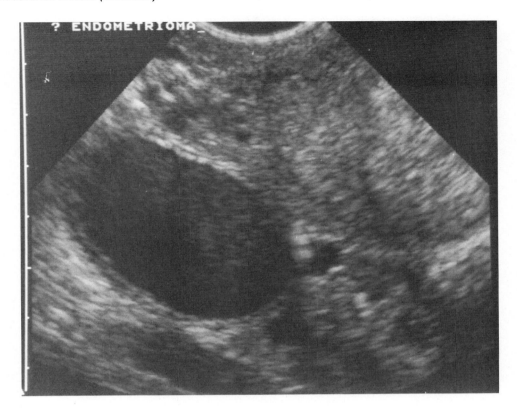

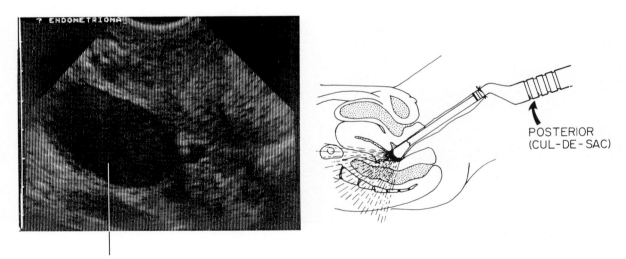

BLOOD WITHIN ENDOMETRIOMA

Figure 3-7B. TVS of an endometrioma containing echogenic material that is layered posteriorly, representing clotted blood.

Adnexal Extraovarian Masses *(Continued)*

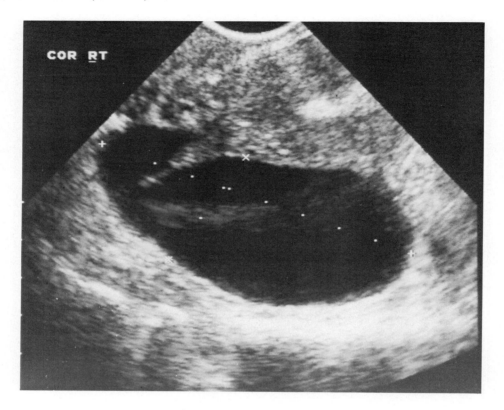

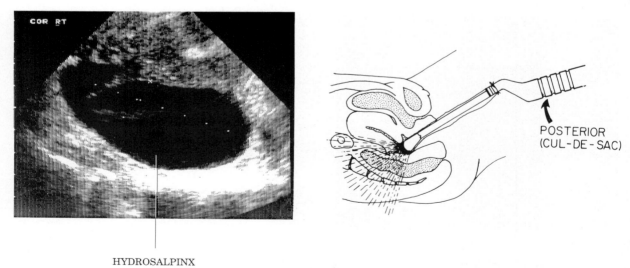

HYDROSALPINX

Figure 3-7C. TVS of a large hydrosalpinx (between cursors) appearing as a fusiform cystic structure posterior to the uterus.

Adnexal Extraovarian Masses *(Continued)*

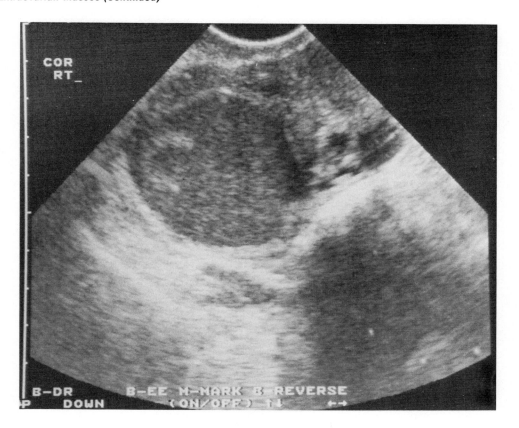

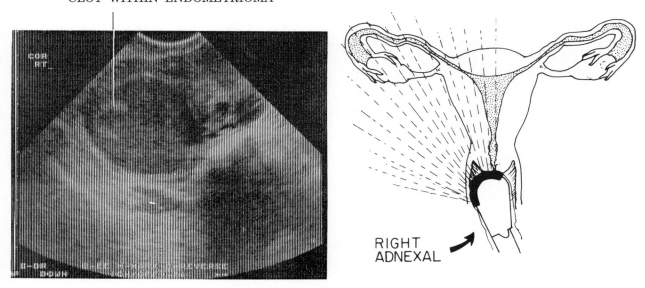

CLOT WITHIN ENDOMETRIOMA

RIGHT ADNEXAL

Figure 3-7D. Endometrioma containing clotted blood and formed clot.

Adnexal Extraovarian Masses *(Continued)*

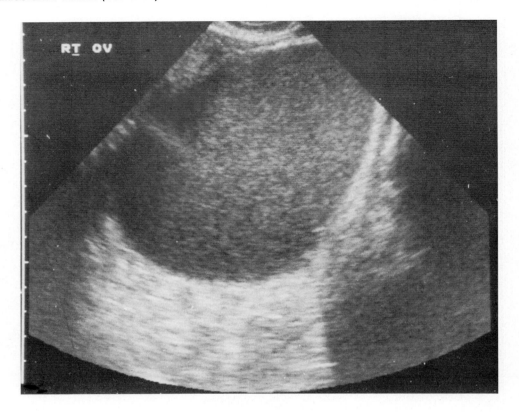

ENDOMETRIOMA

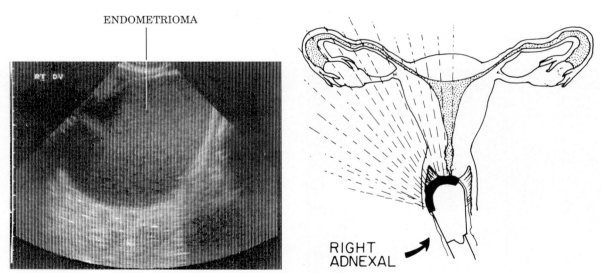

RIGHT
ADNEXAL

Figure 3-7E. Large endometrioma containing clotted blood. Note excellent through transmission, indicating fluid contents of mass.

FIGURE 3-8
Tubal Masses

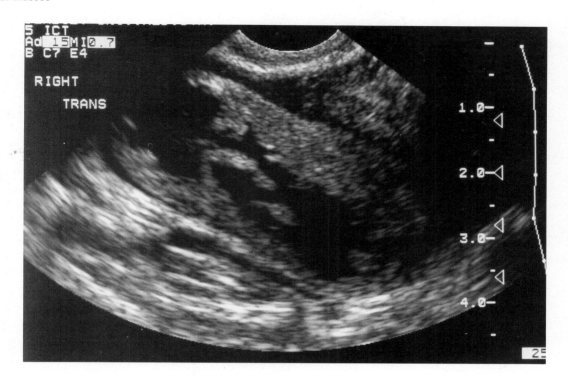

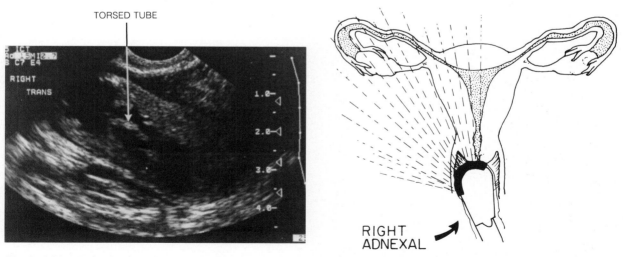

Figure 3-8A. TVS of a torsed hemorrhagic right tube showing a fusiform mass with thick and irregular walls.

Tubal Masses *(Continued)*

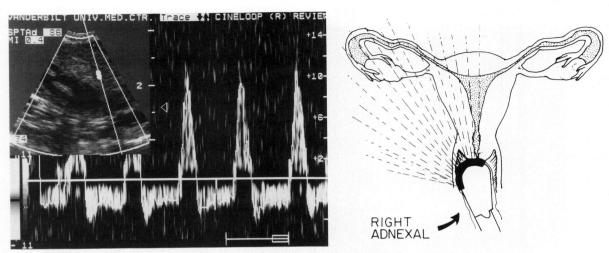

Figure 3-8B. Transvaginal color Doppler sonography showing reversed diastolic flow.

Tubal Masses *(Continued)*

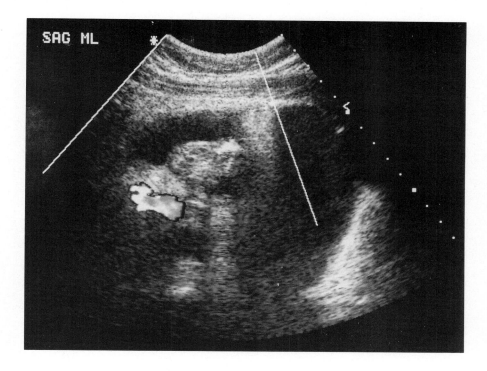

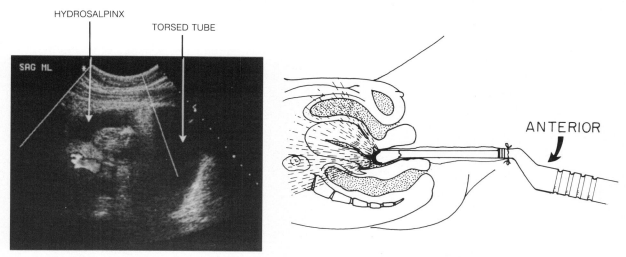

Figure 3-8C. Transvaginal color doppler sonography showing two fusiform masses, one without flow and one smaller one with flow. This represented a gangrenous dilated tube caused by tubal torsion. The other was a simple hydrosalpinx.

Tubal Masses *(Continued)*

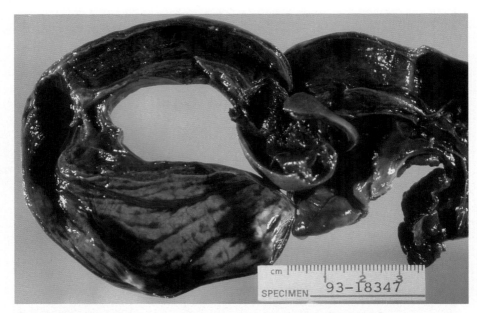

Figure 3-8D.   Resected specimen of gangrenous tube shown in Figure 3-8*C*.

FIGURE 3-9
Uterine Masses

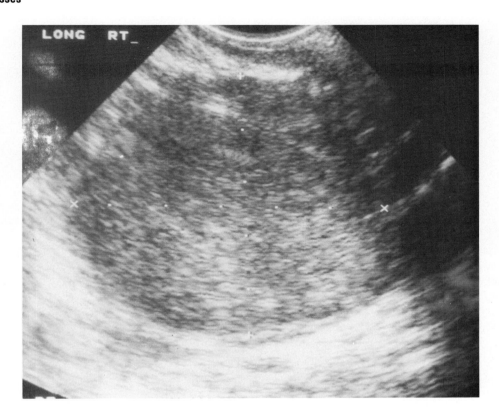

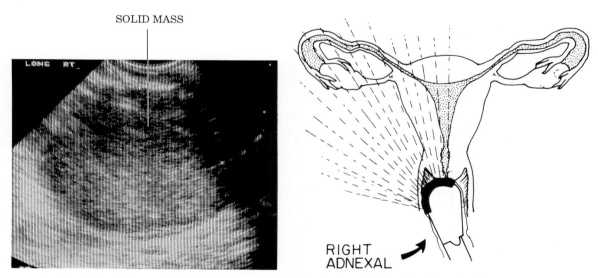

Figure 3-9A. TVS of a large solid pelvic mass (between cursors). It was difficult to determine the origin of the mass by TVS.

Uterine Masses *(Continued)*

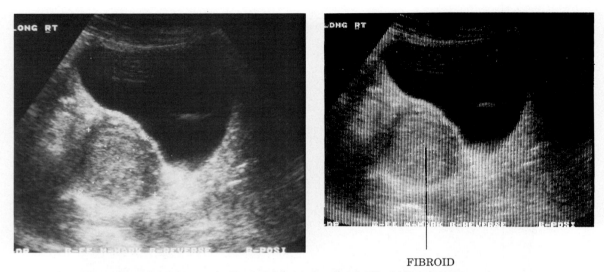

FIBROID

Figure 3-9B. TAS of the same patient as in Figure 3-9*A* showing that the fibroid (between cursors) arises from the posterior corpus of the uterus.

Uterine Masses *(Continued)*

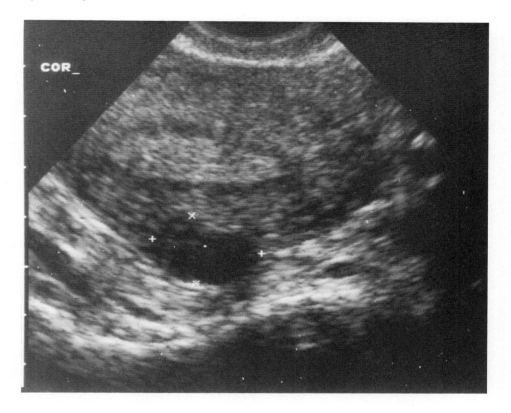

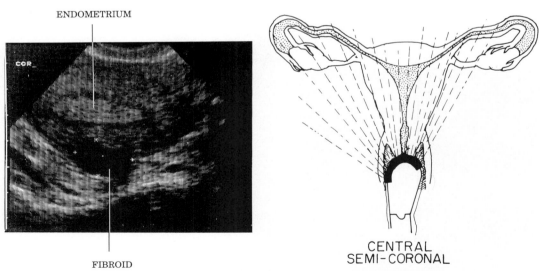

Figure 3-9C. TVS of an intramural fibroid (between cursors). The position of the fibroid relative to the endometrium is shown.

FIGURE 3-10
Bowel Masses

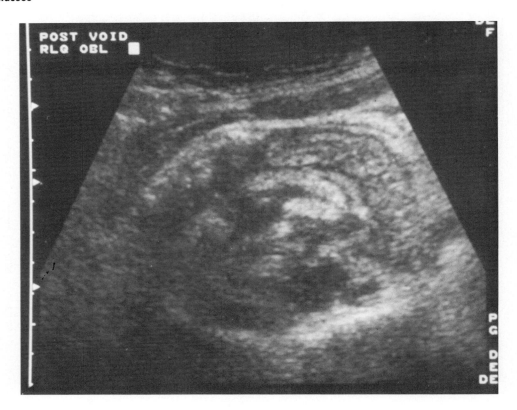

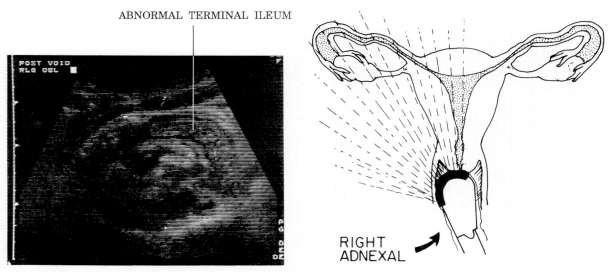

Figure 3-10A. TVS of a thickened loop of small bowel in a patient with Crohn's disease.

Bowel Masses *(Continued)*

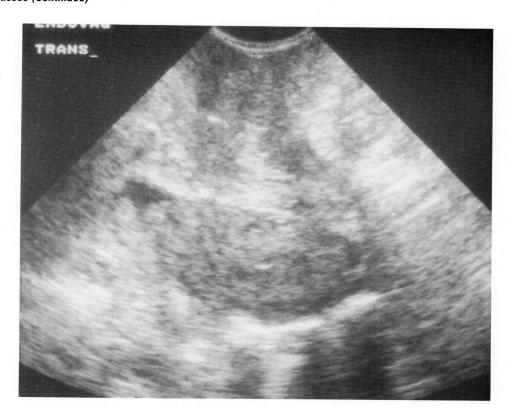

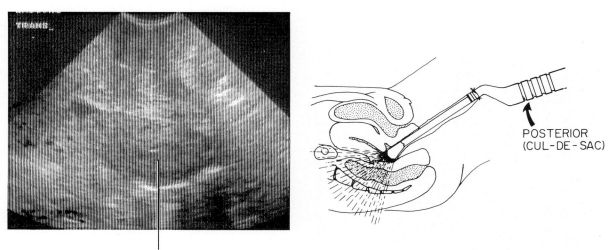

POSTERIOR
(CUL-DE-SAC)

BOWEL MASS

Figure 3-10B. TVS of a markedly thickened bowel loop in a patient with advanced Crohn's disease.

Bowel Masses *(Continued)*

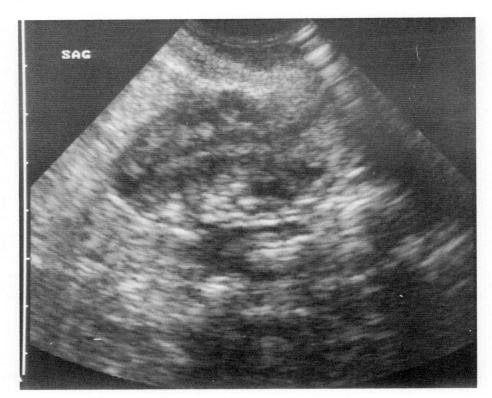

SIGMOID DIVERTICULOSIS

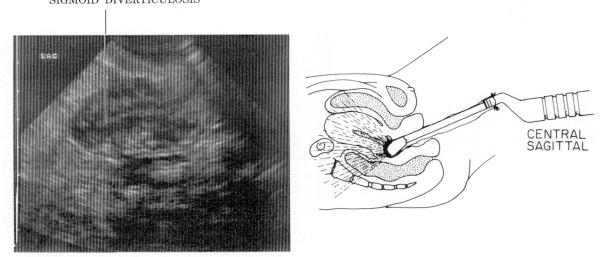

Figure 3-10C. Diverticulosis of sigmoid colon appearing as a multilayered fusiform structure.

Bowel Masses *(Continued)*

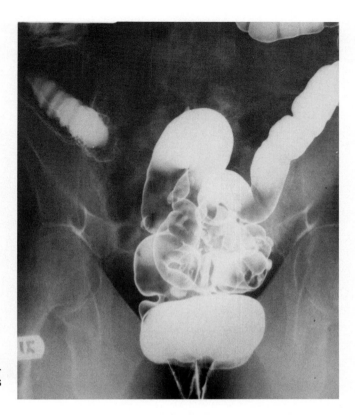

Figure 3-10D. Radiograph taken following a barium enema in the patient in Figure 3-10*C* showing diverticulosis of the sigmoid colon.

Bowel Masses *(Continued)*

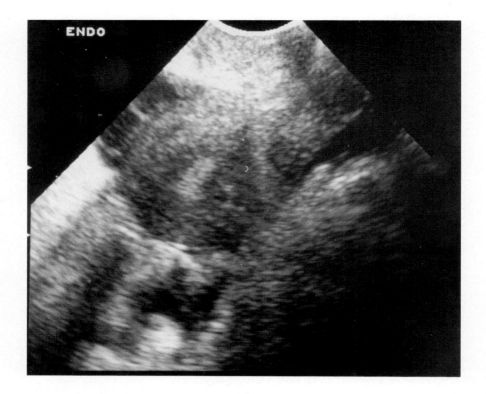

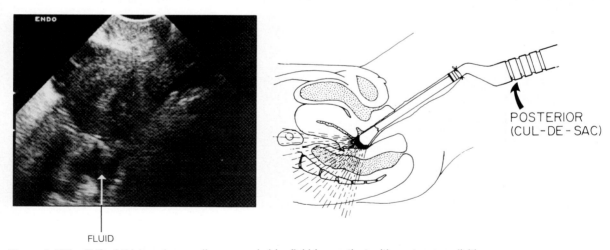

Figure 3-10E. TVS of thickened appendix surrounded by fluid in a patient with acute appendicitis.

Bowel Mass *(Continued)*

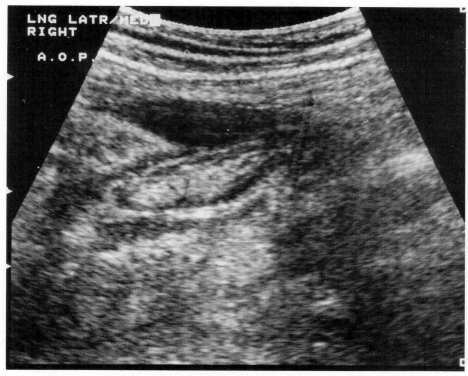

Figure 3-10F. TAS of the same patient in Fig. 3-10E showing a thickened appendix in a patient with acute appendicitis.

Bowel Masses *(Continued)*

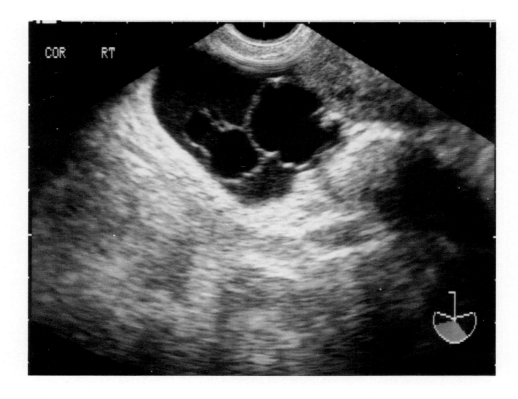

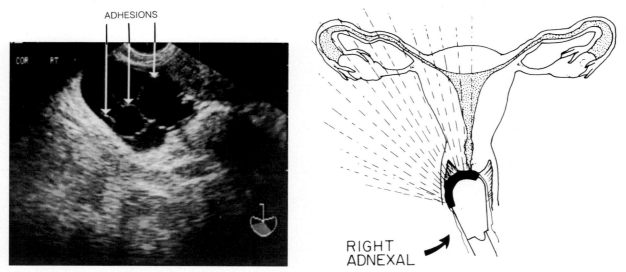

Figure 3-10G. TVS of a pseudomass created by multiple adhesions within a fluid collection in a postoperative patient.

Bowel Masses *(Continued)*

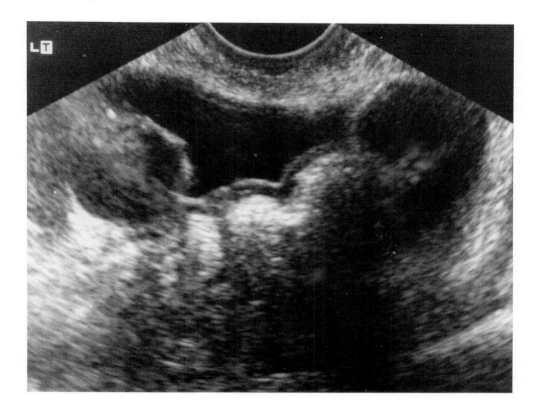

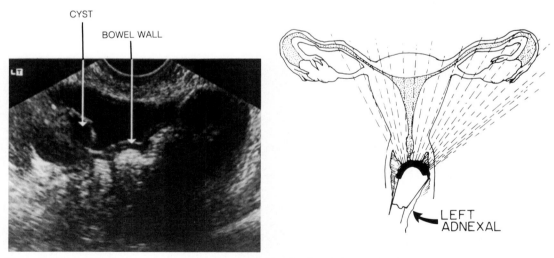

Figure 3-10H. Peritoneal pseudocyst representing fluid collection delineated by the large bowel in a postoperative patient.

Transvaginal Sonography: A Clinical Atlas, Second Edition, edited by Arthur C. Fleischer and Donna M. Kepple. J.B. Lippincott Company, Philadelphia, © 1995.

CHAPTER **4**

Uterine Disorders

Arthur C. Fleischer, MD
Donna M. Kepple, RDMS
Jeanne A. Cullinan, MD

INTRODUCTION

Transvaginal sonography (TVS) affords detailed delineation of the uterus and its myometrium, endometrium, and vessels (Mendelson and coworkers, 1988). Consequently, several uterine disorders may be evaluated by TVS. This chapter discusses normal anatomy and scanning technique as well as the use of TVS in the evaluation of both benign and malignant uterine disorders. The potential applications of transvaginal color Doppler sonography are also presented.

NORMAL ANATOMY AND SCANNING TECHNIQUE

The uterus can be imaged in three major scanning planes with TVS. These include views in long axis, oblique semicoronal or semiaxial plane, and short axis (Fig. 4-1). The long-axis image is obtained when the transducer-probe is introduced into the vagina and the uterus is imaged in the greatest long axis. The semicoronal depiction of the uterus is obtained

when the transducer is turned 90° to the long axis and the greatest longitudinal plane of the uterus is imaged. For anteflexed uteri, the probe handle is held posteriorly with the beam directed anteriorly; the opposite maneuver is used for retroflexed uteri. In the semicoronal scanning plane, the uterus is imaged in its width. The short-axis view is obtained by retracting the transducer-probe into the midvagina and directing it anteriorly through the fornix.

The size and shape of the uterus vary depending on the patient's parity and whether the patient is premenopausal or postmenopausal (Table 4-1). TVS should not be attempted until the patient is in her late teens; therefore, this discussion does not include prepubertal patients. In nulliparous, postpubertal patients, the uterus is approximately 6 cm long and 3 to 4 cm in the anteroposterior (AP) and transverse dimensions. In the parous patient, the uterine long axis can be up to 8 cm long, whereas in the postmenopausal woman, the long axis decreases to approximately 4 to 6 cm.

Variations in the normal anatomy of the central endometrial interfaces can be detected in pa-

Table 4-1
Uterine Size (cm)

	Length	Width	AP	Volume (mL)	Cx: Corpus/ Fundus
Adult (nulliparous)	6–8	3–5	3–5	30–40	1:2
Adult (parous)	8–10	5–6	5–6	60–80	1:2
Postmenopausal	3–5	2–3	2–3	14–17	1:1

From Warwick W, ed. Gray's Anatomy. 35th ed. Philadelphia: WB Saunders, 1973:1356.

tients who have fusion abnormalities of the uterus (Fig. 4-2). Specifically, the bicornuate uterus can be readily identified by the two echogenic endometrial stripes. This is most apparent when these patients are scanned in the secretory phase. Other anatomic variations include prominence of myometrial arcuate vessels and calcification of these vessels in the elderly patient. Small (less than 1 cm) cervical inclusion cysts (Nabothian) may be present within the cervix.

The myometrial fibers are arranged in a specific pattern. They provide effective contraction of the uterus in the normal cycle (de Vries and coworkers, 1990). Occasionally, a sustained contraction can appear as a hypoechoic rounded area. These contractions can be detected on TVS if the study is recorded and played at fast-forward on a videocassette recorder and if the direction and intensity of the contractions can be seen. During menses, these contractions begin at the fundus and extend to the cervix. In midcycle, they are propagated in the opposite direction. Perhaps these contractions affect the efficiency of sperm transport, thereby optimizing the chances of implantation.

Blood is supplied to the uterus by the uterine artery, a branch of the hypogastric artery. Arcuate vessels are present in the outer third of the myometrium. The venous structures are more prominent than the arterial ones (see Fig. 4-2C). Triplex color Doppler sonography of these vessels can be obtained to assess the relative uterine perfusion (see Fig. 12-1).

Transvaginal sonography clearly depicts changes in the endometrial texture and thickness during the menstrual cycle (Fig. 4-3). In the menstrual phase, the endometrium appears as an interrupted interface that is thin and has some hypoechoic areas related to extravasated blood and sloughing tissue (see Fig. 4-3A). In the proliferative phase, the endometrium appears as isoechoic to the myometrium (see Fig. 4-3B and C). During the periovulatory phase, the endometrium may have a multilayered appearance with an inner hypoechoic layer and an echogenic outer layer (see Fig. 4-3D).

The inner hypoechoic layer probably represents the inner endometrium, which is relatively edematous.

The outer echogenic endometrium most likely represents the basalis layer. In the secretory phase, the thickness measures between 8 and 14 mm, and the endometrium is echogenic (see Fig. 4-3E through H). This is probably related to mucous and glycogen stored in the endometrial glands and the echogenic interfaces provided by the tortuous glands and stromal edema. Table 4-2 includes the relative thicknesses of the endometrium throughout the cycle. The thickness of the endometrium is listed as an endometrial "width" that includes both layers measured in the greatest AP dimension.

In women on hormone replacement therapy, the endometrium can be slightly thicker than in those not on any medication. Women on unopposed estrogen may have thicker endometria than those on combined estrogen/progesterone therapy. In addition, women on tamoxifen may have a thick endometrium due to the estrogen-agonist effect of the medication on the endometrium. The response of the endometrium to medications varies. In some women, the endometrium thickens rapidly and, in others, it remains thin (Lin and coworkers, 1992).

LEIOMYOMA

Leiomyomas are common tumors consisting of smooth muscle and connective tissue arising from the soft tissue and smooth muscle covering the in-

Table 4-2
Endometrial Thickness with TVS

	Bilayer thickness (mm)
Proliferative phase	4–8
Secretory phase	7–14
Postmenopausal (no HRT)	4–8
Postmenopausal (HRT)	6–10

HRT, hormone replacement therapy.

tramyometrial arcuate vessels. They can remain intramural. If they extend into the uterine lumen or submucosa, or if they extend outward, they become pedunculated and subserosal. Leiomyomas have a variety of sonographic textures, ranging from hypoechoic to echogenic with a definite border (Fig. 4-4A through C). These tumors have varying amounts of smooth muscle and connective tissue.

Transvaginal sonography can be used to monitor the size of leiomyomas. Color Doppler sonography may help identify those leiomyomas that are vascular and may be responsive to gonadotropin-releasing hormone analog (Lupron) treatment (Friedman and coworkers, 1987). TVS is particularly helpful in identifying intraligamentous fibroids and the pedicle of pedunculated subserosal fibroids, thereby differentiating these from intramural fibroids (see Fig. 4-4D and E).

Sonohysterography, which involves fluid instillation into the lumen, is useful in differentiating polyps from submucosal fibroids (Fig. 4-5) (Syrop and Sahakian, 1993; Goldstein, 1994). For this technique, a 5 French insemination catheter is fed up into the cervix and 5 to 10 mL of sterile saline is infused. Submucosal fibroids tend to expand into the lumen from the myometrium, whereas polyps tend to have a well-defined pedicle. This distinction is helpful in differentiating women who are best treated by hysteroscopic removal of the polyp versus those who may have to undergo wire loop resection of the fibroid (Fedele and coworkers, 1991).

ENDOMETRIAL HYPERPLASIA

Bleeding in the postmenopausal woman is fairly common, but could be an indicator of endometrial carcinoma. The differential diagnosis includes atrophic endometrium, which is prone to hemorrhagic ulceration or estrogen-induced hyperplasia of the endometrium.

Several large studies have set the upper limits of the thickness of the endometrium in healthy postmenopausal women to be between 6 and 8 mm in AP dimension (see Fig. 4-5) (Goldstein and coworkers, 1990; Osmers and coworkers, 1991; Nasri and Coast, 1991; Granberg and coworkers, 1991). The endometrium may be slightly thicker in patients on hormone replacement therapy (Zalud and coworkers, 1993; Lin, 1992).

Transvaginal sonography is used in the evaluation of postmenopausal women who have vaginal bleeding. Endometrial thickening greater than 8 mm in the AP dimension in patients who are postmenopausal usually indicates either hyperplasia or carcinoma (Goldstein and coworkers, 1990). TVS

can assess the amount of tissue within the endometrium and is predictive in cases in which there is scant (less than 6 mm in width) endometrium, but these samples might have insufficient tissue for diagnosis or scant cellular material. The relative amount of tissues that will be retrieved by dilation and curettage can be predicted by the appearance of the endometrium on TVS. Measuring the endometrium in length, AP dimension, and width enables estimation of endometrial volume (Fleischer, 1990).

Transvaginal sonography is not a screening procedure in patients with endometrial hyperplasia because the evaluation of these patients is based on a histopathologic diagnosis. TVS can supply information concerning the relative amount of endometrial hyperplasia, however. Sonographic images of endometrial thickening may result from hyperplasia but actually represent polyps larger than 5 to 10 mm in diameter. Because these are usually compressed, however, individual polyps may not be discernible with TVS. Sonohysterography enhances the delineation of polyps (see Fig. 4-5G and H) (Parsons and Lense, 1993; Kupfer, 1994).

Transvaginal sonography may detect a thickened endometrium in patients being evaluated for an adnexal mass. If the endometrium is larger than 10 mm in the AP dimension or more than 5 to 10 cm^3 in volume, an endometrial biopsy may be indicated, especially if there is a history of bleeding, because hyperplasia is a known precursor to carcinoma (Ferenczy, 1988). Women taking tamoxifen should be carefully studied because they are prone to hyperplasia and cancer (Hulka and Hall, 1993).

ENDOMETRIAL NEOPLASMS

Transvaginal sonography aids in the assessment of the depth of invasion in patients with histologically proven endometrial carcinoma (Gordon and coworkers, 1989). In most cases, the extent of invasion can be detected and classified as superficial, intermediate, or deep, depending on the extent of the tumor invasion relative to the myometrial thickness (>50% = deep) (Fig. 4-6) and extension into the cervix (Fig. 4-7).

Most endometrial tumors are echogenic, although less well-differentiated tumors may be hypoechoic (see Fig. 4-6B and C) (Gordon and coworkers, 1989). Difficulties arise in tumors that are exophytic or those that stretch the myometrium but do not invade it. Microscopic invasion is also not detectable, and preexisting conditions such as leiomyoma and adenomyoma may make it difficult to precisely delineate the extent of myometrial invasion. Contrast enhanced magnetic resonance imaging may be used to evaluate the extent of myometrial invasion in difficult or equivocal cases.

OTHER CONDITIONS

Transvaginal sonography can also evaluate patients with suspected adenomyosis in which the sonographic findings range from normal sonographic appearances to echogenic myometrium caused by multiple adenomyomas. Endometritis may also demonstrate an echogenic pattern and thickening of the endometrium.

Retained secretions, either mucous or serous, can simulate endometrial pathology. Occasionally, TVS can detect adhesions as hypoechoic bands that cross the endometrium (Narayan and Goswamy, 1993). These may be detected even without the use of fluid instillation in some cases.

SUMMARY

Transvaginal sonography is the diagnostic modality of choice for evaluating most uterine disorders (Atri, 1994). It is particularly useful in identifying the exact location and size of leiomyomas and other uterine tumors.

REFERENCES

Atri M. Transvaginal US appearance in endometrial abnormalities. Radiographics 1994;14:453.

de Vries K, Lyons E, Ballard G. Contractions of the inner fluid of the myometrium. Am J Obstet Gynecol 1990; 62:679.

Fedele L, Bianchi S, Dorta M, Brioschi D, Zanotti F, Vercellini P. Transvaginal ultrasonography versus hysteroscopy in the diagnosis of uterine submucous myomas. Obstet Gynecol 1991;77:745.

Ferenczy A. Endometrial hyperplasia and neoplasia: A two disease concept. In: Berkowitz RL, Cohen CJ, Kase NG, eds. Obstetric Ultrasonography/Gynecologic Oncology. New York: Churchill-Livingstone, 1988;197.

Fleischer A, Gordon A, Entman S, Kepple D. Transvaginal sonography of the endometrium: Current and potential clinical applications. Crit Rev Diagn Imaging 1990; 30:85.

Friedman AJ, Barbieri RL, Benacerraf BR, Schiff I. Treatment of leiomyomata with intranasal or subcutaneous leuprolide, a gonadotropin-releasing hormone agonist. Fertil Steril 1987;48:560.

Goldstein SR. Use of ultrasonohysterography for triage of perimenopausal patients with unexplained bleeding. Am J Obstet Gynecol 1994;170:565.

Goldstein SR, Nachtigall M, Snyder JR, Nachtigall L. Endometrial assessment by vaginal ultrasonography before endometrial sampling in patients with postmenopausal bleeding. Am J Obstet Gynecol 1990; 163:119.

Gordon AN, Fleischer AC, Reed GW. Depth of myometrial invasion in endometrial cancer: Preoperative assessment by transvaginal ultrasonography. Gynecol Oncol 1989;34:175.

Granberg S, Wikland M, Karlsson B, Norstrom A, Friberg LG. Endometrial thickness as measured by endovaginal ultrasonography for identifying endometrial abnormality. Am J Obstet Gynecol 1991;164:47.

Hulka C, Hall D. Endometrial abnormalities associated with tamoxifen therapy for breast cancer: Sonographic and pathologic correlation. AJR 1993;160:809.

Kupfer M, Schiller V, Hansen G, Tessler R. Transvaginal somographic evaluation of endometrial polyps. J Ultrasound Med 1994;13:535.

Lin M, Gisink B, Wolf S. Endometrial thickness after menopause: Effect of hormone replacement. Radiology 1993;180:427.

Mendelson EB, Bohm-Velez M, Joseph N, Neiman HL. Endometrial abnormalities: Evaluation with transvaginal sonography. AJR 1988;150:139.

Narayan R, Goswamy R. Transvaginal sonography of the uterine cavity with hysteroscopic correlations in the investigation of infertility. Ultrasound in Ob/Gyn 1993;3:129.

Nasri MN, Coast GJ. Correlation of ultrasound findings and endometrial histopathology in postmenopausal women. Br J Obstet Gynaecol 1989;96:1333.

Osmers R, Volksen M, Schauer A. Vaginosonography for early detection of endometrial carcinoma. Lancet 1990;335:1569.

Parsons A, Lense J. Sonohysterography for endometrial abnormalities: Preliminary results. J Clin Ultrasound 1993;21:82.

Syrop CH, Sahakian V. Transvaginal sonographic detection of endometrial polyps with fluid contrast augmentation. Obstet Gynecol 1992;79:1041.

Zalud I, Conway C, Schulman H, Trinca D. Endometrial and myometrial thickness and uterine blood flow in postmenopausal women: The influence of hormonal replacement therapy and age. J Ultrasound Med 1993; 12:737.

FIGURE 4-1
Normal Uterus

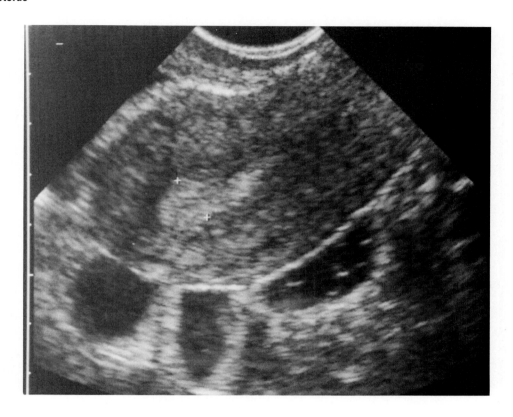

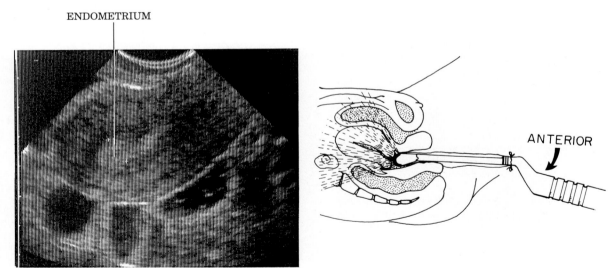

ENDOMETRIUM

ANTERIOR

Figure 4-1A. Normal uterus in long axis.

Normal Uterus *(Continued)*

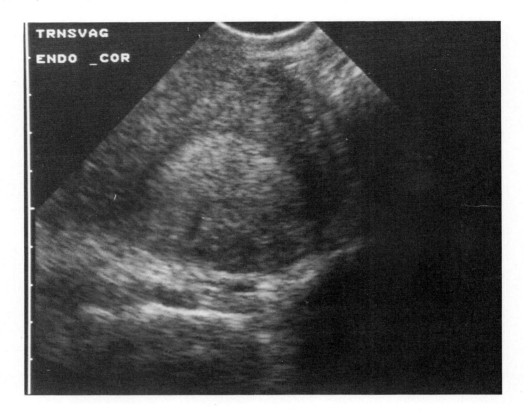

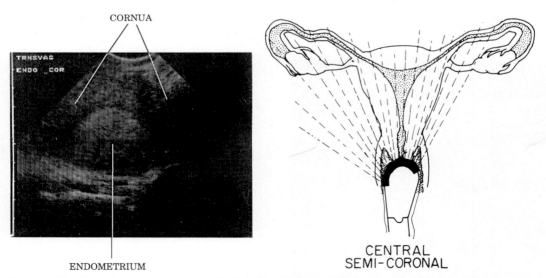

Figure 4-1B. Normal uterus in semicoronal plane. Note the invagination of endometrium into tubal ostia within the uterine cornua.

Normal Uterus *(Continued)*

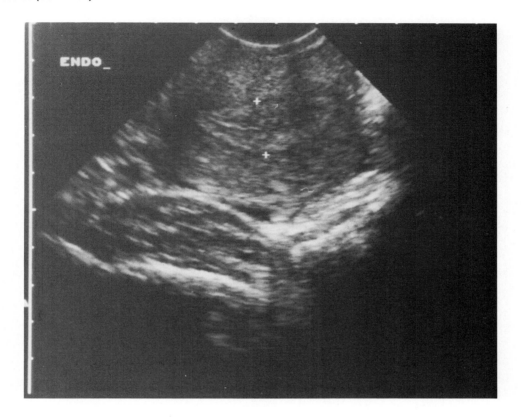

SECRETORY ENDOMETRIUM

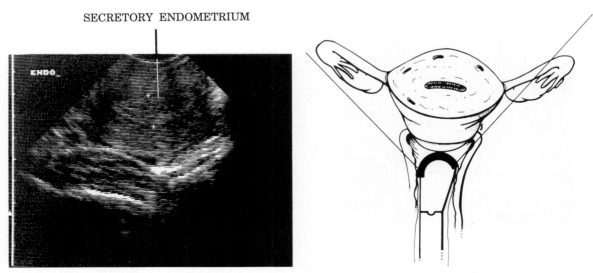

Figure 4-1C. Normal uterus in short axis showing secretory phase endometrium. Note where the endometrium invaginates into the area of tubal ostia.

Normal Uterus *(Continued)*

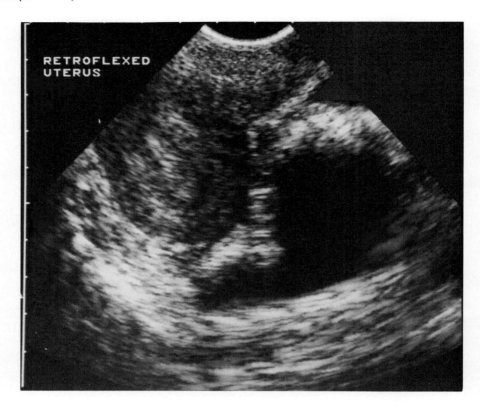

ENDOMETRIUM

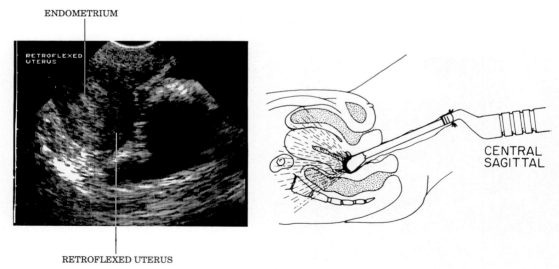

RETROFLEXED UTERUS

Figure 4-1D. Retroflexed uterus in long axis.

Normal Uterus *(Continued)*

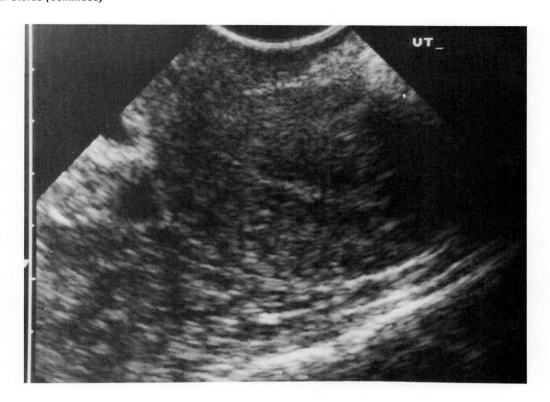

ATROPHIC ENDOMETRIUM

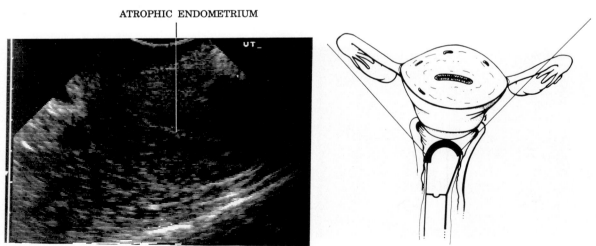

Figure 4-1E. Normal atrophic endometrium in postmenopausal woman.

Normal Uterus *(Continued)*

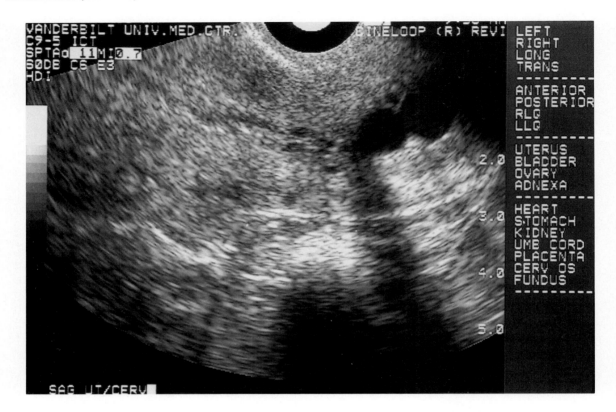

CERVICAL INCLUSION CYST

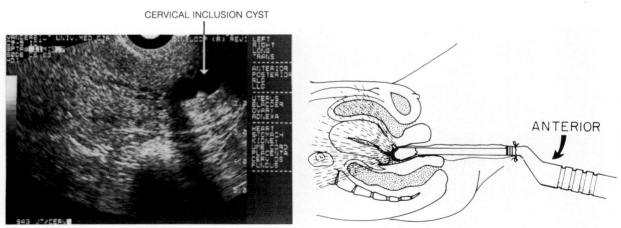

Figure 4-1F. Normal thin endometrium distinct from the multiple cervical inclusion cysts in a postmenopausal woman.

Normal Uterus *(Continued)*

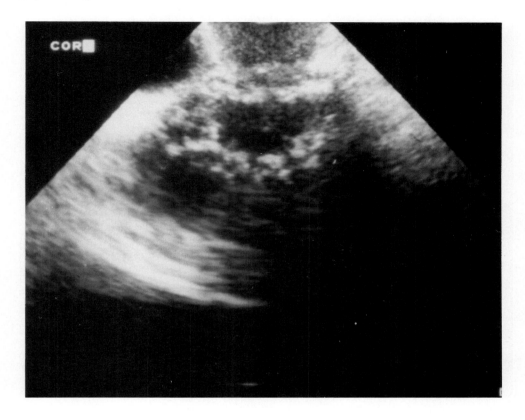

ARCUATE ARTERY CALCIFICATIONS

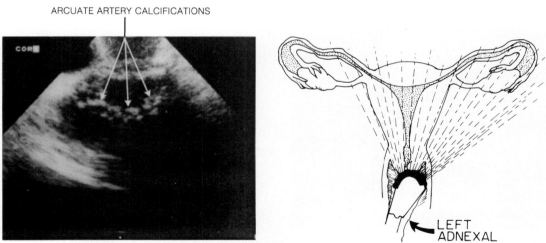

LEFT ADNEXAL

Figure 4-1G. Arcuate artery calcification in an elderly patient.

Normal Uterus *(Continued)*

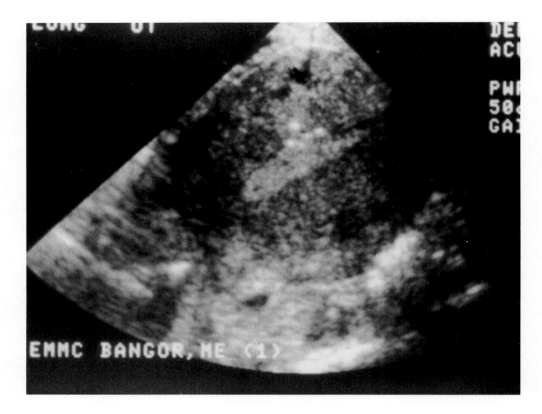

ECHOGENIC FOCI

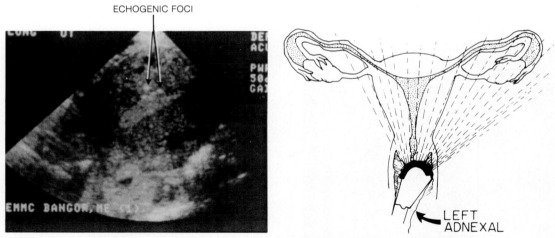

LEFT ADNEXAL

Figure 4-1H. Multiple puncture echogenicities within inner myometrium in a patient S/P dilatation and curettage. (Courtesy of Mary Warner, M.D.)

FIGURE 4-2
Normal Variants

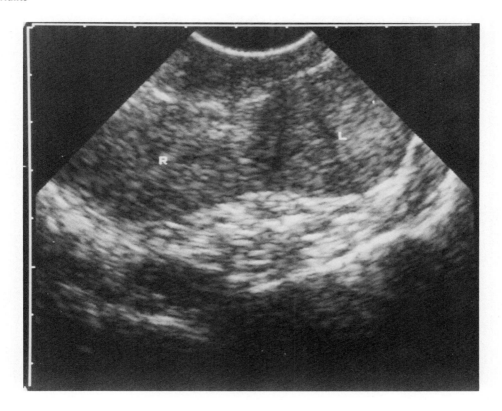

BICORNUATE UTERUS

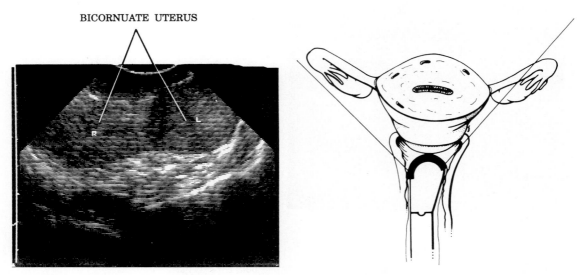

Figure 4-2A. Bicornuate uterus demonstrating two endometria. *R,* right horn; *L,* left horn.

Normal Variants *(Continued)*

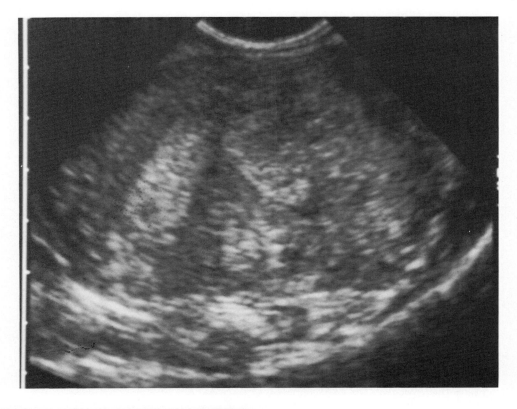

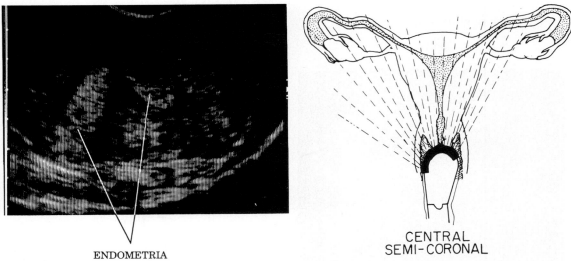

ENDOMETRIA   CENTRAL
                                                       SEMI-CORONAL

Figure 4-2B. Bicornuate uterus in a semicoronal plane showing both endometria.

Normal Variants *(Continued)*

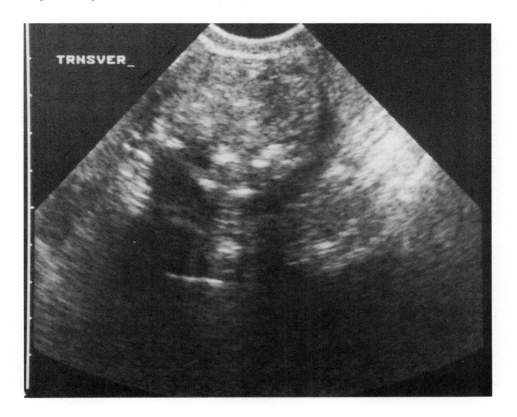

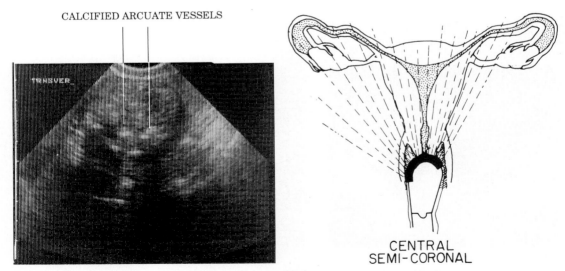

CALCIFIED ARCUATE VESSELS

CENTRAL
SEMI-CORONAL

Figure 4-2C. Calcifications within arcuate artery in an elderly woman.

FIGURE 4-3
Endometrial Changes During a Spontaneous Cycle

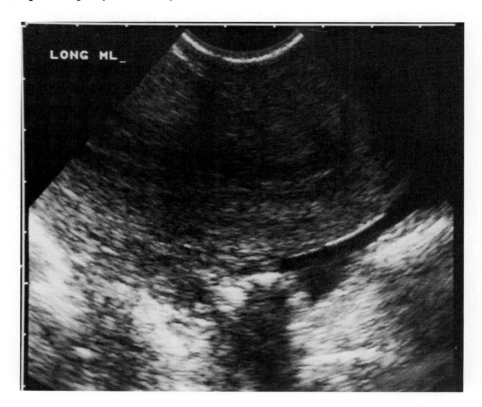

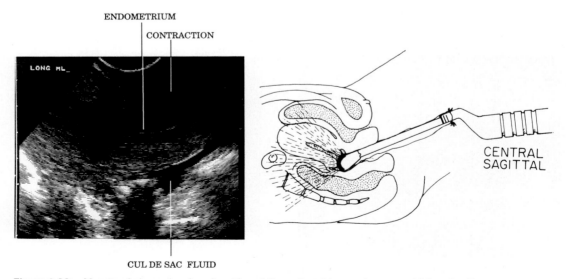

ENDOMETRIUM

CONTRACTION

CENTRAL SAGITTAL

CUL DE SAC FLUID

Figure 4-3A.   Menstrual phase showing sloughing of the endometrium and a myometrial contraction. Cul-de-sac fluid is also present.

Endometrial Changes During a Spontaneous Cycle *(Continued)*

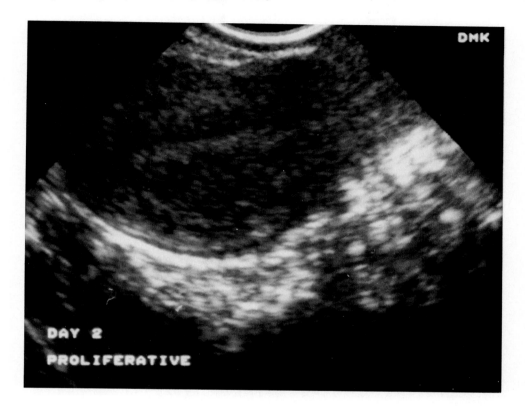

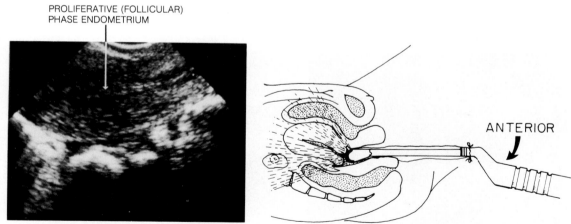

Figure 4-3B. Early proliferative phase showing thin, slightly hyperechoic texture.

Endometrial Changes During a Spontaneous Cycle *(Continued)*

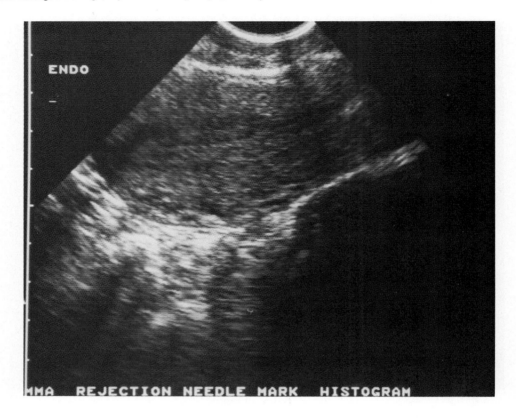

ENDOMETRIUM

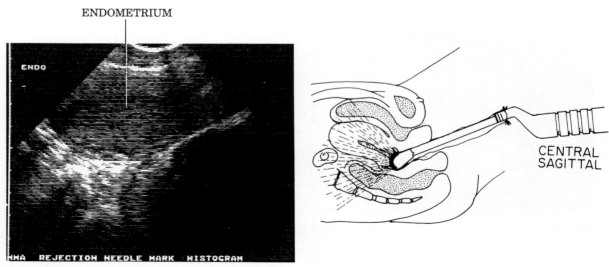

Figure 4-3C. Proliferative phase showing as isoechoic to the myometrium.

Endometrial Changes During a Spontaneous Cycle *(Continued)*

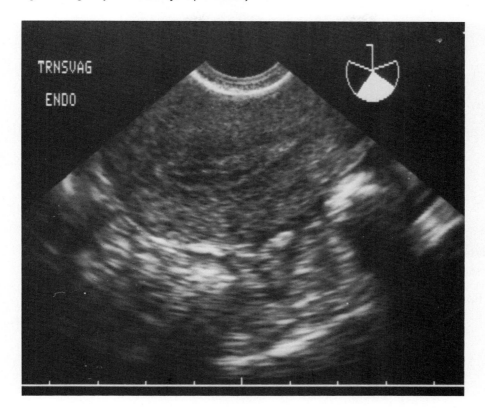

MULTILAYERED ENDOMETRIUM

CENTRAL SAGITTAL

Figure 4-3D. Periovulatory period showing multiple layers due to edema of the compactum layer.

Endometrial Changes During a Spontaneous Cycle *(Continued)*

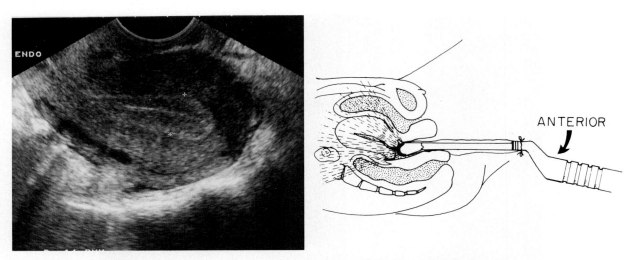

Figure 4-3E. Midsecretory phase in a retroflexed uterus showing multilayered appearance. The outer echogenic layer represents the basalis, the inner, more hypoechoic layer represents the functionalis layer. The median echo arises from intraluminal mucus and trapped fluid.

Endometrial Changes During a Spontaneous Cycle *(Continued)*

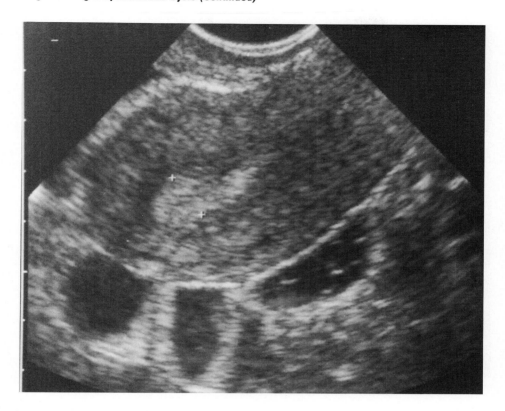

SECRETORY ENDOMETRIUM

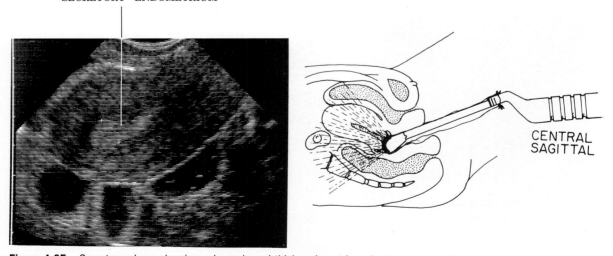

CENTRAL
SAGITTAL

Figure 4-3F. Secretory phase showing echogenic and thick endometrium due to mucus and glycogen stored within glands (between cursors).

Endometrial Changes During a Spontaneous Cycle *(Continued)*

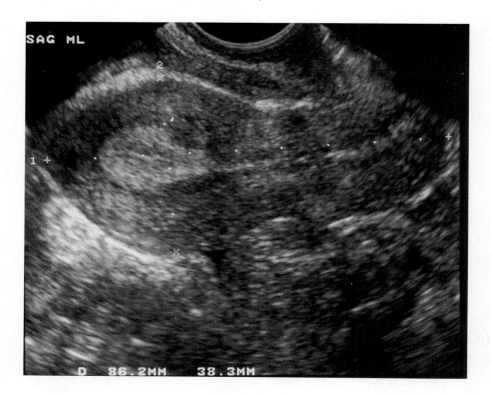

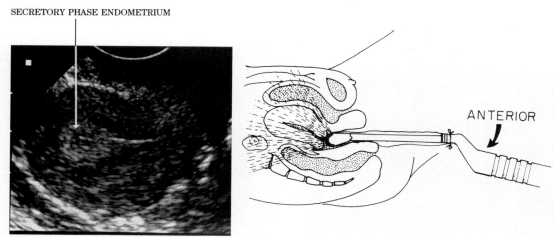

Figure 4-3G. Midsecretory phase showing echogenic texture.

Endometrial Changes During a Spontaneous Cycle *(Continued)*

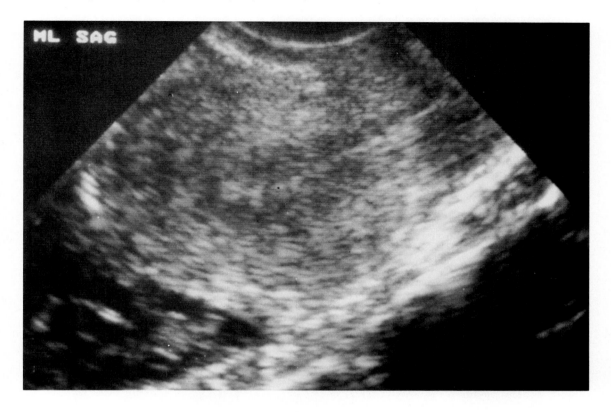

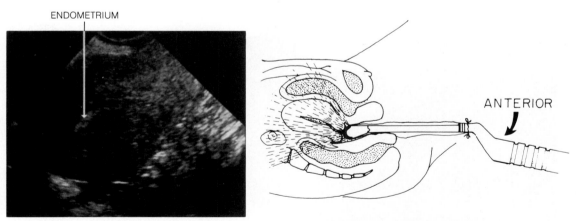

Figure 4-3H. Late secretory phase showing marked thinning and irregularity of the endometrium.

FIGURE 4-4
Leiomyoma

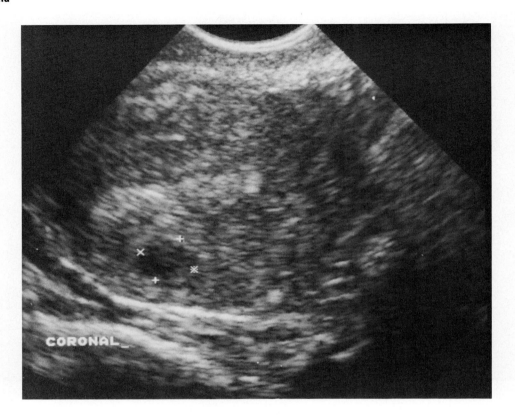

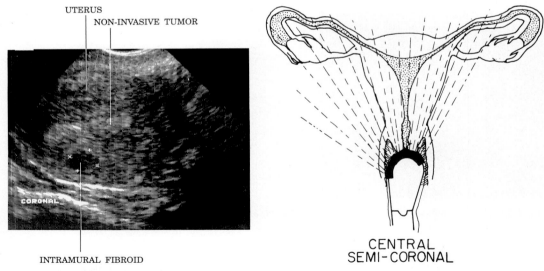

Figure 4-4A. Small hypoechoic intramural fibroid.

Leiomyoma *(Continued)*

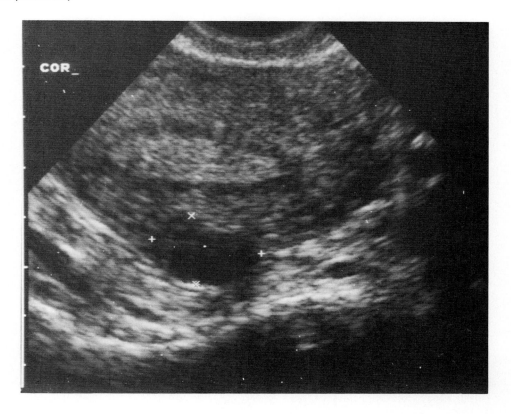

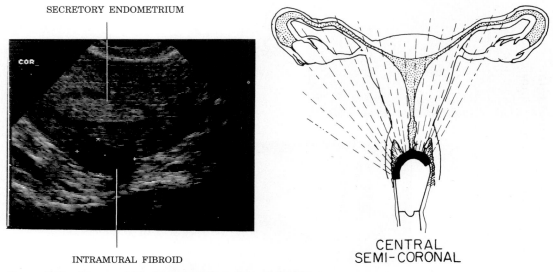

Figure 4-4B. Intramural fibroid separate from the endometrium.

Leiomyoma *(Continued)*

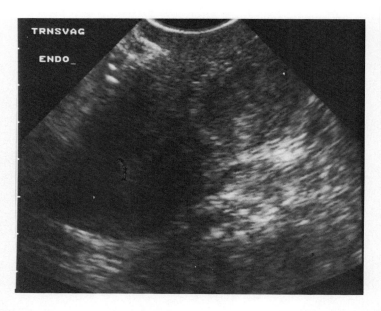

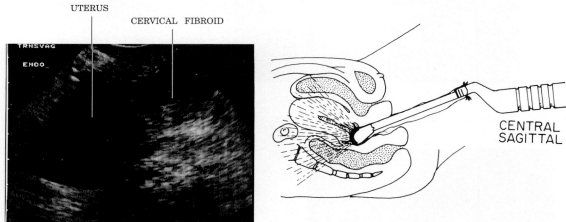

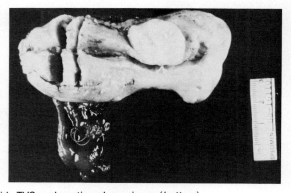

Figure 4-4C. Cervical fibroid. TVS and sectioned specimen (*bottom*).

Leiomyoma *(Continued)*

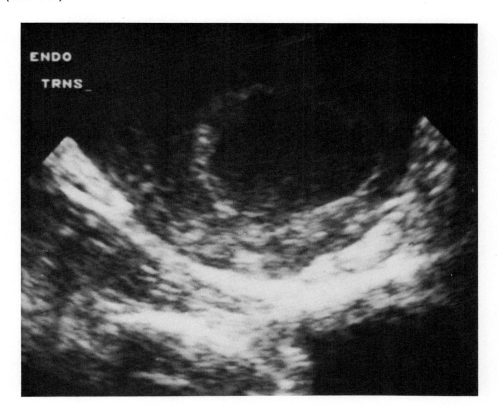

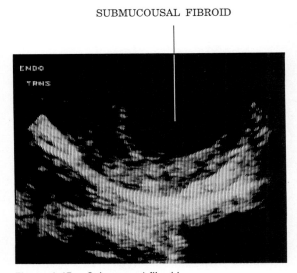

SUBMUCOUSAL FIBROID

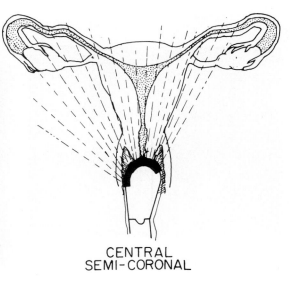

CENTRAL
SEMI-CORONAL

Figure 4-4D. Submucosal fibroid.

Leiomyoma *(Continued)*

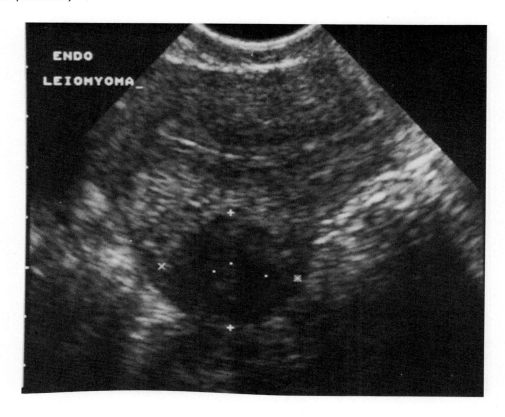

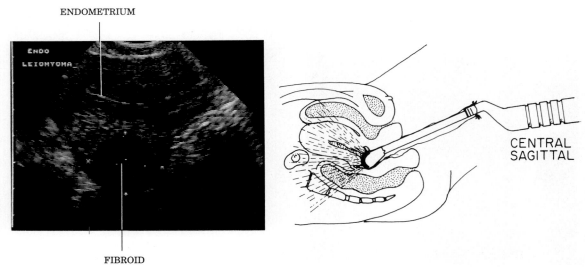

Figure 4-4E.   Subserous fibroid extrinsic to endometrium.

FIGURE 4-5
Endometrial Hyperplasia/Adenomyosis

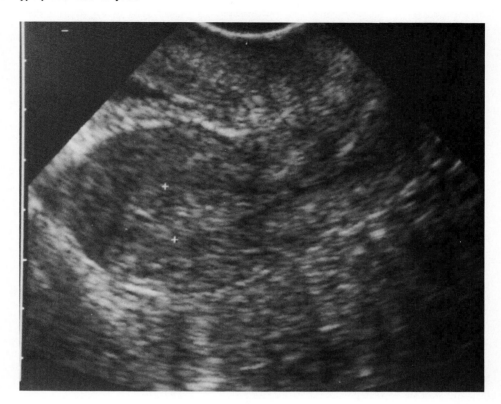

HYPERPLASTIC ENDOMETRIUM

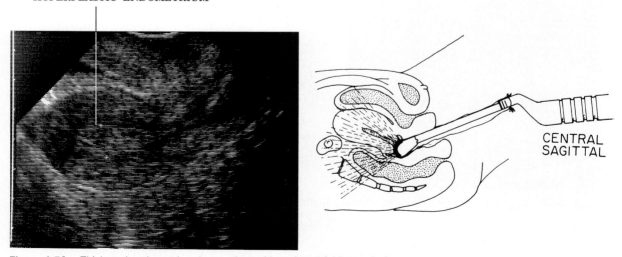

CENTRAL SAGITTAL

Figure 4-5A. Thickened endometrium in a patient with endometrial hyperplasia.

Endometrial Hyperplasia/Adenomyosis *(Continued)*

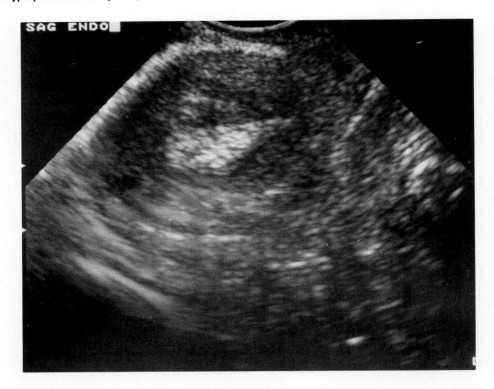

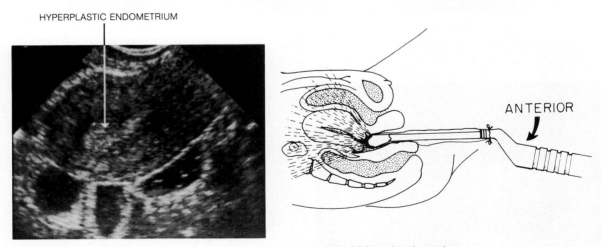

Figure 4-5B. Adenomatous hyperplasia demonstrating an irregularly thickened endometrium.

Endometrial Hyperplasia/Adenomyosis *(Continued)*

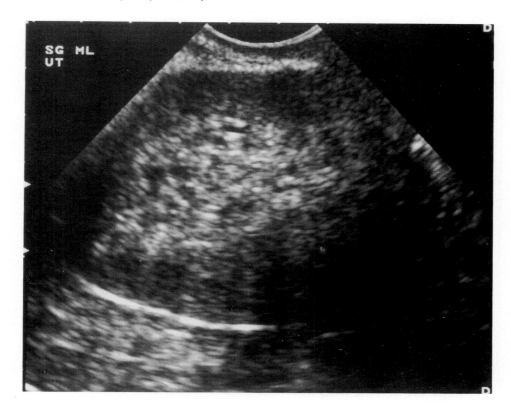

ENDOMETRIAL POLYP

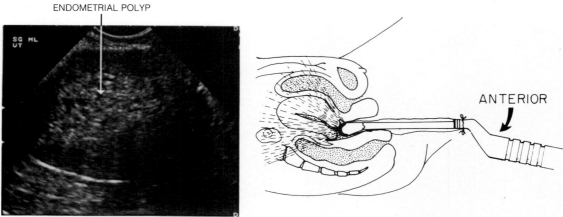

Figure 4-5C. Large polyp with punctate cystic areas within echogenic lesion in a patient on tamoxifen therapy.

Endometrial Hyperplasia/Adenomyosis *(Continued)*

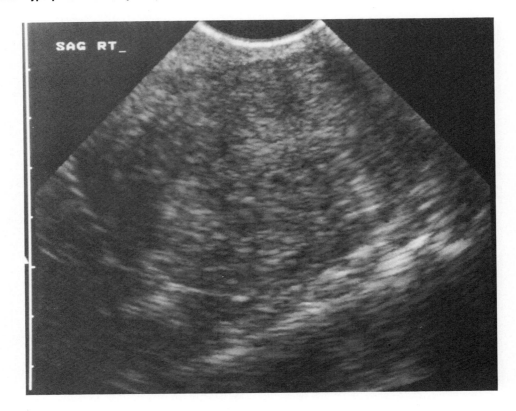

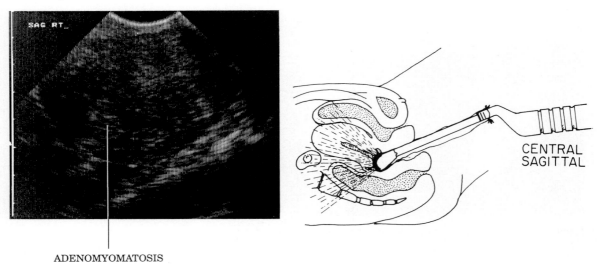

ADENOMYOMATOSIS

Figure 4-5D. Adenomyosis causing increased echogenicity of the myometrium.

Endometrial Hyperplasia/Adenomyosis *(Continued)*

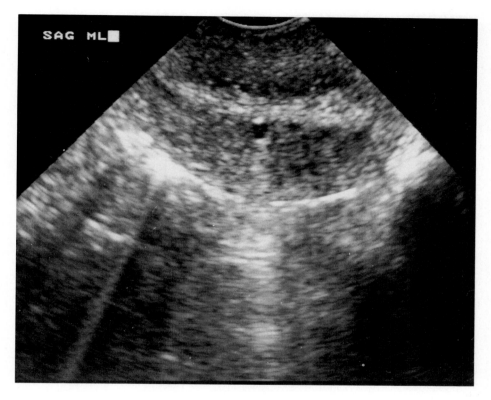

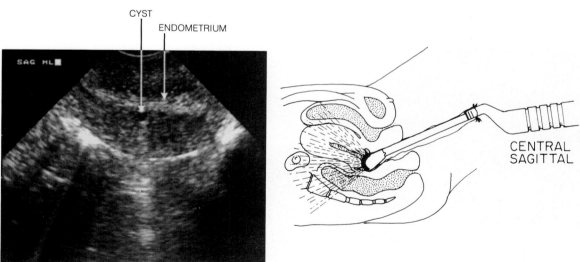

Figure 4-5E. Cystic areas within the inner myometrium in a woman on tamoxifen therapy.

Endometrial Hyperplasia/Adenomyosis *(Continued)*

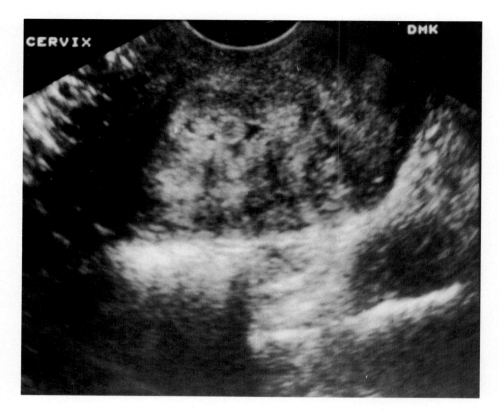

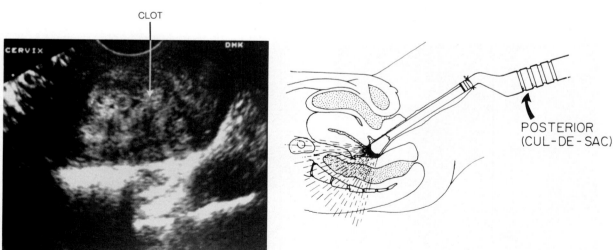

Figure 4-5F. Blood clots within the endometrial lumen.

Endometrial Hyperplasia/Adenomyosis *(Continued)*

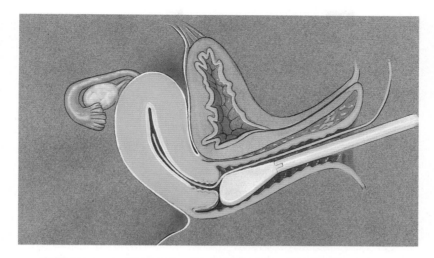

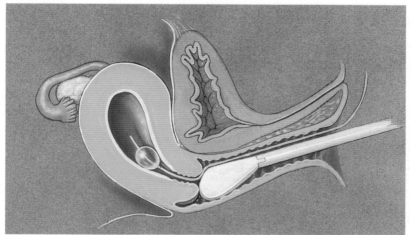

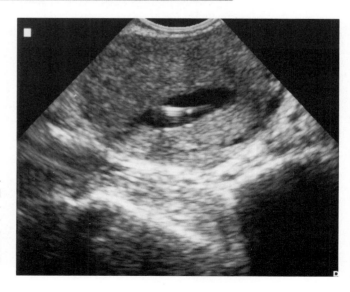

Figure 4-5G. Normal sonohysterography. (*Top*) Diagram of a pediatric feeding tube catheter. The tip should be placed within the fundal portion of the lumen. (*Middle*) Same as *top* using a catheter with an inflated balloon. This device is recommended in parous women to reduce leakage around the catheter. (*Bottom*) Normal sonohysterogram showing fluid on either side of the catheter. The endometrium is thin and regular.

Endometrial Hyperplasia/Adenomyosis *(Continued)*

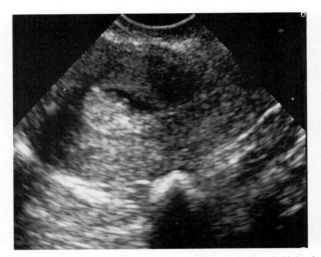 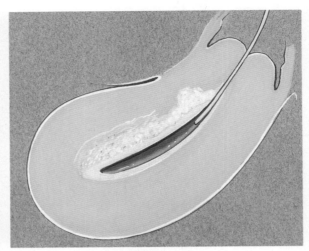

Figure 4-5H. Abnormal sonohysterogram. (*left*) Focal thickening of the endometrium in disordered proliferative endometrium. (*right*) Focal thickening.

Endometrial Hyperplasia/Adenomyosis *(Continued)*

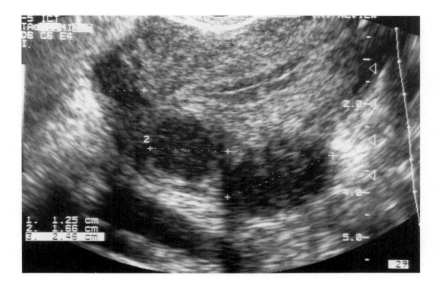

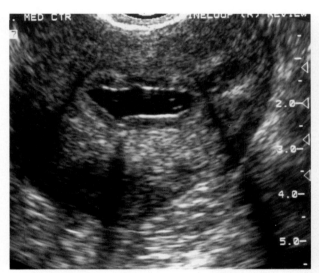

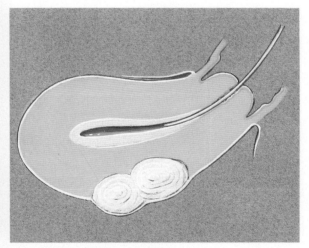

Figure 4-5I. *(top)* Three intramural fibroids (between cursors) not displacing the endometrium. *(bottom left)* Sonohysterogram showing normal endometrium. *(bottom right)* Diagram of intramural fibroids (shown at *top* and *bottom left*).

Endometrial Hyperplasia/Adenomyosis *(Continued)*

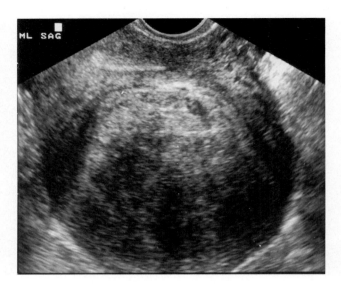

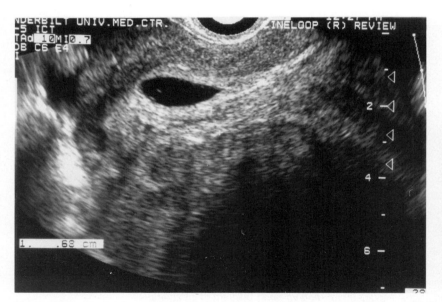

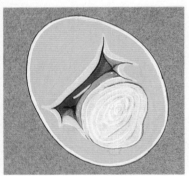

Figure 4-5J. (*top*) Intramural fibroid displaying normal endometrium. (*bottom left*) Sonohysterogram of the patient (shown at *top*) showing normal endometrium overlying the intramural fibroid. (*bottom right*) Diagram of the intramural fibroid (shown at *top* and *bottom left*).

Endometrial Hyperplasia/Adenomyosis *(Continued)*

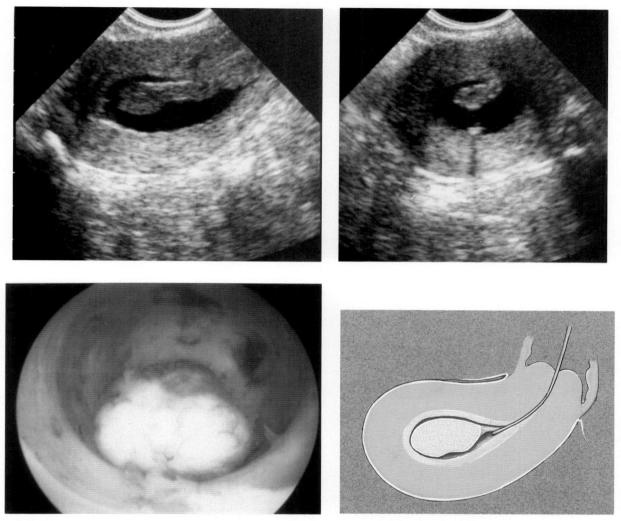

Figure 4-5K. (*top left*) Sonohysterogram in long axis showing a large endometrial polyp. (*top right*) Sonohysterogram in short axis showing a large endometrial polyp. (*bottom left*) Hysteroscopic view of polyps (shown at *top left* and *top right*). (Courtesy of Ester Eisenberg, M.D.). (*bottom right*) Diagram of polyps (shown at *top left, top right,* and *bottom left*).

Endometrial Hyperplasia/Adenomyosis *(Continued)*

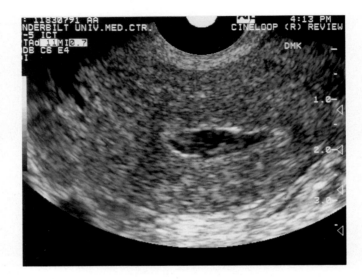

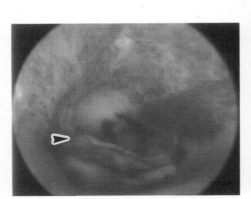
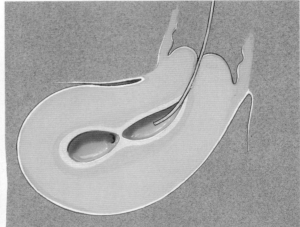

Figure 4-5L. *(top)* Sonohysterogram showing an adhesion crossing the lumen. *(bottom left)* Hysteroscopic view of the adhesion (shown at *top*) *(arrowhead)*. (Courtesy of Ester Eisenberg, M.D.). *(bottom right)* Diagram of adhesion (shown at *top*).

FIGURE 4-6
TVS of Endometrial Carcinoma With Accompanying Sectioned Gross Specimen

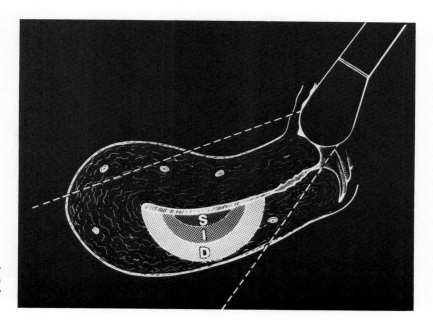

Figure 4-6A. Diagram showing superficial (S), intermediate (I), and deep (D) myometrial invasion as determined by TVS.

TVS of Endometrial Carcinoma With Accompanying Sectioned Gross Specimen *(Continued)*

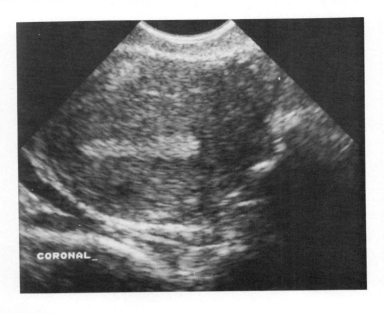

NON-INVASIVE TUMOR

UTERUS

ANTERIOR

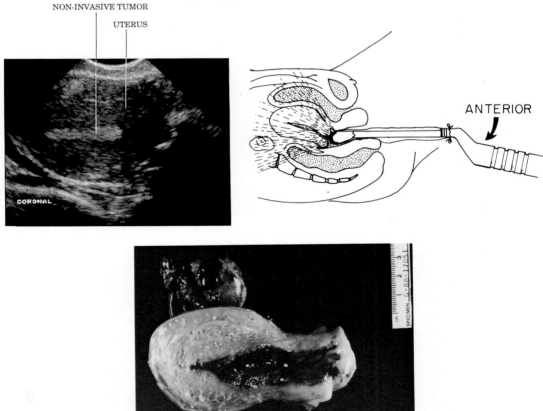

Figure 4-6B. Noninvasive tumor demonstrating distinct endometrial/myometrial interface.

TVS of Endometrial Carcinoma With Accompanying Sectioned Gross Specimen *(Continued)*

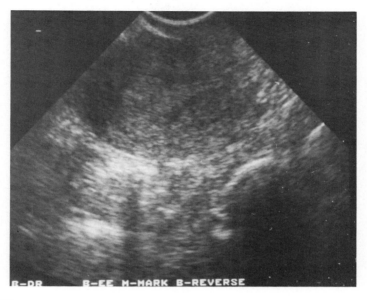

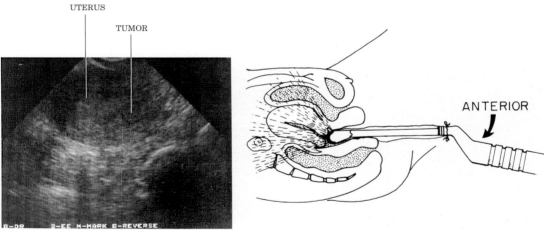

UTERUS

TUMOR

ANTERIOR

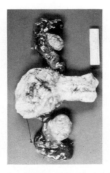

Figure 4-6C.   Superficial myometrial invasion as evidenced by focal discontinuity of subendometrial halo.

TVS of Endometrial Carcinoma With Accompanying Sectioned Gross Specimen *(Continued)*

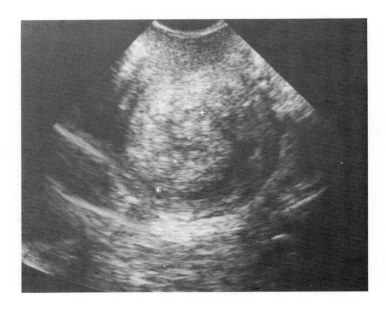

UTERUS

TUMOR

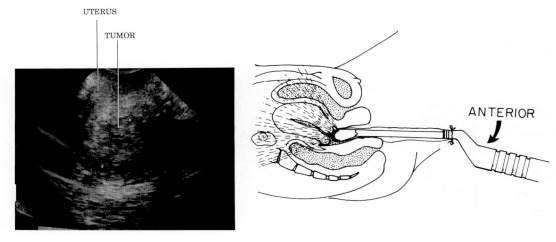

ANTERIOR

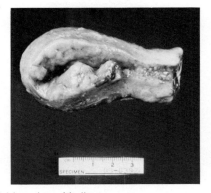

Figure 4-6D. Superficial myometrial invasion of bulky tumor.

TVS of Endometrial Carcinoma With Accompanying Sectioned Gross Specimen *(Continued)*

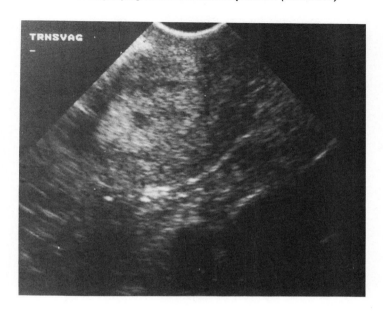

TUMOR

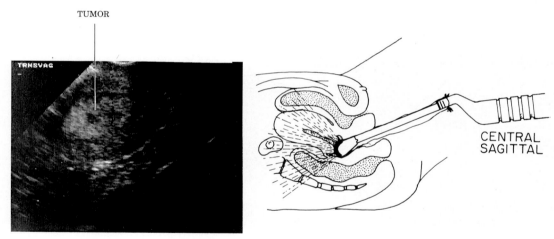

CENTRAL
SAGITTAL

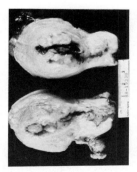

Figure 4-6E. Superficial invasion of a polypoid tumor.

TVS of Endometrial Carcinoma With Accompanying Sectioned Gross Specimen *(Continued)*

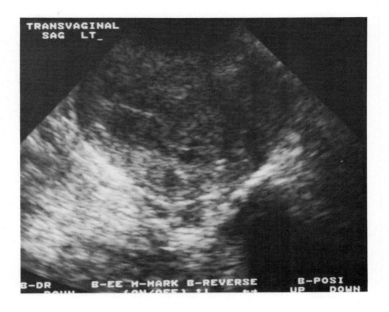

UTERUS

INVASIVE TUMOR

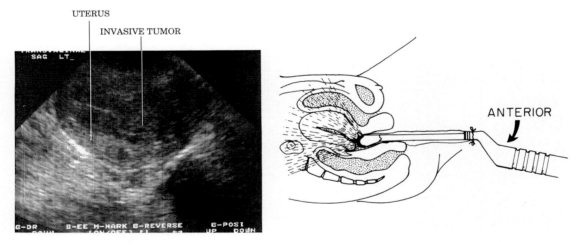

ANTERIOR

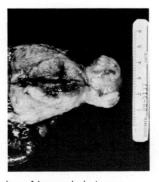

Figure 4-6F. Moderate myometrial invasion of hypoechoic tumor.

TVS of Endometrial Carcinoma With Accompanying Sectioned Gross Specimen *(Continued)*

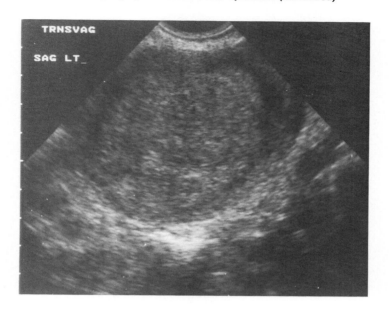

TUMOR

UTERUS

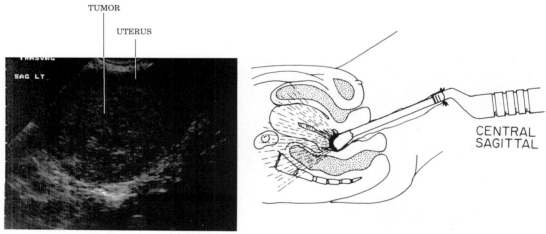

CENTRAL
SAGITTAL

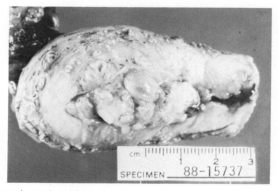

Figure 4-6G. Moderately invasive polypoid tumor.

TVS of Endometrial Carcinoma With Accompanying Sectioned Gross Specimen *(Continued)*

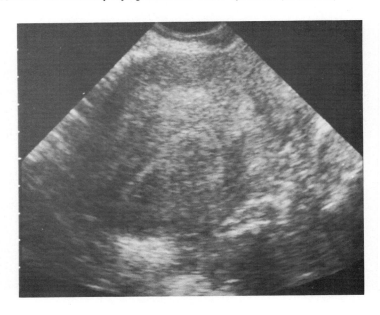

TUMOR

UTERUS

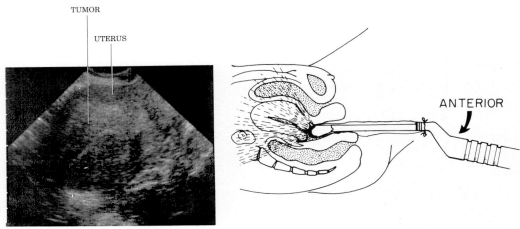

ANTERIOR

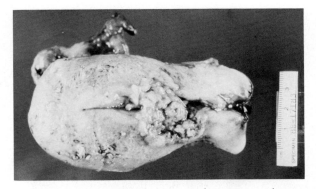

Figure 4-6H.   Deep myometrial invasion within the lower uterine corpus and upper cervix. Because it involves the cervix, this is a stage II tumor.

TVS of Endometrial Carcinoma With Accompanying Sectioned Gross Specimen *(Continued)*

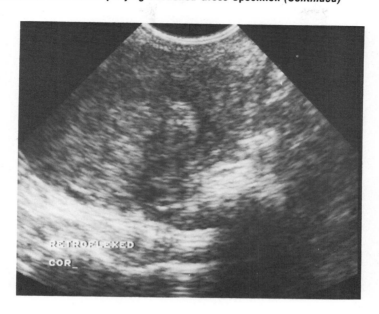

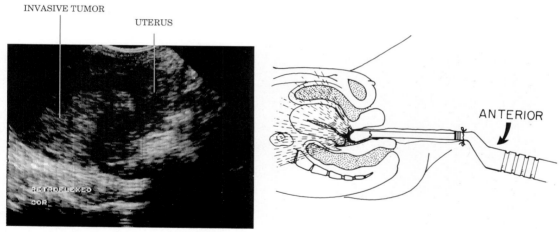

INVASIVE TUMOR

UTERUS

ANTERIOR

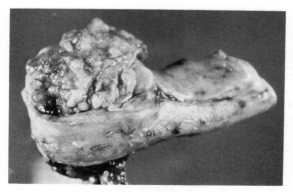

Figure 4-6I. Deep myometrial invasion within uterine fundus.

TVS of Endometrial Carcinoma With Accompanying Sectioned Gross Specimen *(Continued)*

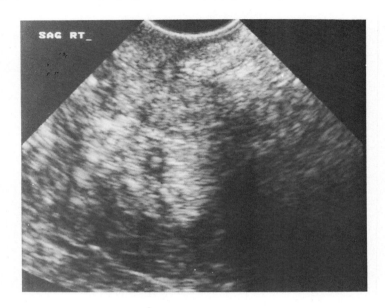

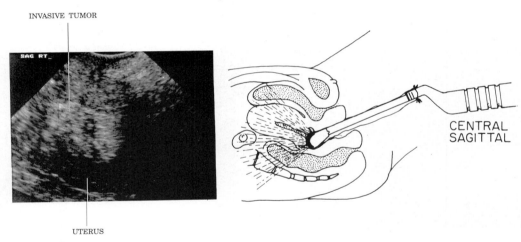

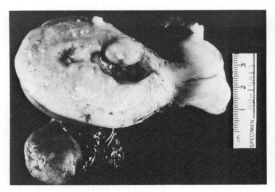

Figure 4-6J. Invasive polypoid tumor.

TVS of Endometrial Carcinoma With Accompanying Sectioned Gross Specimen *(Continued)*

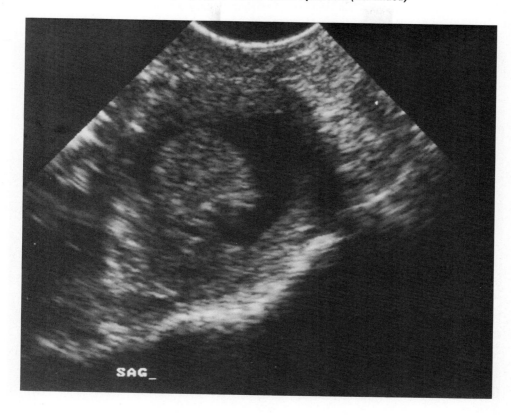

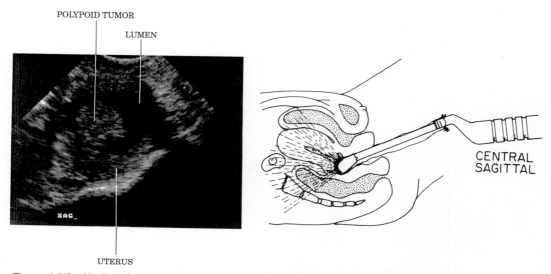

Figure 4-6K. Noninvasive polypoid (papillary serous) tumor on a stalk surrounded by fluid.

FIGURE 4-7
Presumably Invasive Endometrial Tumors That Underwent Radiation Therapy (no surgical confirmation)

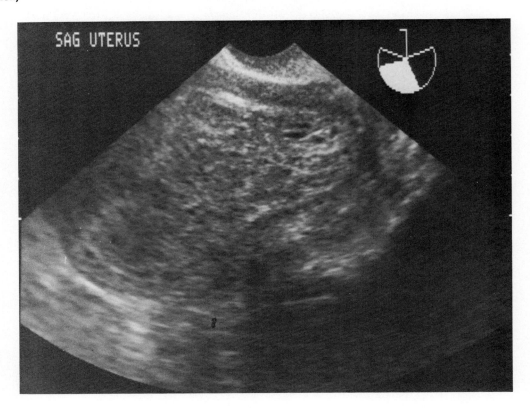

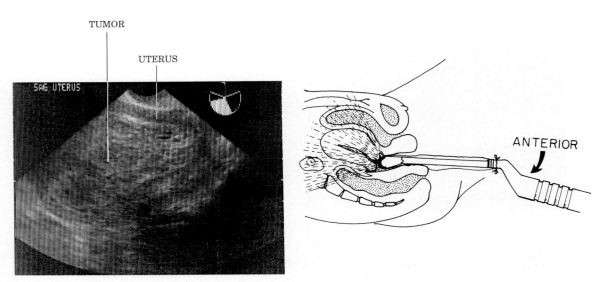

Figure 4-7A. Bulky endometrial tumor extending into the cervix.

Presumably Invasive Endometrial Tumors That Underwent Radiation Therapy (no surgical confirmation) *(Continued)*

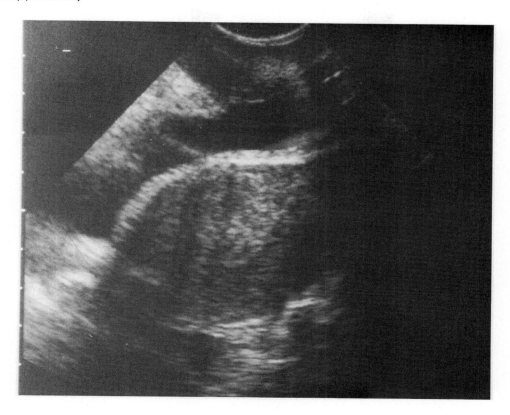

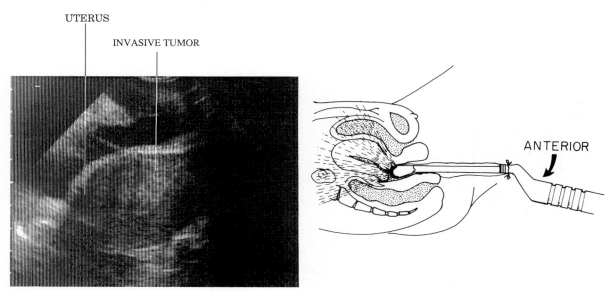

UTERUS

INVASIVE TUMOR

ANTERIOR

Figure 4-7B. Tumor extending to uterine serosa.

Transvaginal Sonography: A Clinical Atlas, Second Edition,
edited by Arthur C. Fleischer and Donna M. Kepple.
J.B. Lippincott Company, Philadelphia, © 1995.

CHAPTER 5

Ovarian Masses

Arthur C. Fleischer, MD

INTRODUCTION

Transvaginal sonography (TVS) affords detailed delineation of the normal ovary as well as masses that
are confined to the true pelvis. Masses larger than
10 cm are best evaluated using conventional transabdominal sonography (TAS), however. This chapter emphasizes both the transvaginal and transabdominal sonographic approaches to evaluation of
the ovarian mass. The discussion is divided into
sonographic categories of ovarian masses.

The probability of malignancy can be estimated
based on certain morphologic features. In general,
the more solid or irregular components of a mass,
the more likely it is to be malignant. Several scoring
systems have been proposed to estimate the chance
of malignancy based on size, internal components,
and wall thickness (Sassone and coworkers, 1991;
DePriest and van Nagell, 1992). Although it is not
necessary to "score" each mass, the complete evaluation of each mass is important.

NORMAL OVARIES

Transabdominal and transvaginal sonography can
identify the ovary in most women. Although the
ovary may be difficult to identify transabdominally
in the postmenopausal patient, both ovaries can be
identified in more than 60% of postmenopausal patients, particularly if scanning transvaginally and
using abdominal palpation (Fleischer and coworkers, 1990; Rodriguez and coworkers, 1988).

In premenopausal women, the normal ovary
typically measures $3 \times 2 \times 1$ cm (Fig. 5-1*A*). It may
be up to 5 cm in length in one dimension, but
should remain oval in shape. Rounded ovaries typically are encountered in patients with polycystic
ovarian disease. Measurement of the long, short,
and anteroposterior dimension of the ovary determines ovarian volume by the prolate ellipsoid for-
mula (length $\times$ height $\times$ width $\times$ 0.5 = volume in
cm^3). In premenopausal women, the normal ovary
ranges from 10 to 12 cm^3 in size, depending on the
presence of a mature follicle, which can account for
up to 2 cm or 4 cm^3 of volume. In postmenopausal
women, however, the normal ovary should be no
larger than 8 cm^3 (Campbell and coworkers, 1982;
Goswamy and coworkers, 1988). The texture should
be relatively featureless without presence of cystic or solid areas within the ovary (see Fig. 1-5*B*
through *D*).

Recent studies have shown that as many as 15%
of asymptomatic postmenopausal women may have
cysts as large as 5 cm in size (Levine and coworkers,
1992; Wolf, 1991). Some of these cysts may regress
completely or enlarge if examined on follow-up
studies (Levine, 1992). Many of these represent "inclusion" cysts.

CYSTIC OVARIAN MASSES

By definition, cystic ovarian masses contain no internal echoes, contain a smooth wall, and demonstrate enhanced through-transmission. Cystic masses occasionally may contain low-level echoes representing blood, pus, or cellular debris. Low-level echoes may also arise from proteinaceous or mucinous material within a predominantly cystic mass. Low-level echoes may be most apparent when the ovarian mass is scanned with higher frequency transducers or by the transvaginal approach.

In premenopausal women, the most common cystic mass is the physiologic ovarian cyst (Fig. 5-2A and B). These may represent either follicular or luteal cysts, depending on when the cyst begins to form during an ovulatory cycle. Luteal cysts tend to have thicker walls than follicular cysts; both measure more than 3 cm in size—greater than that expected for a mature graafian follicle. The intraovarian location of the cyst can be identified on TVS by displacement of ovarian parenchyma forming a "beak" of normal ovarian tissue around the cyst (see Fig. 5-2B).

When hemorrhage occurs within the cyst, low-level echoes or thin internal septa can be identified within the ovarian mass (see Fig. 5-2C). Therefore, hemorrhagic corpus lutea can mimic the appearance of a variety of ovarian masses, such as endometriomas and some epithelial tumors. Hemorrhagic corpus lutea tend to regress, however, whereas ovarian tumors and untreated endometriomas do not. Hemorrhagic cysts may precipitate ovarian torsion. Torsion can be identified using color Doppler transvaginal scanning or transabdominal scanning by the absence of arterial or venous signals from an enlarged ovary.

Other cystic masses near and around the ovary that can be identified on transabdominal or transvaginal scanning include endometriomas, paraovarian cysts, and sactosalpinges. Paraovarian cysts are separate from the ovary and are usually caused by fluid collecting within a remnant of the Gartner's duct located in the mesovarium (Fig. 5-3A). Endometriomas may have a variety of sonographic appearances, ranging from anechoic to echogenic and from loculated to septated, depending on the amount and coagulation of the internal blood components (see Fig. 5-3). Their borders may be irregular because of the fibrosis they incite in the surrounding soft tissue. Peritoneal cysts are typically related to previous surgery; they represent fluid collections that are walled off by the serosa of the pelvic organs.

CYSTIC OVARIAN TUMORS

Ovarian cystic masses may range from 2 to 40 cm in size. If they are completely anechoic and smooth-walled, the masses have a high probability of benignity (Goldstein and coworkers, 1989; Andolf and coworkers, 1986). Even in postmenopausal women in whom ovarian cancer incidence is greatest, an anechoic mass with smooth walls and good through-transmission has a greater than 95% incidence of being benign (Goldstein and coworkers, 1989; Andolf and Jörgensen, 1989). If there is a question of malignancy, a CA-125 assay may be performed to detect the ovarian tumor in a patient with a completely cystic mass.

Ovarian epithelial tumors have a variety of internal consistencies including septation, papillary excrescences, and irregular solid components. Mucinous tumors tend to have thin internal septa and may have areas of echogenic material within them that arise from mucin (Fig. 5-4A). Serous cystadenomas tend to be hypoechoic and unilocular, whereas epithelial carcinomas may demonstrate internal papillary excrescences (see Fig. 5-4B and C). Echogenic internal material that is mobile may be the result of either hemorrhage, cellular debris, or, in dermoid cysts, sebum that layers above the serous content of the dermoid cyst.

The presence of papillary excrescenses has high predictive value indicating malignancy (Fig. 5-4D and E) (Granberg and Norstrom, 1990).

COMPLEX OVARIAN MASSES

Complex ovarian masses represent lesions that contain both cystic and solid components. The most common of these is the dermoid cyst, although ovarian epithelial tumors, when large, frequently have a complex appearance.

Dermoid cysts demonstrate a variety of sonographic appearances, ranging from anechoic to echogenic. Anechoic dermoid cysts tend to arise from neuroectoderm and are encountered in young girls, whereas solid dermoid cysts tend to represent teratomas, some of which can be malignant, particularly in adolescents. The most common appearance of a dermoid cyst is a mass that has cystic and solid components (Fig. 5-5). The solid areas represent hair follicles and solid tissue combined with echogenic foci that represent calcified elements within the dermoid cysts. Some dermoid cysts contain sebum, a buttery material that tends to layer anteriorly within dermoid cysts because of its low specific gravity (see Fig. 5-5D).

Complex ovarian masses most frequently arise from masses containing hemorrhage such as the hemorrhagic corpus luteum (Fig. 5-6). Endometriomas may also demonstrate this appearance, as do some types of hemorrhagic ovarian masses in patients with bleeding disorders.

SOLID OVARIAN TUMORS

Compared with cystic ovarian tumors, solid ones are relatively uncommon (Fig. 5-7). Solid ovarian tumors typically arise from either primary or secondary adenocarcinoma of the ovary or the less differentiated ovarian tumors. Solid ovarian tumors may be differentiated from pedunculated fibroids by the transvaginal route. When pelvic or abdominal pressure is applied to the mass, the examiner should be able to separate a uterine from an ovarian lesion. Metastases to the ovary are not uncommon and usually present as solid ovarian masses.

ADNEXAL TORSION

Ovarian torsion usually occurs when it is associated with an increase in weight of the ovary due to hemorrhage, edema, or a mass. Degrees of torsion and chronicity are reflected on the morphologic and color Doppler findings. The ovary is usually enlarged and may contain several irregular areas due to hemorrhage. Transvaginal color Doppler sonography may show a lack of flow or very high resistance flow in complete torsion. Venous flow may be absent as an early finding in ovarian torsion, but further studies are needed to evaluate the sonographic findings relative to chronicity and extent of torsion.

EARLY DETECTION OF OVARIAN CARCINOMA

Several reports on the possible use of TAS and TVS in the screening and early detection of patients with ovarian carcinoma are encouraging. Campbell's series of more than 5000 women demonstrates the efficacy of a program using TAS (Campbell and coworkers, 1989). Five patients with primary ovarian cancer were identified, all with stage I tumors. Higgins' study involving 500 patients demonstrates the efficacy of TVS in the early detection of ovarian tumors (Higgins and coworkers, 1989). Jacobs' study and Finkler's work demonstrate the efficacy of using both TAS and the CA-125 assay as early detec-

tion programs (Jacobs and coworkers, 1988; Finkler and coworkers, 1988).

Although ovarian carcinoma occurs in 1 of 70 women in the United States, its detection in its early stages is worthwhile because most ovarian tumors are discovered in later stages if left to clinical discovery. Our study shows that TVS has significant negative predictive value, in that, if an ovarian mass is not shown, the patient most likely does not have an ovarian tumor (Fig. 5-8) (Fleischer and coworkers, 1990).

Transvaginal color Doppler sonography helps detect ovarian lesions, particularly those that incite significant neovascularization (Fleischer and coworkers, 1990; Bourne and coworkers, 1989; Kurjak, 1991; Kurjak and Predanic, 1992; Kurjak and coworkers, 1993; Kurjak, 1994; Weiner and coworkers, 1993; Timor-Tritsch and coworkers, 1992; Tekay and Jouppila 1992; Kawai and coworkers, 1992; Hamper and coworkers, 1993). Because there is such a large number of women who need to be screened, the best method for early detection seems to be a combination of sensitive serum assay and sonography.

When combined with the detection of endometrial disorders in asymptomatic women, transvaginal color Doppler sonography detected four stage I ovarian cancers and six endometrial cancers in 5000 asymptomatic women screened (Kurjak, 1994; Kurjak and coworkers, 1994). This detection rate approaches that for breast carcinoma, which is of unquestionable established efficacy in detecting breast cancer in asymptomatic women. (Fleischer and Emerson, 1993; Kurjak and coworkers, 1994.) Further improvements in ovarian cancer early detection will include identifying women at greater risk by genetic history or laboratory means. Women with a history of ovarian carcinoma, breast, or colonic cancer are at greater risk for ovarian cancer.

PARAOVARIAN MASSES

Some paraovarian masses may appear to arise from the ovaries, especially when the compressed rim of ovarian tumor, which usually surrounds an intraovarian mass, cannot be detected (Fig. 5-9). These masses normally represent endometriosis that is attached to the ovarian serosa or paraovarian masses that arise from the meso-ovarium.

GUIDED CYST ASPIRATION

Transvaginal sonographically guided cyst aspiration can be used in certain patients who may not be surgical candidates (Fig. 5-10). Its accuracy in distinguishing benign from malignant cystic masses is limited by difficulties in establishing a cytologic diagnosis of cancer.

SUMMARY

This chapter outlines the sonographic appearances of most ovarian tumors using both transabdominal and transvaginal sonography. The use of transabdominal and transvaginal sonography for the early detection of ovarian carcinoma seems promising and should be pursued by several institutions in clinical trials.

REFERENCES

Andolf E, Jörgensen C. Cystic lesions in elderly women, diagnosed by ultrasound. Br J Obstet Gynaecol 1989; 96:1076.

Andolf E, Svalenius E, Astedt B. Ultrasonography for early detection of ovarian carcinoma. Br J Obstet Gynaecol 1986;93:1286.

Bourne T, Campbell S, Steer C, Whitehead MI, Collins WP. Transvaginal colour flow imaging: A possible new screening technique for ovarian cancer. BMJ 1989;299:1367.

Campbell S, Bhan V, Royston P, Whitehead MI, Collins WP. Transabdominal ultrasound screening for early ovarian cancer. BMJ 1989;299:1363.

Campbell S, Goessens L, Goswamy R, Whitehead MI. Realtime ultrasonography for the determination of ovarian morphology and volume: A possible early screening test for ovarian cancer. Lancet 1982;1:425.

DePriest P, van Nagell J. Transvaginal ultrasound screening for ovarian cancer. Clin Obstet Gynecol 1992; 35:40.

Finkler NJ, Benacerrat B, Wojciechowski C, Lavin PT, Knapp RC. Comparison of serum CA 125, clinical impression, and ultrasound in the preoperative evaluation of ovarian masses. Obstet Gynecol 1988; 72:659.

Fleischer A, Emerson D. Color Doppler Sonography in Obstetrics and Gynecology. New York: Churchill-Livingstone, 1993.

Fleischer AC, Gordon A, McKee M, et al. Transvaginal sonography of postmenopausal ovaries with pathologic correlation. J Ultrasound Med 1990;9:637.

Fleischer AC, Kepple DM, Rao BK, Jeanty P. Transvaginal color Doppler sonography: Preliminary experience. Dynamic Cardiovasc Imaging 1990;3:52.

Goldstein SR, Subramanyam B, Snyder JR, Beller U, Raghavendra BN, Beckman EM. The postmenopausal cystic adnexal mass: The potential role of ultrasound in conservative management. Obstet Gynecol 1989;74:8.

Goswamy RK, Campbell S, Royston JP, et al. Ovarian size in postmenopausal women. Br J Obstet Gynaecol 1988;95:795.

Granberg S, Norstrom A. Tumors of the lower pelvis as imaged by vaginal sonography. Gynecol Oncol 1990; 37:224.

Hamper UM, Sheth S, Abbas FM, Rosenshein NB, Aronson D, Kurman RJ. Transvaginal color Doppler sonography of adnexal masses: Differences in blood flow impedance in benign and malignant lesions. AJR 1993;160:1225.

Higgins RV, van Nagell JR Jr, Donaldson ES, et al. Transvaginal sonography as a screening method for ovarian cancer. Gynecol Oncol 1989;34:402.

Jacobs I, Stabile I, Bridges J, et al. Multimodal approach to screening for ovarian cancer. Lancet 1988;1:268.

Kawai M, Kano T, Kikkawa F, Maeda O, Oguchi H, Tomoda Y. Transvaginal Doppler ultrasound with color flow imaging in the diagnosis of ovarian cancer. Obstet Gynecol 1992;79:163.

Kurjak A. Transvaginal Color Doppler. 2nd ed. London: Parthenon Press, 1994.

Kurjak A, Predanic M. New scoring system for prediction of ovarian malignancy based on transvaginal color Doppler sonography. J Ultrasound Med 1992;11:631.

Kurjak A, Shalam H, Kupesic S. An attempt to screen asymptomatic women for ovarian and endometrial cancer with transvaginal color and pulsed Doppler sonography. J Ultrasound Med 1994;13:295.

Kurjak A, Shalan H, Kupesic S, et al. Transvaginal color Doppler sonography in the assessment of pelvic tumor vascularity. Ultrasound Obstet Gynecol 1993; 3:137.

Kurjak A, Zalud I, Alfirevic Z. Evaluation of adnexal masses with transvaginal color ultrasound. J Ultrasound Med 1991;10:295.

Levine D, Gosink BB, Wolf SI, Feldesman MR, Pretorius DH. Simple adnexal cysts: The natural history in postmenopausal women. Radiology 1992;184:653.

Rodriguez MH, Platt LD, Medearis AL, Lacarra M, Lobo RA. The use of transvaginal sonography for evaluation of postmenopausal ovarian size and morphology. Am J Obstet Gynecol 1988;159:810.

Sassone A, Timor-Tritsch I, Artner A. Transvaginal sonographic characterization of ovarian disease: Evaluation of a new scoring system to predict ovarian malignancy. Obstet Gynecol 1991;78:90.

Tekay A, Jouppila P. Validity of pulsatility and resistance indices in classification of adnexal tumors with transvaginal color Doppler ultrasound. Ultrasound Obstet Gynecol 1992;2:338.

Timor-Tritsch IE, Lerner JP, Monteagudo A, Santos R. Transvaginal ultrasonographic characterization of ovarian masses by means of color flow-directed Doppler measurements and a morphologic scoring system. Am J Obstet Gynecol 1993;168:909.

Weiner Z, Beck D, Shteiner M, et al. Screening for ovarian cancer in women with breast cancer with transvaginal sonography and color flow imaging. J Ultrasound Med 1993;12:387.

Wolf SI, Gosink BB, Feldesman MR, Lin MC, Stuenkel CA, Braly PS, Pretorius DH. Prevalence of simple adnexal cysts in postmenopausal women. Radiology 1991;180:65.

FIGURE 5-1
Normal Ovaries

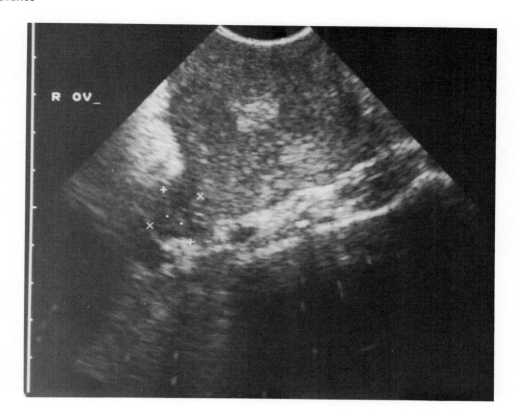

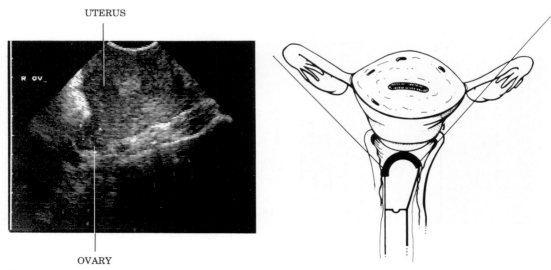

UTERUS

OVARY

Figure 5-1A. TVS of a postmenopausal woman demonstrating a normal right ovary (between cursors).

Normal Ovaries *(Continued)*

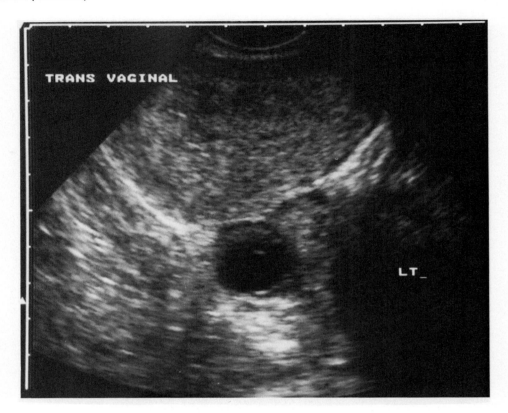

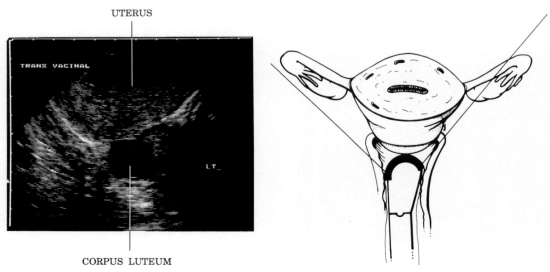

Figure 5-1B. Fresh corpus luteum within the left ovary.

Normal Ovaries *(Continued)*

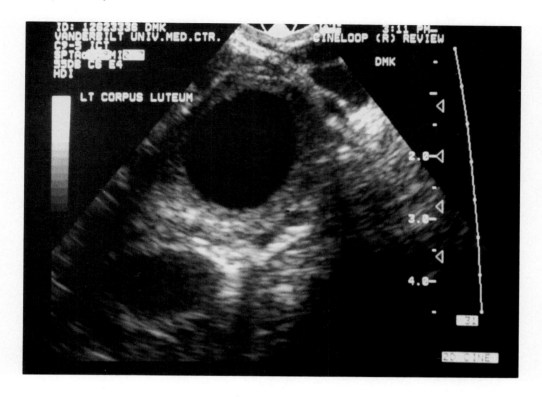

"FRESH" CORPUS LUTEUM

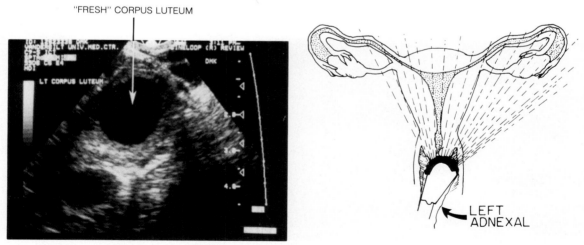

LEFT
ADNEXAL

Figure 5-1C. Fresh corpus luteum appearing as a hypoechoic area within the left ovary.

Normal Ovaries *(Continued)*

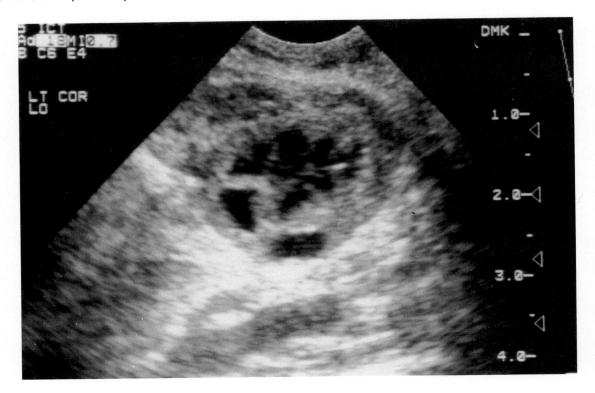

HEMORRHAGIC CORPUS LUTEUM

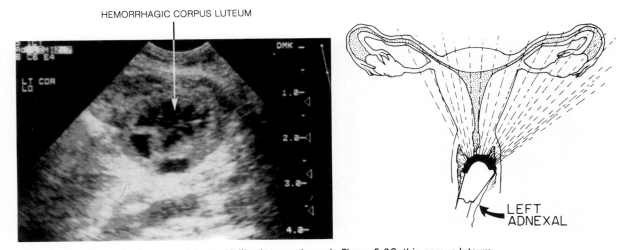

LEFT
ADNEXAL

Figure 5-1D. Hemorrhagic corpus luteum. Unlike the one shown in Figure 5-3C, this corpus luteum has a crenated thickened wall and areas of internal hemorrhage.

Normal Ovaries *(Continued)*

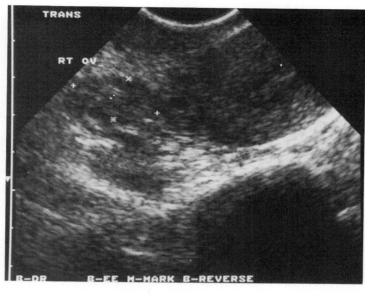

OVARY

UTERUS

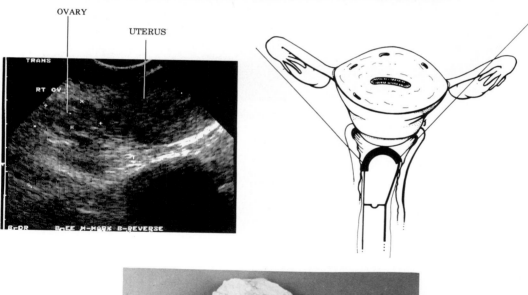

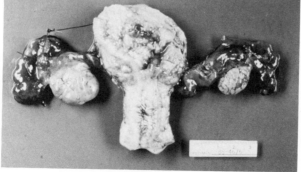

Figure 5-1E. Normal right ovary in perimenopausal woman. The resected uterus and ovaries show that the right ovary was twice the size of the left.

FIGURE 5-2
Cystic Masses

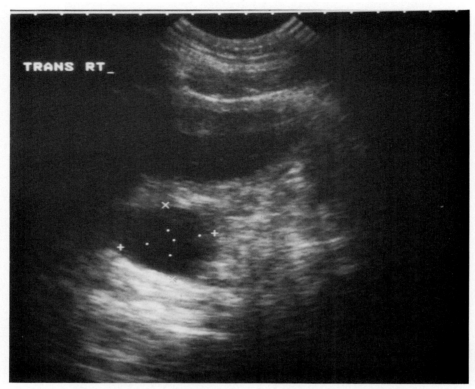

Figure 5-2A. Transabdominal sonogram demonstrating the appearance of a nonspecific right adnexal cystic mass (between cursors).

Cystic Masses *(Continued)*

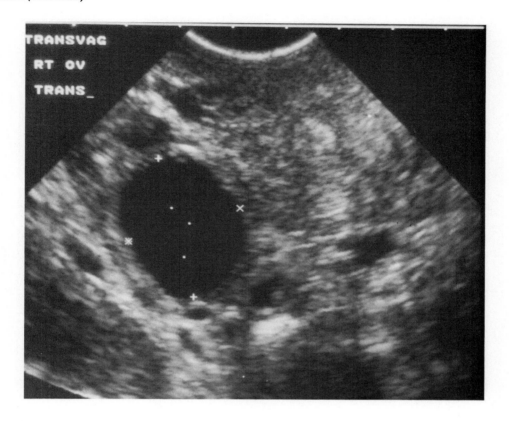

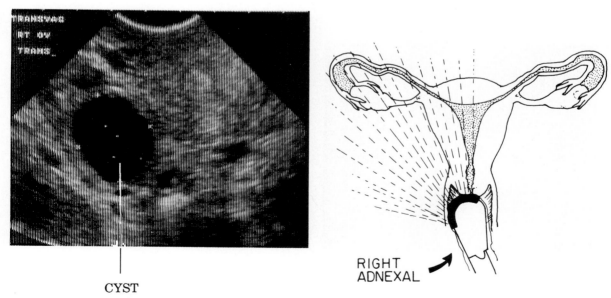

CYST

RIGHT
ADNEXAL

Figure 5-2B. TVS of the patient in Figure 5-2*A* demonstrating an intraovarian cyst (between cursors). Note the displacement of normal ovarian tissue surrounding the cyst.

Cystic Masses *(Continued)*

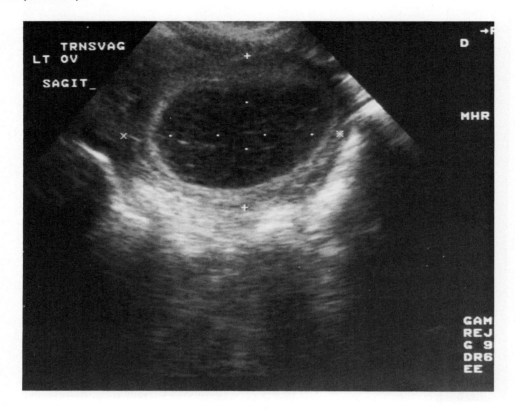

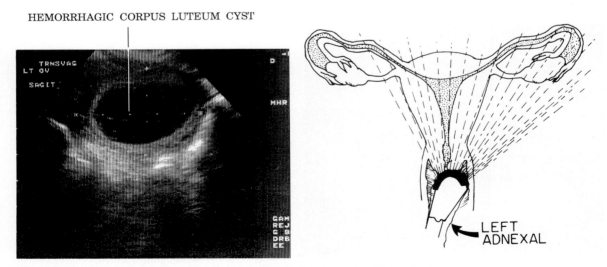

Figure 5-2C. TVS of hemorrhagic corpus luteum demonstrating low-level internal echoes.

FIGURE 5-3
Extraovarian Adnexal Masses

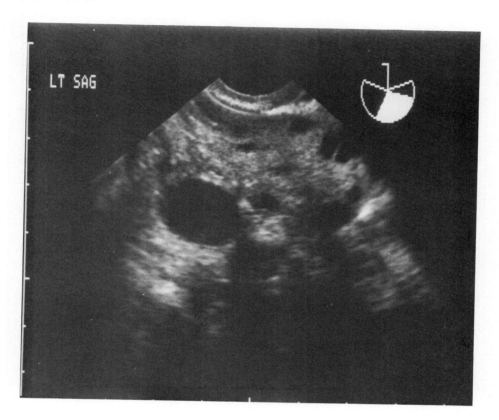

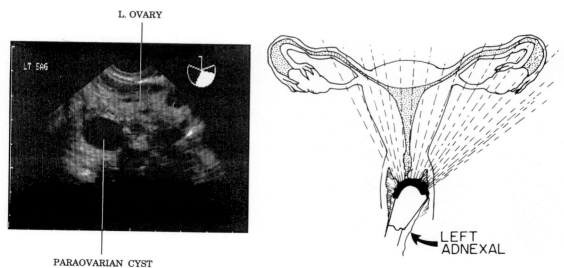

L. OVARY

PARAOVARIAN CYST

LEFT ADNEXAL

Figure 5-3A. TVS of a paraovarian cyst adjacent to the left ovary.

Extraovarian Adnexal Masses *(Continued)*

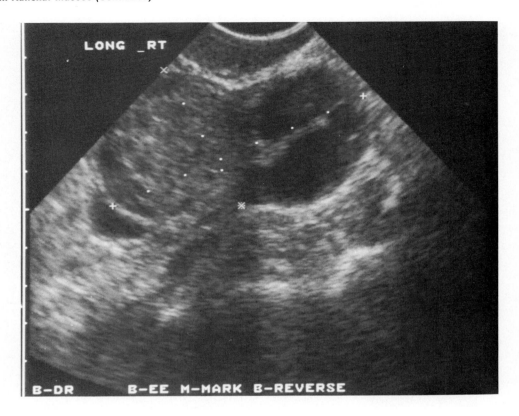

ENDOMETRIOMA   R. OVARY

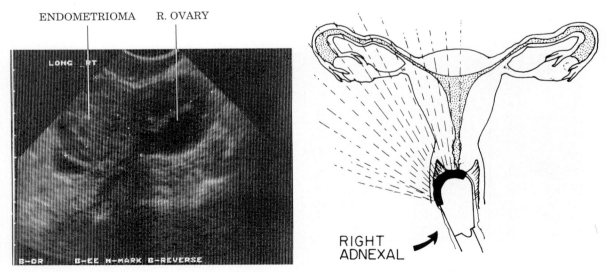

Figure 5-3B. TVS of endometrioma, adjacent to the right ovary, containing echogenic organized blood.

Extraovarian Adnexal Masses *(Continued)*

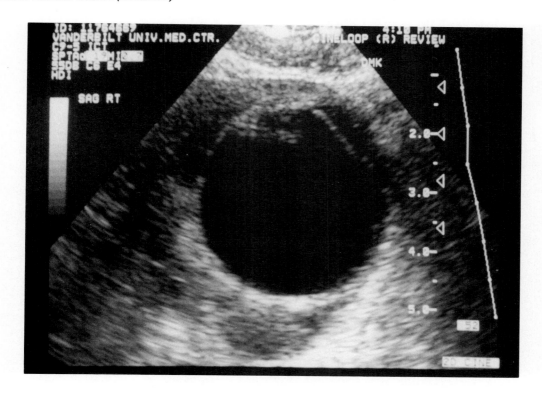

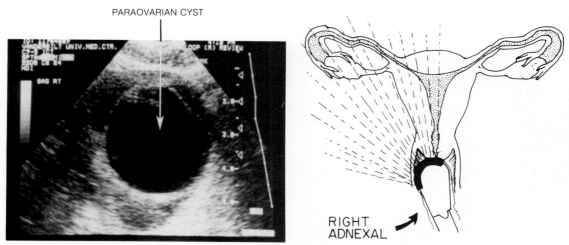

Figure 5-3C. TVS of a paraovarian cyst separate from the right ovary.

Extraovarian Adnexal Masses *(Continued)*

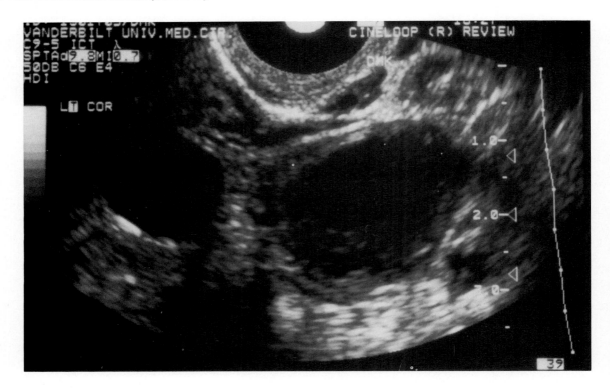

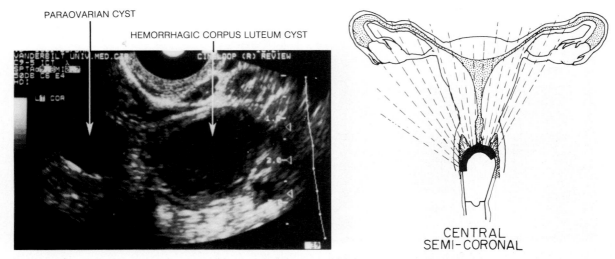

Figure 5-3D. TVS of a paraovarian cyst adjacent to the left ovary which had contained a hemorrhagic corpus luteum.

FIGURE 5-4
Predominately Cystic Ovarian Tumors

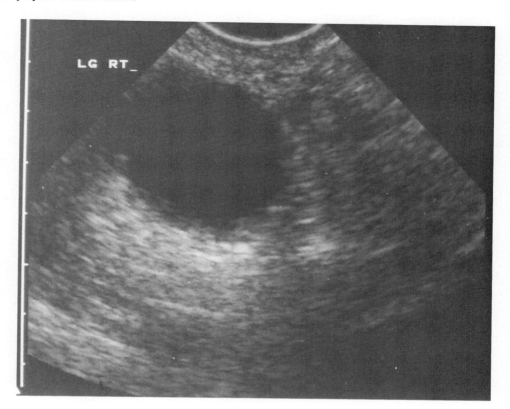

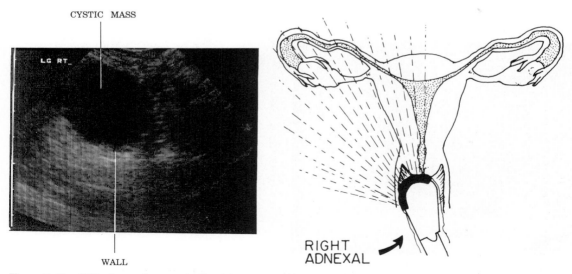

Figure 5-4A. TVS of a cystic mass in the right ovary, which has a slightly irregular wall.

Predominately Cystic Ovarian Tumors *(Continued)*

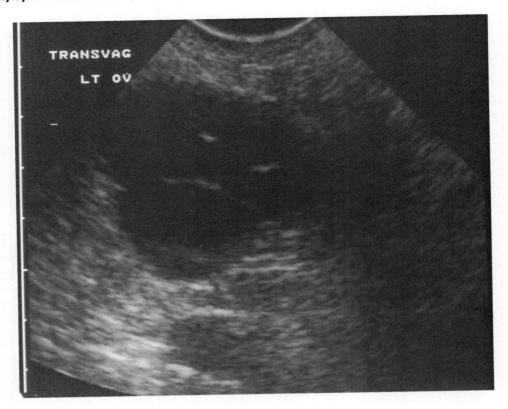

CYSTADENOMA

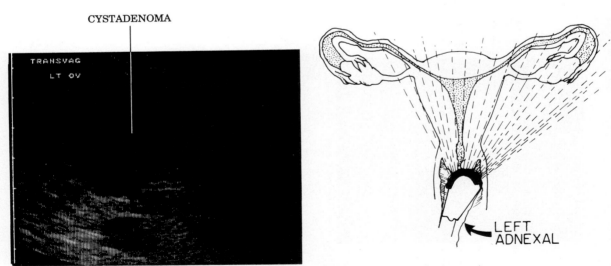

LEFT
ADNEXAL

Figure 5-4B. TVS of the same patient as in Figure 5-4*A* demonstrating a 3-cm septated mass in the left ovary. This patient had bilateral serous cystadenomas.

Predominately Cystic Ovarian Tumors *(Continued)*

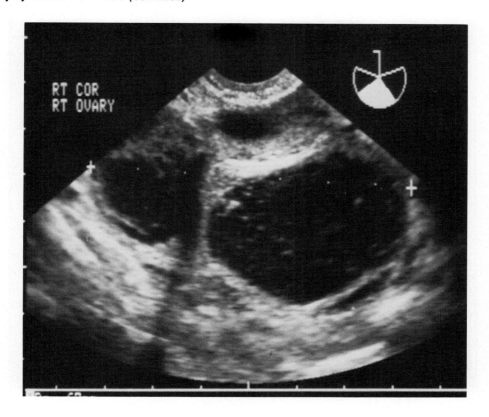

OVARIAN CYSTADENOMAS

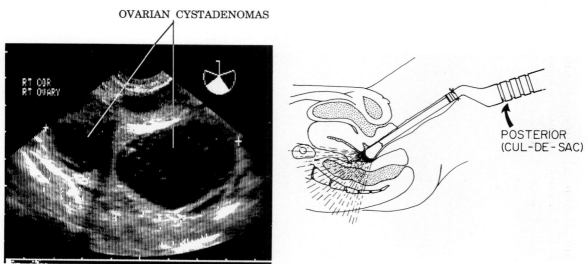

Figure 5-4C. TVS demonstrating bilateral cystic masses containing septae and solid components representing bilateral mucinous cystadenomas.

Predominately Cystic Ovarian Tumors *(Continued)*

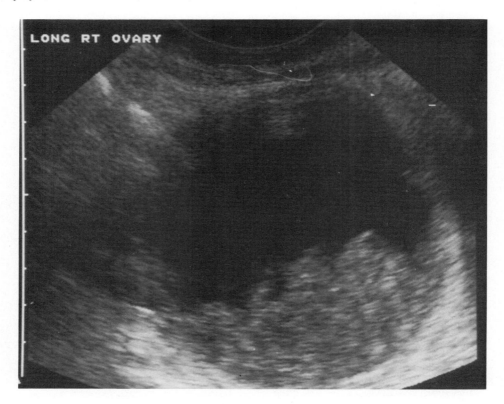

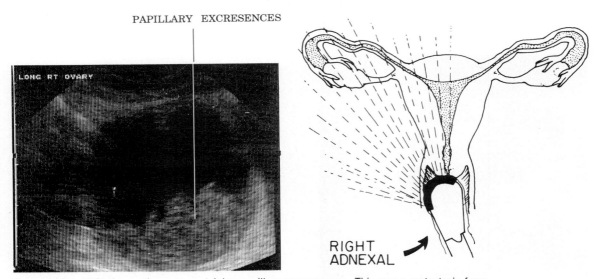

Figure 5-4D. TVS of a cystic mass containing papillary excrescences. This was a metastasis from a gastrointestinal tract tumor.

Predominately Cystic Ovarian Tumors *(Continued)*

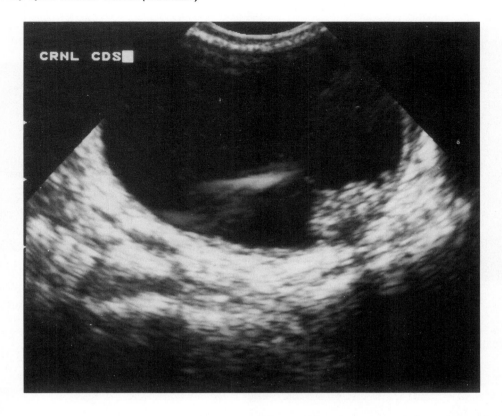

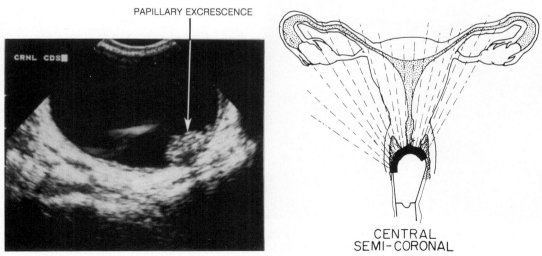

Figure 5-4E. TVS of a cystic ovarian mass containing a large papillary excrescence. This was a papillary serous cystadenocarcinoma.

FIGURE 5-5
Dermoid Cyst

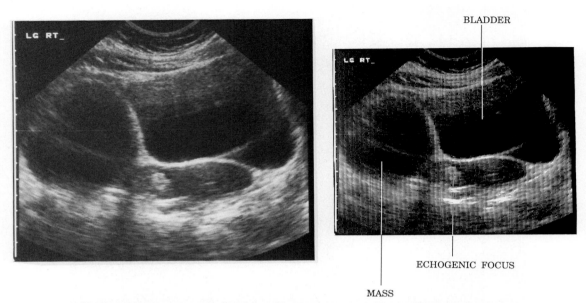

Figure 5-5A. Transabdominal sonogram demonstrating cystic mass superior to the right ovary, which contains an echogenic focus.

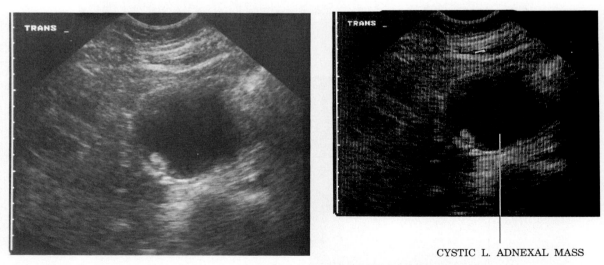

Figure 5-5B. Transabdominal sonogram of the same patient in Figure 5-5*A* demonstrating a cystic mass in the left adnexa with an echogenic internal component.

Dermoid Cyst *(Continued)*

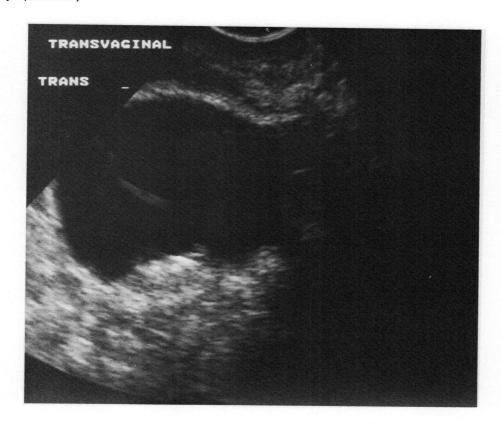

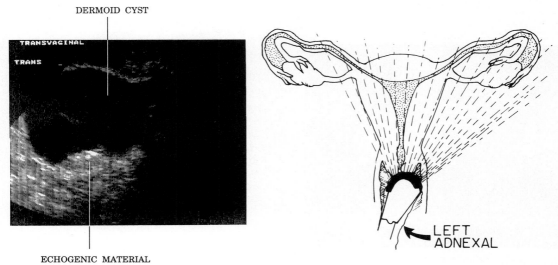

Figure 5-5C. TVS of the same patient as in Figure 5-5*B* showing a left adnexal mass with echogenic mobile material. This patient had bilateral dermoid cysts.

Dermoid Cyst *(Continued)*

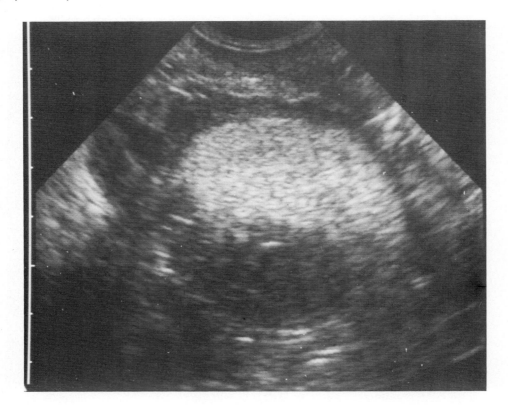

SEBUM

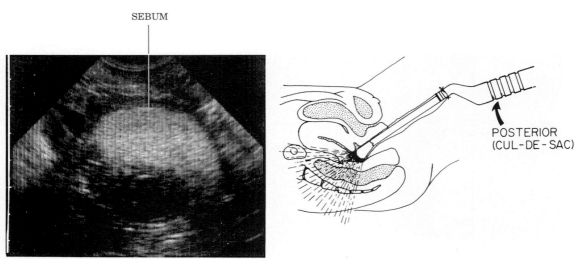

POSTERIOR
(CUL-DE-SAC)

Figure 5-5D. TVS of a dermoid cyst with a layer of sebum.

Dermoid Cyst *(Continued)*

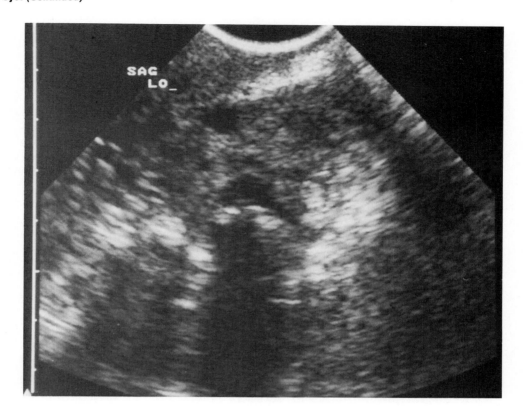

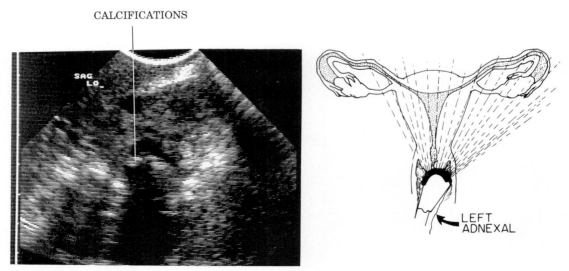

Figure 5-5E. TVS of a dermoid cyst containing echogenic teeth.

Dermoid Cyst *(Continued)*

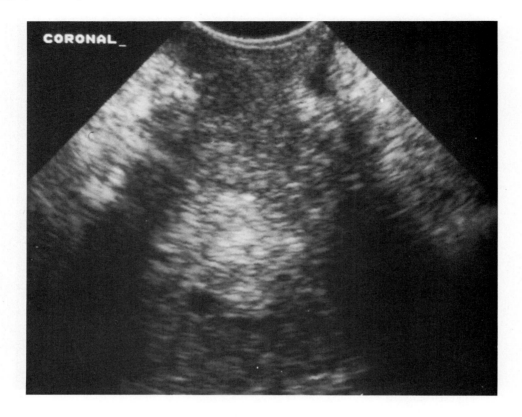

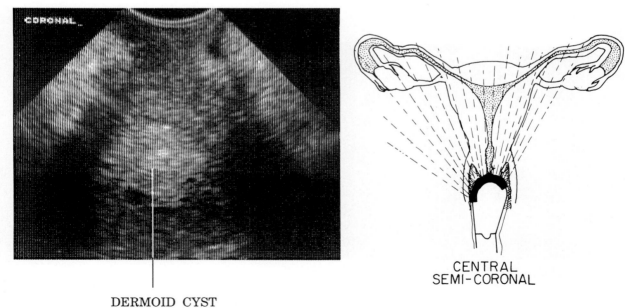

DERMOID CYST

CENTRAL
SEMI-CORONAL

Figure 5-5F. TVS of a nonspecific echogenic area found to represent a dermoid cyst at surgery.

Dermoid Cyst *(Continued)*

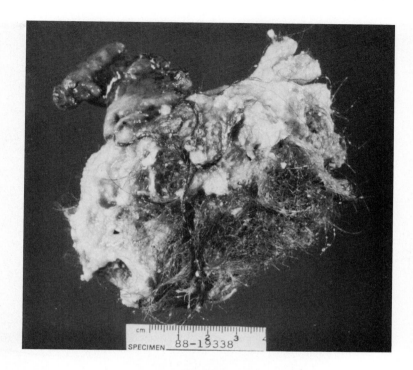

Figure 5-5G. Opened specimen of dermoid cyst shown in Figure 5-5F. Note abundant hair.

Dermoid Cyst *(Continued)*

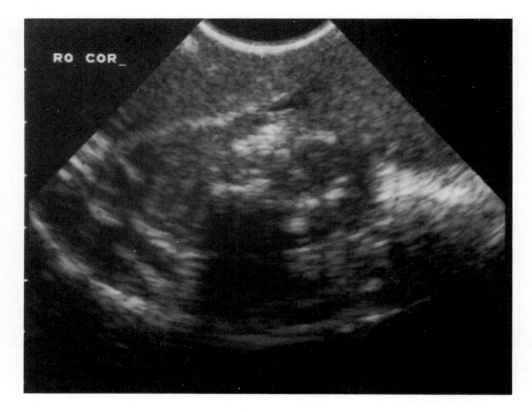

DERMOID CYST

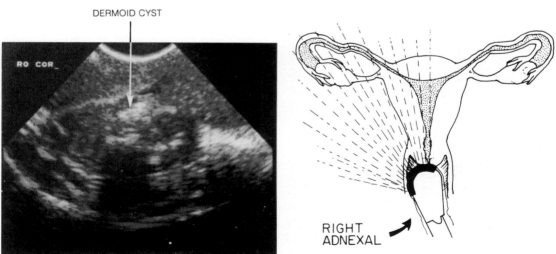

RIGHT
ADNEXAL

Figure 5-5H. TVS of a dermoid cyst containing several calcifications. Note shadowing.

Dermoid Cyst *(Continued)*

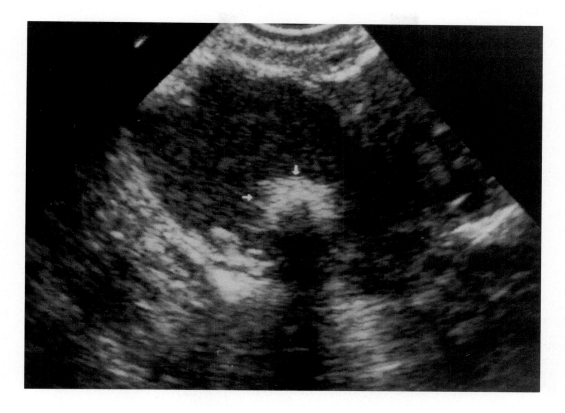

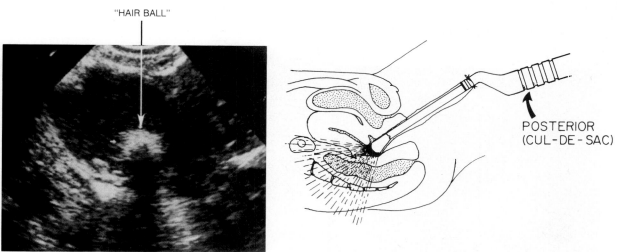

"HAIR BALL"

POSTERIOR
(CUL-DE-SAC)

Figure 5-5I. TVS of a dermoid cyst containing a "hair ball" and having several areas of irregular wall.

FIGURE 5-6
Complex Ovarian Masses

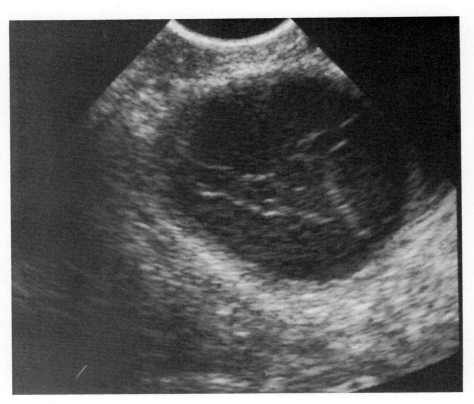

HEMORRHAGIC CORPUS LUTEUM CYST

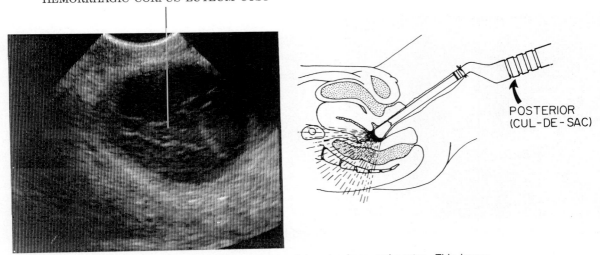

POSTERIOR
(CUL-DE-SAC)

Figure 5-6A. TVS of a 10-cm complex mass containing internal echoes and septae. This image represents a hemorrhagic corpus luteum cyst.

Complex Ovarian Masses *(Continued)*

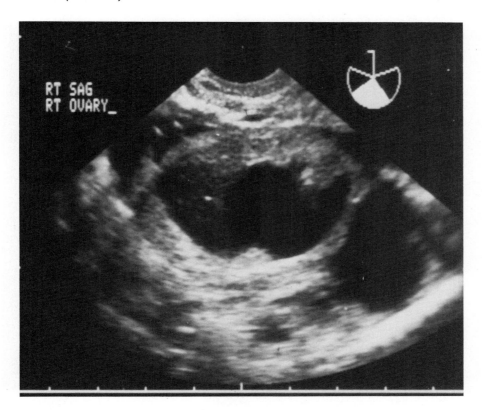

OVARIAN METASTASIS

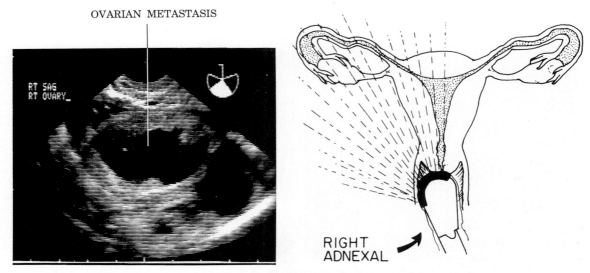

RIGHT
ADNEXAL

Figure 5-6B. TVS showing a complex mass with an irregular solid wall, representing an ovarian metastasis.

Complex Ovarian Masses *(Continued)*

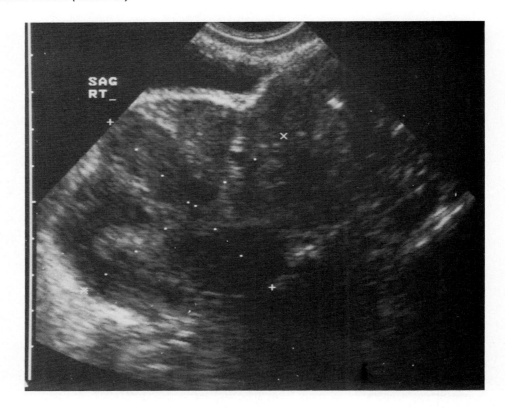

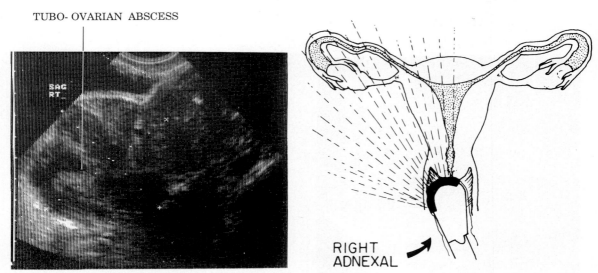

TUBO- OVARIAN ABSCESS

RIGHT ADNEXAL

Figure 5-6C. TVS of an enlarged ovary containing a tubo-ovarian abscess.

Complex Ovarian Masses *(Continued)*

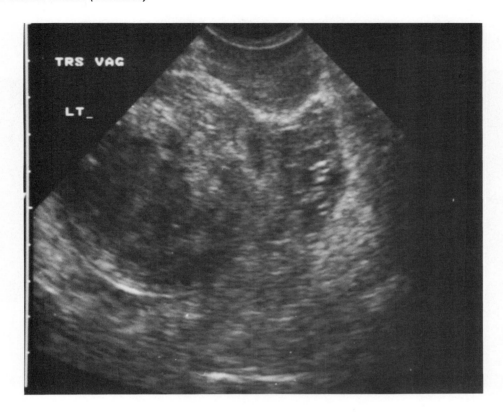

HEMORRHAGIC OVARIAN CYST

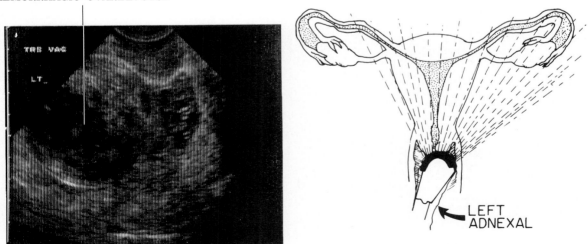

Figure 5-6D. TVS of a large solid mass representing a hemorrhagic ovarian cyst compressing the remaining normal portion of the left ovary.

FIGURE 5-7
Solid Ovarian Masses

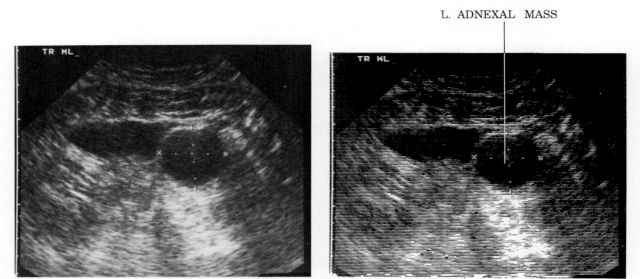

Figure 5-7A. Transabdominal sonogram showing a hypoechoic mass in the left adnexa (between cursors).

Solid Ovarian Masses *(Continued)*

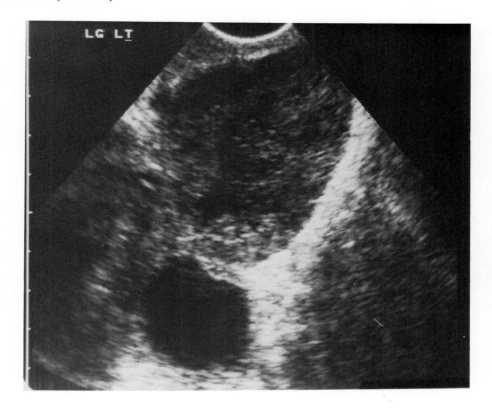

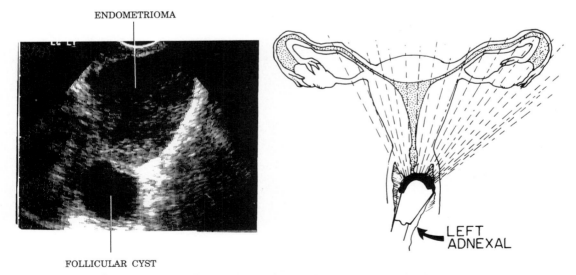

ENDOMETRIOMA

FOLLICULAR CYST

LEFT ADNEXAL

Figure 5-7B. TVS of the patient in Figure 5-7*A* showing a solid ovarian mass adjacent to the cystic one. A torsed endometrioma was identified, as was a physiologic ovarian cyst in the left ovary.

Solid Ovarian Masses *(Continued)*

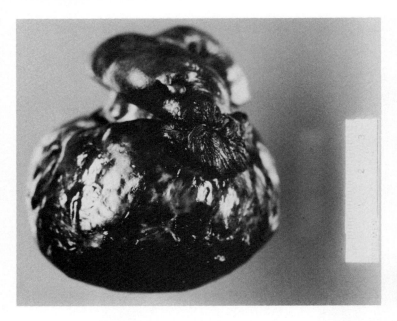

Figure 5-7C. Gross specimen of *A* and *B* show-ing torsed endometrioma within the gangrenous ovary of the patient in Figure 5-7*A*.

Solid Ovarian Masses *(Continued)*

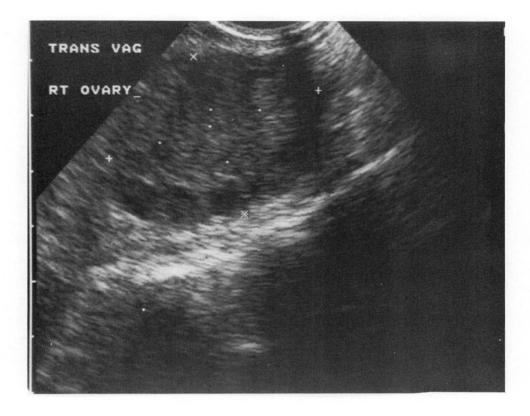

HEMORRHAGE

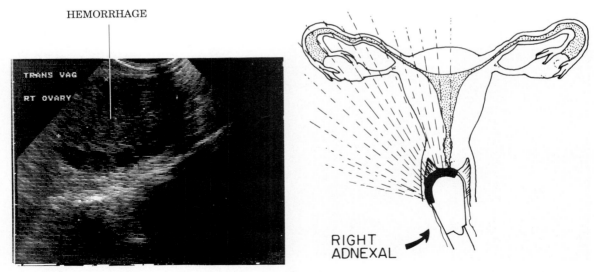

RIGHT
ADNEXAL

Figure 5-7D. TVS of an enlarged right ovary with a hemorrhagic area.

Solid Ovarian Masses *(Continued)*

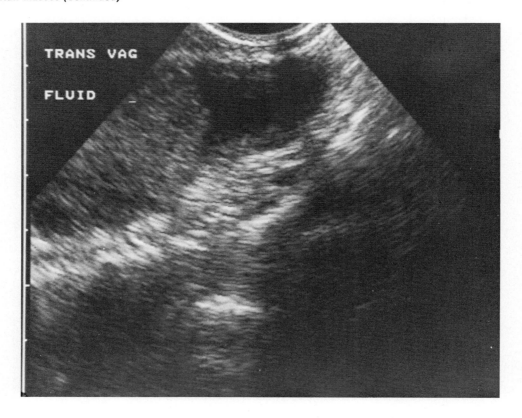

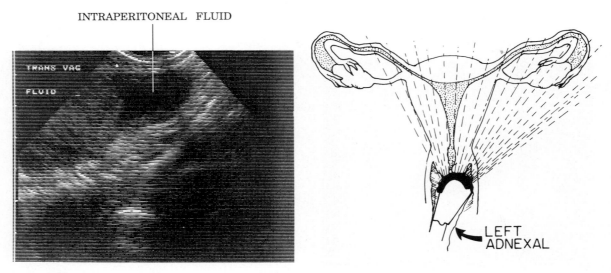

Figure 5-7E. TVS of the patient in Figure 5-7*D*. Loculated cul-de-sac fluid is seen. A torsed right ovary was found at surgery.

Solid Ovarian Masses *(Continued)*

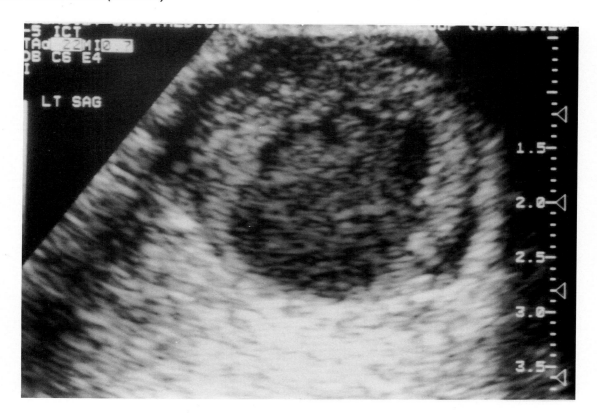

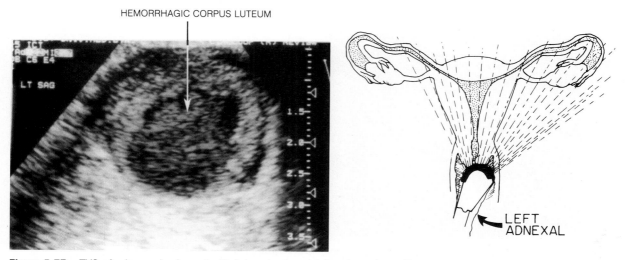

Figure 5-7F. TVS of a hemorrhagic cyst with internal echoes and an irregular wall.

Solid Ovarian Masses *(Continued)*

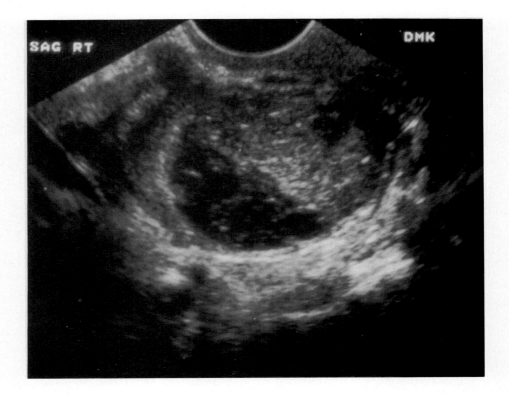

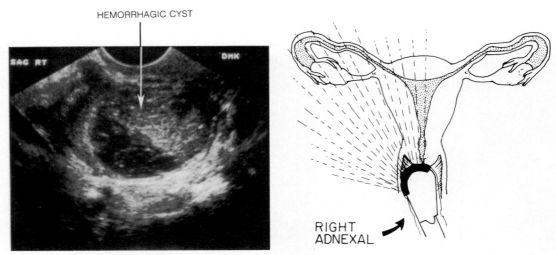

Figure 5-7G. TVS of a hemorrhagic cyst containing a layer of clotted blood.

Solid Ovarian Masses *(Continued)*

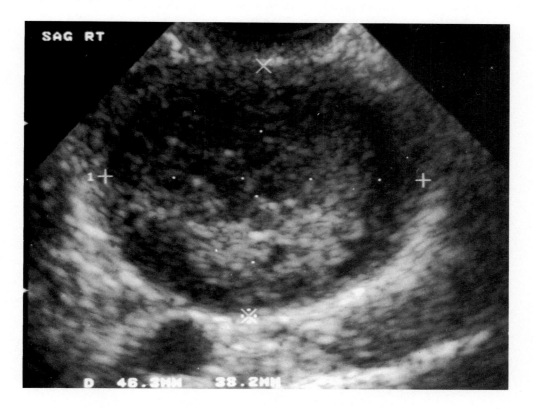

HEMORRHAGIC CYST

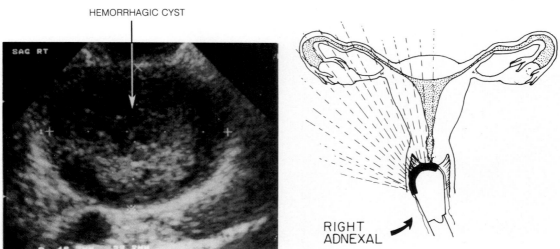

RIGHT ADNEXAL

Figure 5-7H. TVS of a hemorrhagic cyst with focal areas of echogenicity corresponding to clotted blood.

FIGURE 5-8
Small (<5 cm) Ovarian Lesions in Postmenopausal Women With Nonpalpable Ovaries

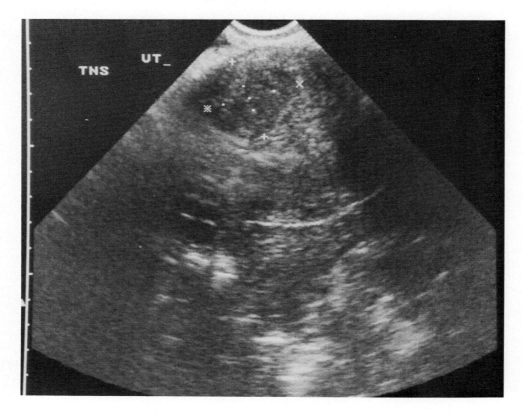

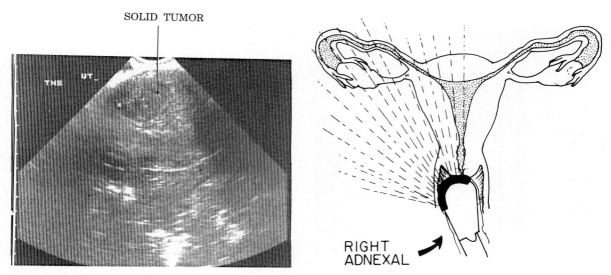

Figure 5-8A. TVS of a right ovary showing a small solid area (between cursors).

Small (<5 cm) Ovarian Lesions in Postmenopausal Women With Nonpalpable Ovaries *(Continued)*

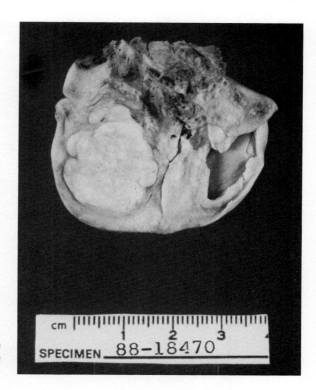

Figure 5-8B. Sectioned specimen of the ovary shown in Figure 5-8*A* showing an 18-mm Sertoli's cell tumor adjacent to a simple cyst.

Small (<5 cm) Ovarian Lesions in Postmenopausal Women With Nonpalpable Ovaries
(Continued)

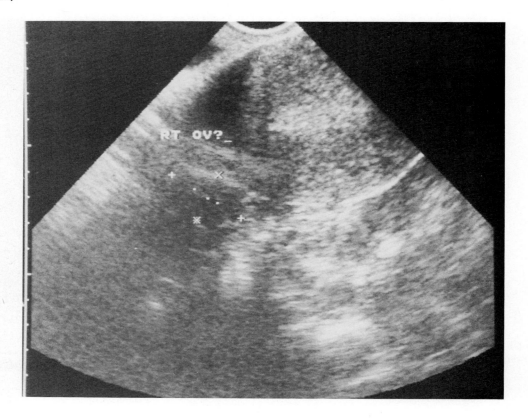

R. OVARY

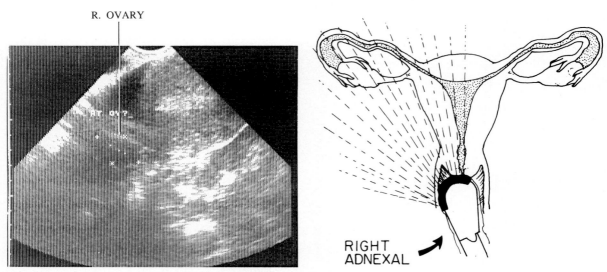

RIGHT
ADNEXAL

Figure 5-8C. TVS of a right ovary with cystic area (between cursors).

Small (<5 cm) Ovarian Lesions in Postmenopausal Women With Nonpalpable Ovaries
(Continued)

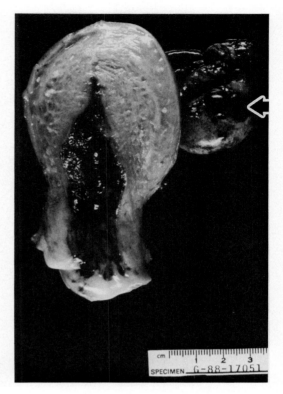

Figure 5-8D. Resected ovary in Figure 5-8C showing a 2-cm cystade-noma (*arrow*).

Small (<5 cm) Ovarian Lesions in Postmenopausal Women With Nonpalpable Ovaries
(Continued)

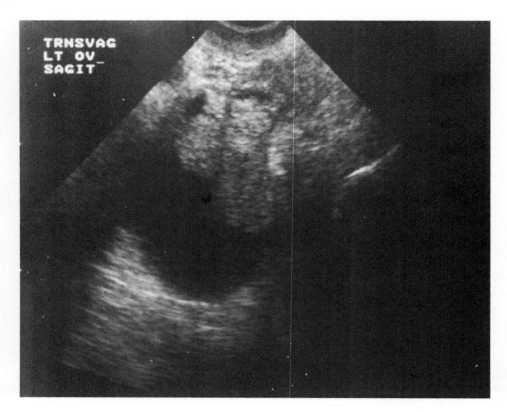

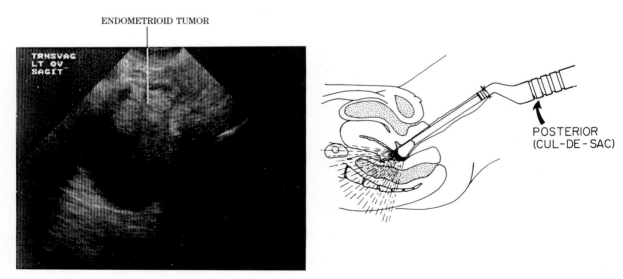

Figure 5-8E. TVS of a left ovary showing complex mass with cystic and solid components.

Small (<5 cm) Ovarian Lesions in Postmenopausal Women With Nonpalpable Ovaries *(Continued)*

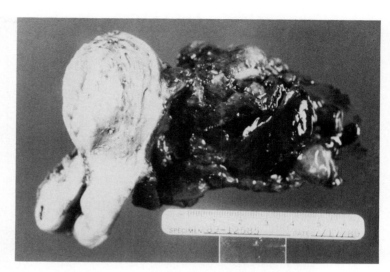

Figure 5-8F. Sectioned specimen showing endometrioid tumor containing solid areas.

FIGURE 5-9
Paraovarian and Tubal Lesions

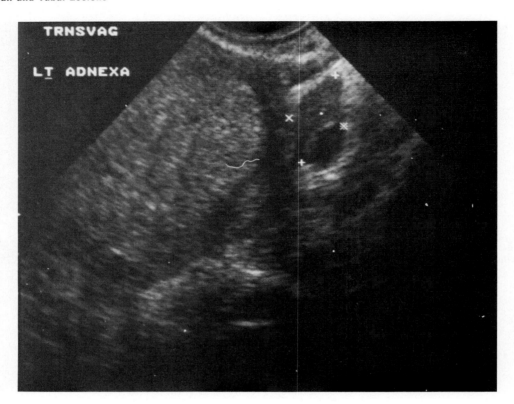

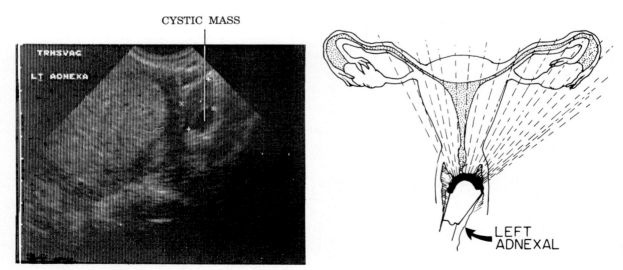

Figure 5-9A. TVS showing cystic area adjacent to the left ovary.

Paraovarian and Tubal Lesions *(Continued)*

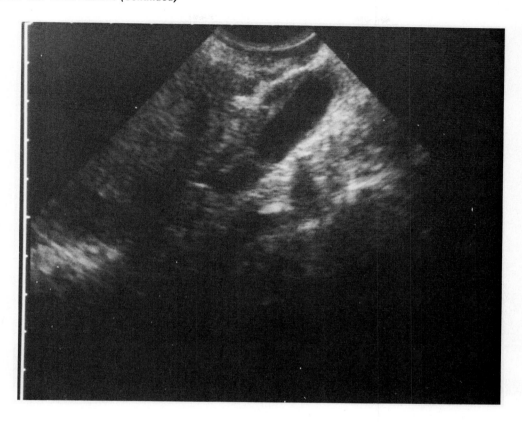

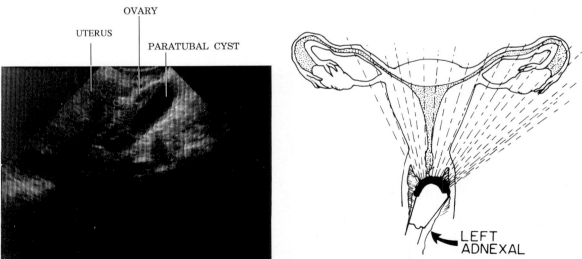

Figure 5-9B. TVS of the area shown in Figure 5-9*A*. The cystic structure appears as a tubular mass when imaged in its long axis.

Paraovarian and Tubal Lesions *(Continued)*

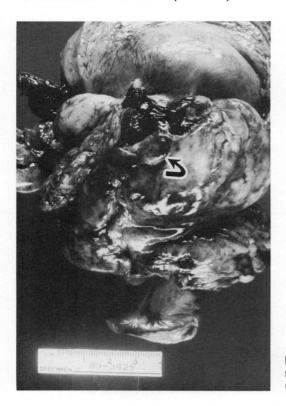

Figure 5-9C. Gross specimen of area shown in Figure 5-9*A* and 5-9*B* showing opened paraovarian cyst adjacent to a normal atrophic left ovary (*curved arrow*).

Paraovarian and Tubal Lesions *(Continued)*

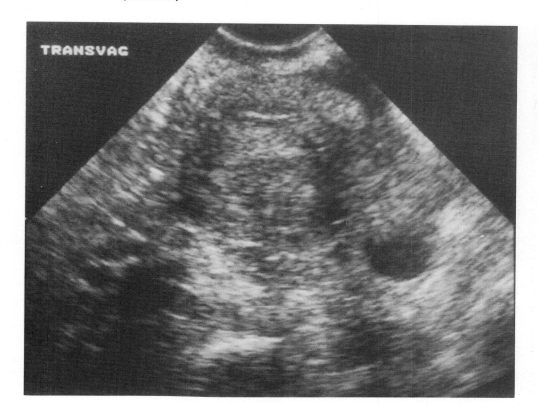

UTERUS

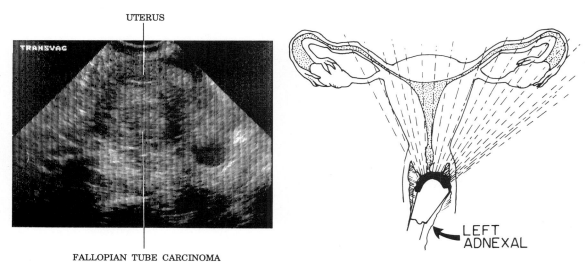

FALLOPIAN TUBE CARCINOMA

LEFT
ADNEXAL

Figure 5-9D. TVS of a fusiform solid mass adjacent to a fibroid uterus.

Paraovarian and Tubal Lesions *(Continued)*

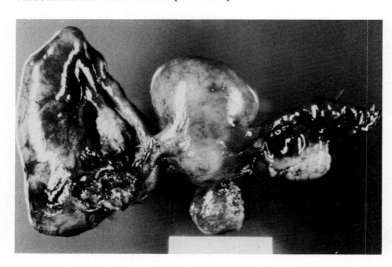

Figure 5-9E. Resected specimen showing fallopian tube carcinoma.

FIGURE 5-10.
TVS Guided Aspiration of Ovarian Cysts

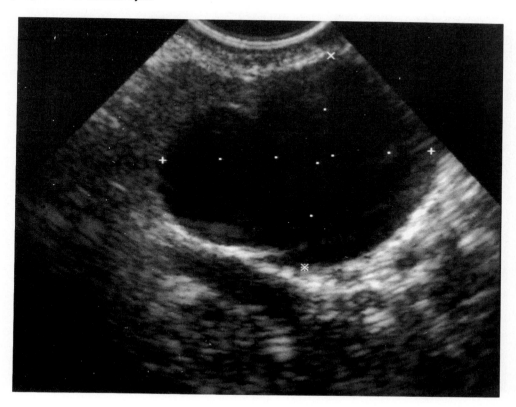

PAPILLARY PROJECTION

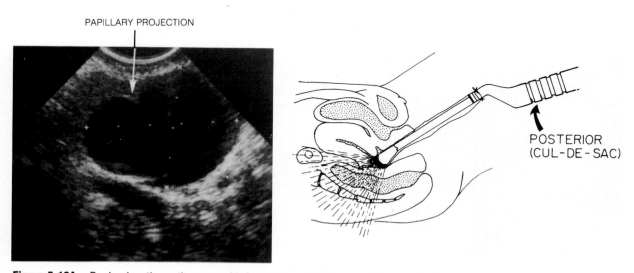

POSTERIOR
(CUL-DE-SAC)

Figure 5-10A. Predominantly cystic mass with focal area containing a papillary projection.

TVS Guided Aspiration of Ovarian Cysts *(Continued)*

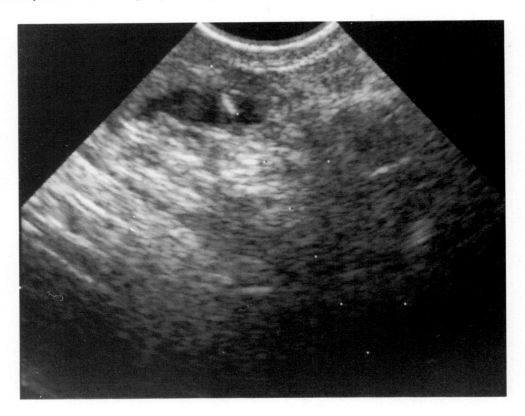

NEEDLE TIP

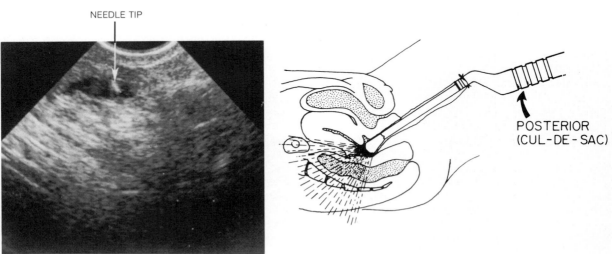

POSTERIOR
(CUL-DE-SAC)

Figure 5-10B. Under TVS guidance, the mass in Figure 5-10*A* was completely aspirated. No malignant cells were found in the aspirate.

Transvaginal Sonography: A Clinical Atlas, Second Edition,
edited by Arthur C. Fleischer and Donna M. Kepple.
J.B. Lippincott Company, Philadelphia, © 1995.

CHAPTER **6**

Infertility

Arthur C. Fleischer, MD
Donna M. Kepple, RDMS
Jaime Vasquez, MD

INTRODUCTION

The increased use and availability of transvaginal transducer-probes has had a major impact on the management and treatment of patients with gynecologic infertility (Winfield and coworkers, 1990). Transvaginal sonography (TVS) has its greatest clinical impact in precise monitoring of follicular development, guided follicular or cyst aspiration, and guided transcervical cannulization of the fallopian tube. Additional applications of transvaginal sonography include assessment of tubal patency or intrauterine synechiae by sonohysterography. Other applications of TVS include evaluation of the adequacy of endometrial development and evaluation of vascular perfusion of the ovary and uterus with duplex or color Doppler sonography.

FOLLICULAR MONITORING

Transvaginal sonography has a vital role in depicting follicular development in patients treated for infertility that can be traced to disorders of ovulation (Fleischer and coworkers, 1983). Although the maturity of the oocyte is indirectly inferred by the size of the follicle, the sonographic information can be coupled with serum estradiol values to provide an accurate assessment of the presence and number of mature follicles (Ritchie, 1986; Tarlatizis and coworkers, 1984). The anatomic information obtained with TVS concerning the size and development of maturing follicles and corpora lutea can be used to distinguish physiologic from insufficient or abnormal menstrual cycles (McArdle and coworkers, 1983; Geisthovel and coworkers, 1983). For example, the maximal follicle size in insufficient cycles has been reported to be significantly less than in normal ones, and the absence of a corpus luteum was found more often in insufficient (luteal phase inadequate) cycles (Geisthovel and coworkers, 1983). In addition, the undesirable development of multiple immature follicles rather than development of a single dominant follicle can be seen in patients with polycystic ovaries (Hann and coworkers, 1984).

Although its contribution to infertility is controversial, some infertility specialists describe an abnormality in ovulation called luteinized unruptured follicle (LUF) syndrome as a cause of unexplained infertility (Liukkonen and coworkers, 1984). In LUF, there is failure of extrusion of the oocyte, which remains trapped within the follicle. The presence of this abnormality can be confirmed only by laparoscopic observation of the absence of a stigma (i.e., the healed rent where ovulation occurred) in the ovarian capsule. Because this stigma may not be present before 2 hours after ovulation, the presence of this syndrome is difficult to confirm. With TVS, failure of the follicle to deflate and the absence of intraperitoneal fluid associated with ovulation can be observed. This syndrome may be more common in women with endometriosis and may not be present in consecutive cycles (Geisthovel and coworkers, 1983; Liukkonen and coworkers, 1984).

In the empty follicle syndrome, a cumulus cannot be identified within the follicle (Hilgers and Dvorak, 1989). Although TVS can be used to assess the presence of an oocyte, documentation of the cumulus does not have sufficient reliability to confidently diagnose this entity.

In normal cycles, TVS demonstrates an increase in peak systolic velocity in arterioles surrounding the developing follicle (Steer and coworkers, 1992).

With development of the corpus luteum, there is a low-impedance, high-diastolic velocity flow within the wall of the corpus luteum (Kupesic and Kurjack, 1993). In LUF syndrome, there is a lack of this increase in maximum systolic velocity.

SPONTANEOUS OVULATION

At the time of birth, the female neonate has approximately 2 million primary oocytes within each ovary. When menarche begins, approximately 200,000 per ovary remain. During the childbearing years, approximately 200 oocytes are ovulated. This indicates that approximately 99.9% of primary oocytes become atretic or do not develop.

Maturation of the oocyte and follicle is responsive primarily to changes in follicle stimulating hormone (FSH), luteinizing hormone (LH), and circulating levels of estrogen (E_2). With the elaboration and release of FSH in the late secretory phase, there is development of several follicles. Only one and sometimes two become dominant, however; the remainder become atretic. The follicle begins its maturation process several months before ovulation of the oocyte. It is not uncommon to observe two follicles developing to approximately 10 mm, with one becoming dominant and growing and the other regressing. LH reinitiates meiosis of the oocyte and, typically, ovulation occurs within 36 hours of its surge in circulating levels. Estradiol is synthesized

by the granulosa cells and provides feedback to the pituitary in the production of FSH and LH.

Transvaginal sonography can depict the developing follicles starting when they measure between 3 and 5 mm. In the spontaneous cycle, is usually one or, at most, two follicles that develop to approximately 10 mm. As the follicle matures, more fluid is elaborated into its center, and the number of granulosa cells lining the inner wall of the follicle increases. The oocyte, which is less than 0.01 mm, is surrounded by a cluster of granulosa cells. This complex is termed the ''cumulus oophorus.'' It measures approximately 1 mm and occasionally can be depicted along the wall of some mature follicles with TVS. Immediately before ovulation, the cumulus separates from the wall and floats freely within the center of the follicle. Even with the enhanced resolution afforded by TVS, the attached or floating cumulus is only rarely visualized.

Mature follicles (ones that contain a mature oocyte) typically measure between 17 and 25 mm in average inner dimension (Fig. 6-1) (Fleischer and coworkers, 1981). Within the same individual, however, the size of a mature follicle is relatively constant from cycle to cycle. Intrafollicular echoes may be observed with mature follicles, probably arising from clusters of granulosa cells that shear off the wall near the time of ovulation. After ovulation, the follicular wall becomes irregular as the follicle becomes ''deflated'' (Figs. 6-2 and 6-3). The fresh corpus luteum usually appears as a hypoechoic structure with an irregular wall and may contain some internal echoes corresponding to hemorrhage. As the corpus luteum develops 4 to 8 days after ovulation, it appears as an echogenic structure of approximately 15 mm. Its wall is thickened by the process of luteinization (see Fig. 6-3).

In addition to delineation of changes in follicle size and morphology, TVS can depict the presence of intraperitoneal fluid (Fig. 6-4). It is normal to have approximately 1 to 3 mL of such fluid in the cul-de-sac throughout the cycle. When ovulation occurs, there is typically between 4 and 5 mL of fluid within the cul-de-sac. The intraperitoneal fluid resulting from ovulation may be loculated outside of the posterior cul-de-sac, surrounding bowel loops in the lower abdomen and upper pelvis, or in the anterior cul-de-sac superior to the uterine fundus.

INDUCED OVULATION

In patients whose infertility can be attributed to an ovulation abnormality, ovulation induction is indicated. Ovulation induction is also used for in vitro fertilization–embryo transfer (IVF-ET) to increase the number of oocytes aspirated, which, in turn, increases the number of fertilized concepti that may be transferred and increasing the chance of pregnancy.

The two medications most commonly used for ovulation induction include clomiphene citrate (CC) and human menopausal gonadotropin (hMG). Although both medications result in the development of multiple follicles, they act by different mechanisms. TVS has a vital role in monitoring follicular development in women receiving ovulation-induction medication (Ritchie, 1986; Tarlatizis and coworkers, 1984). Leuprolide acetate, a GnRH agonist, is given to block the neurologic–hypothalamic axis.

Patients undergoing ovulation induction are usually examined every other day beginning between days 7 and 9 of their menstrual cycle. Patients undergoing IVF-ET are examined by TVS earlier in their cycles and usually daily to carefully monitor their follicular development.

Clomiphene citrate is an estrogen antagonist that binds estrogen receptor sites in the pituitary and hypothalamus. This leads to increased FSH secretion by the pituitary, thereby recruiting more follicles. Because the process of selection and dominance may be overridden, multiple, relatively synchronous follicles usually develop (Fig. 6-5). Although the preovulatory E_2-LH feedback may be intact in CC-treated patients with an intact hypothalamus, some patients are given human chorionic gonadotropin (hCG) to induce final follicular and oocyte maturation.

Follicular development with CC can be different than that observed in spontaneous cycles. Specifically, each follicle seems to develop at an individual rate and, at times, may be accelerated or decelerated. Therefore, the largest follicle on a given date may not be the same 2 days later and may not even be the one that is most mature. Furthermore, correlation of E_2 and follicle size is poor, and the maximal preovulatory diameter can range from 19 to 24 mm.

Unlike treatment with CC, treatment with hMG does not require an intact hypothalamus or pituitary. In hMG-treated patients, there are two apparent patterns of follicular development (Ritchie, 1986). In those amenorrheic women with no exogenous estrogen, no estrogenic activity, and dormant ovaries, the response to endogenous gonadotropin is to develop a small number of large follicles (see Fig. 6-4). The growth rate and E_2 secretion are linear, correlate well, and are of equal predictive value. A high pregnancy rate is achieved in this group. In contrast, patients with estrogenic activity who harbor antral follicles at different stages of development react differently (Fig. 6-6). Stimulation of these patients requires less hMG and usually results in the rapid recruitment of many follicles with different growth rates in varying degrees of E_2 secretory capacity. Also, the rate at which E_2 levels increase is exponential, increasing the risk of hyperstimulation. Thus, there is a dissociation between follicle size and E_2 levels, suggesting that growth rate and functional maturity are asynchronous. This group of women particularly benefits from combined E_2 and follicular monitoring with TVS. Because hMG contains both FSH and LH and a spontaneous LH surge is less frequent when inducing follicular development with hMG, hCG may be required to induce final follicular maturation. TVS delineation of follicle size is crucial because hCG is best administered once follicles reach 15 to 18 mm.

For in vitro fertilization, follicles are typically aspirated when they reach 15 to 18 mm in average dimension and when there is evidence by estradiol values of a mature follicle (approximately 400 pg/mL/mature follicle) (Marrs and coworkers, 1983). Another sonographic sign of a mature follicle is the presence of low-level, intrafollicular echoes. These echoes probably arise from clumps of granulosa cells that have separated from the follicular wall. In one study involving patients who underwent ovulation induction and were scanned transabdominally, a higher pregnancy rate was achieved in those patients whose follicles demonstrated these intrafollicular echoes (Mendelson and coworkers, 1985).

Transvaginal sonography has an important role in decreasing the likelihood of ovarian hyperstimulation. Ovarian hyperstimulation disorder occurs in most patients who undergo ovulation induction. Its severity ranges from mild abdominal discomfort (probably due to the distension of the ovarian capsule) to severe circulatory compromise and electrolyte imbalance (probably secondary to ascites or pleural effusions). The more severe form, ovarian hyperstimulation syndrome (OHSS), is usually associated with massive stromal edema of the ovary. The enlarged ovaries may be prone to torsion. The symptoms associated with OHSS usually begin 5 to 8 days after hCG is given but can be most severe in patients who actually achieve pregnancy. Studies have shown that hyperstimulation is unlikely in women whose ovaries contain several large (over 15 mm) follicles and tends to occur when there are several small or intermediately sized follicles (Blankstein and coworkers, 1987).

Although sonographic findings of bilaterally enlarged ovaries that have multiple immature follicles with the presence of intraperitoneal fluid may suggest the possibility of hyperstimulation, this syndrome can be more accurately predicted by extremely high levels of E_2 (more than 3000 pg/mL). Despite the superovulation required for IVF, hyperstimulation is only rarely encountered. This is probably a reflection of the close monitoring that these patients receive but also may be secondary to drainage and collapse of the aspirated follicles.

On TVS, patients with OHSS usually have bilaterally enlarged ovaries (over 10 cm) that may contain several hypoechoic areas (Fig. 6-7). The hypoechoic areas may correspond to atretic follicles or regions of hemorrhage within the ovary. Because it demonstrates lack of arterial and venous flow, color Doppler sonography may be useful in the detection of ovarian torsion (see Fig. 6-7). However, the ovary has a dual blood supply, one arises from the adnexal branch of the uterine artery, the other courses through the infundibulopelvic ligament (Fig. 6-8). Torsion may affect one arterial blood supply more than the other, resulting in the presence of arterial flow on color Doppler sonography. In the hyperstimulated ovary, venous flow usually loses phasicity with respiration.

The pregnancies that occur with OHSS may be early (<4 weeks), and no definitive sonographic findings may be found. Intraperitoneal fluid is usually present and is a consequence of the serum osmotic imbalance. With supportive medical therapy, this syndrome usually spontaneously regresses.

After induced ovulation, the stimulated follicles usually undergo regression but may persist and enlarge over the remainder of the cycle. This seems to be most commonly seen in patients on gonadotropin releasing hormone (GnRH) analogs. The presence of physiologic ovarian cysts (over 3 cm) may preclude attempts at ovulation induction during that cycle because the previously induced follicles may not have totally regressed and the remaining ovarian tissue may not be as responsive to ovulation-induction medication. Theoretically the risk of torsion and rupture may also be increased in these women.

Transvaginal sonography can also detect other adrexal masses such as a hydrosalpinx, endometriomas, paraovarian cysts, or peritoneal cysts that may mimic physiologic cysts or follicles that are either totally anechoic or contain low-level homogeneous echoes. These masses can be differentiated from ovarian cysts because they are extraovarian.

Sonographic monitoring of follicular development is also helpful in decreasing the likelihood of multiple gestations that may occur with fertilization of multiple ova. It is difficult, however, to predict which pregnancies will result in multiple births, but when there are more than four mature follicles, the chance for multiple gestation beyond twinning is more probable than if only two or three mature follicles are induced.

GUIDED PROCEDURES

Needle guides that can be attached to transvaginal probes greatly facilitate guided follicular aspiration. After the probe is draped with a condom, these needle guides can be placed directly on the transducer-probe, allowing for a direct and continuous visualization of the aspirating needle as it is advanced into the ovary (Fig. 6-9). The line of sight is generated on the video monitor and closely approximates the needle path to be traversed.

Follicular Aspiration

Transvaginal sonographically guided follicular aspiration is the preferred procedure for oocyte retrieval over the previously used laparoscopic techniques. Advantages of this technique include decreased exposure to general anesthesia, lower chance for operative complications, and feasibility of performing this procedure in an outpatient setting. The success rate, as determined by the number of fertilizable oocytes retrieved and pregnancies produced, is comparable with the laparoscopic technique (Table 6-1) (Feldberg and coworkers, 1988). The procedure is also advantageous in patients with pelvic adhesions because laparoscopic access to the ovary may be hampered (Taylor and coworkers, 1986). Most importantly, patient acceptance of the procedure is high (Schulman and coworkers, 1987; Feichtinger and Kemeter, 1986; Hammarberg and coworkers, 1987).

There are several methods for follicular aspiration that involve sonographic guidance (Fig. 6-10) (Schulman and coworkers, 1987; Feichtinger and Kemeter, 1986; Hammarberg and coworkers, 1987; Dellenbach and coworkers, 1985; Parsons and coworkers, 1985; Marrs, 1986). These include TVS for guidance of transvaginal aspiration, transabdominal sonography (TAS) for guidance of transvaginal aspiration, TAS for guidance of transvesical aspiration, and TAS for guidance of transurethral aspiration. Although TVS with transvaginal aspiration is used most frequently, the method used may be tailored to each patient according to the anatomic position of the ovary and other structures. For example, the transvaginal aspiration is the preferred route when

TABLE 6-1
Results of Ovum Pickup by Three Methods

	Laparoscopic	Transvesical	Transvaginal
Oocytes recovered/patient	6.4 ± 0.9	6.2 ± 0.3	5.7 ± 0.6
Oocytes recovered/follicle (%)	93.0	86.0	82.0
Fertilization rate (%)	73.6	72.3	70.9
Cleavage rate (%)	82.6	79.4	81.6
Number of embryos transferred	3.9 ± 0.6	3.2 ± 6.4	3.6 ± 0.3
Pregnancy rate/per pickup (%)	23.7	22.3	21.6
Pregnancy rate/transfer (%)	26.6	26.7	25.9
Pregnancy rate/cycle (%)	20.2	22.6	21.1

From Feldberg D, Goldman JA, Ashkenazi J, et al. Transvaginal oocyte retrieval controlled by vaginal probe for in vitro fertilization: A comparative study. J Ultrasound Med 1988; 7:339–343.

the ovaries are in the cul-de-sac, whereas the per urethral approach may be used for aspiration of follicles in ovaries located near the dome of the bladder.

With all of these aspiration techniques, use of a long (30 cm) 16- or 18-gauge needle that is scored at the tip results in enhanced sonographic visualization (see Fig. 6-9D). The aspiration procedure is performed under local anesthesia with supplemental intravenous or intramuscular medication.

For transvaginal aspiration with transvaginal transducers, a needle guide is attached to the transducer-probe (see Fig. 6-9). This allows the needle to traverse the beam path of the transducer. The cursor is displayed on the scanner's screen, which indicates the path of the needle. After a condom containing sterile gel is placed over the transducer and the sterile needle guide is attached, the operator manipulates the transducer to optimally delineate the ovary (see Fig. 6-10A). The desired follicle is brought into the line of sight and the needle is introduced into the needle guide. After the initial aspiration, the follicle is filled with buffered media and flushed so that chances for retrieving a mature oocyte are maximized (see Fig. 6-10B and C).

This aspiration technique is associated with a low complication rate. One complication that has been described is inadvertent introduction of the needle into a vessel (usually the internal iliac vein) in the pelvis (Feldberg and coworkers, 1988). To avoid this complication, the operator should carefully examine any round structure in both the long and short axis to distinguish a vascular structure from a follicle.

The use of GnRH analogs (leuprolide acetate) may be associated with the development of follicular cysts. It is thought that the presence of the cysts may impair folliculogenesis because of either the elaboration of hormones or a direct affect on reducing perfusion by parenchymal compression by the cyst itself. In these cases, TVS-guided aspiration affords direct visualization and monitoring of guidance for aspiration of these physiologic cysts (Fig. 6-11).

Guided Tubal Cannulation

Transvaginal sonography is being used for transcervical cannulation of the uterine and tubal lumen (Jansen and Anderson, 1987). A technique for sonographic guidance of placement of a catheter into the fallopian tubes for gamete intrafallopian transfer (GIFT) procedure has been described (Fig. 6-12) and has several advantages over hysteroscopically guided tubal cannulation (Jansen and Anderson, 1987). For this procedure, a catheter is placed transcervically and manipulated into the area of the uterine cornu. The catheter is slowly introduced under sonographic guidance into the tubal ostia. Once the catheter is in the distal isthmic portion of the fallopian tube, the sperm and ova may be introduced through the cannula directly into the tube.

TUBAL PATENCY ASSESSMENT

Transvaginal sonography can be used with saline or positive contrast solutions to evaluate tubal patency (Schlief and Deichert, 1991; Stern and coworkers, 1992). When using positive contrast, the tube can be definitively outlined relative to the ovary. Passage of saline may be difficult to identify within the tube itself but collection within the cul-de-sac can be observed with tubal patency.

ENDOMETRIAL ASSESSMENT

The developmental state of the endometrium may be a factor influencing the probability of conception (Rabinowitz and coworkers, 1986). Because the endometrium can also be delineated during examinations performed for follicular monitoring, several investigators have evaluated this specialized mucus membrane to study whether there is an optimal thickness or texture (Fleischer and coworkers, 1986; Thickman and coworkers, 1986; Glissant and coworkers, 1985; Fleischer and coworkers, 1984). There is a clear association of the sonographic texture of the endometrium and the circulating levels of E_2 and progesterone (Rabinowitz and coworkers, 1986).

In spontaneous and induced cycles, the sonographic appearance of the endometrium varies according to its specific phases of development. In the menstrual phase, the endometrium appears as a thin, broken echogenic interface. In the proliferative phase, it thickens and becomes isoechoic, measuring 3 to 5 mm in anteroposterior width. Its relative hypoechogenicity is related to the relatively orderly organization of the glandular elements within the endometrium. As ovulation approaches, the endometrium becomes more echogenic; this is probably related to development of secretions within the endometrial glands and the numerous interfaces that arise from distended and tortuous glands. In the periovulatory period, there usually is a hypoechoic area within the inner endometrium that most likely represents edema of the compactum layer. This finding has been described as a means of confirming that ovulation has occurred; however, this finding has been observed with TVS both before and immediately after ovulation. During the secretory phase, the endometrium achieves its greatest thickness (between 6 and 12 mm) and echogenicity. In addition to the echogenic endometrium, a hypoechoic band beneath the endometrium can be identified, probably arising from the inner layer of the myometrium.

Both sonographic and histologic studies have shown that medications used for ovulation induction may alter the development of the endometrium (Fleischer and coworkers, 1984). The importance of these changes relative to the success of achieving pregnancy is speculative. One study evaluating the endometrial thickness (includes both layers) in the secretory phase showed that conception was unlikely in endometrium measuring less than 13 mm at 11 days after ovulation (Fleischer and coworkers, 1984). Other studies indicate that the texture of the endometrium may be related to the success or failure of pregnancy, but there is no statistical pre-

dictive value applicable to these various patterns (Rabinowitz and coworkers, 1986; Glissant and coworkers, 1985). Other studies involved in sonographic evaluation of endometrium during ovulation induction have failed to demonstrate any specific changes in its thickness associated with success of achieving pregnancy (Rabinowitz and coworkers, 1986; Glissant and coworkers, 1985). Our studies using TVS have indicated that there is a statistically significant difference in the pregnancy rate when the endometrium has a multilayered appearance (Fig. 6-13). In two groups of 20 patients that underwent similar but not identical stimulations, 27% of the nonconception group showed a multilayered endometrium versus 79% of the group that conceived. This was statistically different even though the number of mature follicles, E_2 values, and transferred embryos were not (Table 6-2, see Fig. 6-13).

Transvaginal sonography may have a role in further evaluation of patients who have luteal inadequacy. These patients may have underdeveloped endometria that could be characterized sonographically as thinner and less echoic than expected.

Color Doppler sonography affords evaluation of the relative flow to the myometrium and endometrium during normal and abnormal menstrual cycles. One study indicated that the chance of implantation was markedly reduced with high-impedance type flow. This information may be used to postpone embryo transfer.

Uterine synechiae can be detected with TVS outlined with sonohysterography (Narayan and Goswamy, 1993). This procedure involves placement of an insemination catheter within the lumen and injection of 3 to 5 mL of sterile saline solution. The shape and regularity of the endometrium and endometrial cavity can be assessed. Synechiae usually appear as echogenic projections into the lumen. Submucosal fibroids and polyps can also be detected using sonohysterography.

OTHER APPLICATIONS

Transvaginal sonography has a role secondary to hysterosalpingography in the evaluation of certain uterine malformations and tubal disorders. Malformed uteri can be characterized sonographically by delineation of the echogenic secretory phase endometrium within the uterine lumen. Hematometra may result from cervical or lower uterine malformations. Bicornuate uterus may be difficult to distinguish from septated uterus in the nongravid state.

TABLE 6-2
Conception Versus Nonconception IVF Groups

	Endometrial Width (mm) (mean ± SD)	Change Over 4 days (mm)	Percent Multi-layered	Mature Number of Follicles >1.5 cm	E$_2$ (pg/mL)	Number of Retrieved Ova	Number of Embryo Transferred
Nonconception	9.5 ± 1.0	3.1	27	3.1	1,157	3.3	2.3
Conception	9.8 ± 0.9	1.6	74	3.1	1,137	4.1	2.1
P value	NS	.05	.0001	NS	NS	.05	NS

NS, not significant.

Uterine septa are readily apparent as thick intraluminal interfaces in a gravid uterus, which sometimes separate the fetus and placenta.

The precise location of an intrauterine contraceptive device (IUCD) relative to the uterine lumen can also be determined sonographically, particularly with the use of TVS (Fig. 6-14A and B). The location of the IUCD relative to a gestational sac may be a factor in the decision to remove the IUCD. If an IUCD is inferior to the sac, attempts at removal may be feasible.

Transvaginal sonography can be used to delineate enlarged and dilated fallopian tubes and establish their relationship to the ovary (Fig. 6-14C and D). The nondistended fallopian tube can be recognized only occasionally. On TVS, the area of the proximal tube can be identified by the endometrium that projects into the area of the uterine cornu. An injectable contrast medium has been developed that clearly demonstrates tubal patency, especially when monitored with color Doppler sonography.

Sonography also has an important role in evaluating women with infertility who eventually become pregnant. These women have a higher incidence of ectopic pregnancy, anembryonic pregnancy, and spontaneous abortion. Clinical suspicion of these conditions is clearly an indication for TVS evaluation.

FUTURE APPLICATIONS

The transducer used for TVS can be used for simultaneous imaging and pulsed Doppler assessment of uterine and adnexal vasculature. Specifically, the ascending branch of the uterine artery can be assessed with pulsed Doppler sonography. The information obtained can reveal uterine and adnexal perfusion and is important in excluding the possibility of adnexal torsion. As in other parenchymal organs,

the waveform and resistance can be related to physiologic activity. For example, corpus luteum function is characterized by diastolic flow, rather than the sharp systolic peaks and no diastolic flow characteristic of ovaries that do not contain corpus luteum. The adequacy of corpus luteum development may be assessed using this method. Similarly, pulsed Doppler capabilities within the vaginal probe may allow assessment of uterine perfusion, which may be related to relative chance of conception.

Fingertip probes may allow more enhanced visualization of the uterus and ovary than that afforded by conventional TVS imaging.

SUMMARY

Transvaginal sonography affords accurate follicular monitoring and guidance for follicular aspiration. It can also assess endometrial development and provide a means for physiologic assessment of adnexal and uterine blood flow.

REFERENCES

Blankstein J, Shalev J, Saadon T, et al. Ovarian hyperstimulation syndrome: Prediction by number and size of preovulatory ovarian follicles. Fertil Steril 1987; 47:597.

Dellenbach P, Nisand I, Moreau L, et al. Transvaginal sonographically controlled follicle puncture for oocyte retrieval. Fertil Steril 1985;44:656.

Feichtinger W, Kemeter P. Ultrasound-guided aspiration of human ovarian follicles for in vitro fertilization. In: Sanders RC, Hill M. eds. Ultrasound Annual. New York: Raven Press, 1986:25.

Feldberg D, Goldman JA, Ashkenazi J, et al. Transvaginal oocyte retrieval controlled by vaginal probe for in vitro fertilization: A comparative study. J Ultrasound Med 1988;7:339.

Fleischer AC, Daniell JF, Rodier J, et al. Sonographic monitoring of ovarian follicular development. J Clin Ultrasound 1981;9:275.

Fleischer AC, Herbert CM, Sacks GA, et al. Sonography of the endometrium during conception and nonconception cycles of in vitro fertilization and embryo transfer. Fertil Steril 1986;46:442.

Fleischer AC, Pittaway DE, Wentz AC, et al. The uses of sonography for monitoring ovarian follicular development. In: Sanders RC, Hill M, eds. Ultrasound Annual. New York: Raven Press, 1983:163.

Fleischer AC, Pittaway DE, Beard LA, et al. Sonographic depiction of endometrial changes occurring with ovulation induction. J Ultrasound Med 1984;3:341.

Geisthovel F, Skubsch U, Zabel G. et al. Ultrasonographic and hormonal studies in physiologic and insufficient menstrual cycles. Fertil Steril 1983;39:277.

Glissant A, de Mouzon J, Frydman R. Ultrasound study of the endometrium during in vitro fertilization cycles. Fertil Steril 1985;44:786.

Hammarberg K, Eak L, Nilsson L, et al. Oocyte retrieval under the guidance of a vaginal transducer: Evaluation of patient acceptance. Hum Reprod 1987;2:487.

Hann LE, Hall DA, McArdle CR, et al. Polycystic ovarian disease: Sonographic spectrum. Radiology 1984;150:531.

Hilgers TW, Dvorak AD, Tamisiea DF, et al. Sonographic definition of the empty follicle syndrome. J Ultrasound Med 1989;8:411.

Jansen RPS, Anderson JC. Catheterisation of the fallopian tubes from the vagina. Lancet 1987;2:309.

Kupesic S, Kurjak A. Uterine and ovarian perfusion during the periovulatory period assessed by transvaginal color Doppler. Fertil Steril 1993;60:439.

Liukkonen S, Koskimies AI, Tenhunen A, et al. Diagnosis of luteinized unruptured follicle (LUF) syndrome by ultrasound. Fertil Steril 1984;41:26. Abstract.

Marrs RP. Does the method of oocyte collection have a major influence on in vitro fertilization? Fertil Steril 1986;46:193.

Marrs RP, Vargyas JM, March CM. Correlation of ultrasonic and endocrinologic measurements in human menopausal gonadotropin therapy. Am J Obstet Gynecol 1983;145:417.

McArdle CR, Seibel M, Weinstein F, et al. Induction of ovulation monitored by ultrasound. Radiology 1983;148:809.

Mendelson EB, Friedman H, Neiman HL, et al. The role of imaging in infertility management. AJR 1985;144:415.

Narayan R, Goswamy RK. Transvaginal sonography of the uterine cavity with hysteroscopic correlation in the investigation of infertility. Ultrasound in Obstet Gynecol 1993;3:129.

Parsons J, Booker M, Goswamy R, et al. Oocyte retrieval for in-vitro fertilisation by ultrasonically guided needle aspiration via the urethra. Lancet 1985;1:1076.

Rabinowitz R, Laufer N, Lewin A, et al. The value of ultrasonographic endometrial measurement in the prediction of pregnancy following in vitro fertilization. Fertil Steril 1986;45:824.

Ritchie WGM. Sonographic evaluation of normal and induced ovulation. Radiology 1986;161:1.

Schlief R, Deichert U. Hysterosalpingo–contrast sonography of the uterus and fallopian tubes: Results of a clinical trial of a new contrast medium in 120 patients. Radiology 1991;178:213.

Schulman JD, Dorfmann AD, Jones SL, et al. Outpatient in vitro fertilization using transvaginal ultrasound-guided oocyte retrieval. Obstet Gynecol 1987;69:665.

Steer CV, Campbell S, Tan SL, Crayford T, Mills C, Mason BA, Collins WP. The use of transvaginal color flow imaging after in vitro fertilization to identify optimum uterine conditions before embryo transfer. Fertil Steril 1992;57:372.

Stern J, Peters AJ, Coulam CB. Color Doppler ultrasonography assessment of tubal patency: A comparison study with traditional techniques. Fertil Steril 1992; 58:897.

Tarlatizis BC, Laufer N, DeCherney AH. The use of ovarian ultrasonography in monitoring ovulation induction. J In Vitro Fert Embryo Transf 1984;1:226.

Taylor PJ, Wiseman D, Mahadevan M, et al. "Ultrasound rescue": A successful alternative form of oocyte recovery in patients with periovarian adhesions. Am J Obstet Gynecol 1986;154:240.

Thickman D, Arger P, Tureck R, et al. Sonographic assessment of the endometrium in patients undergoing in vitro fertilization. J Ultrasound Med 1986;5:197.

Winfield AC, Fleischer AC, Moore DE. Diagnostic imaging in infertility. Curr Probl Diagn Radiol 1990;19:1.

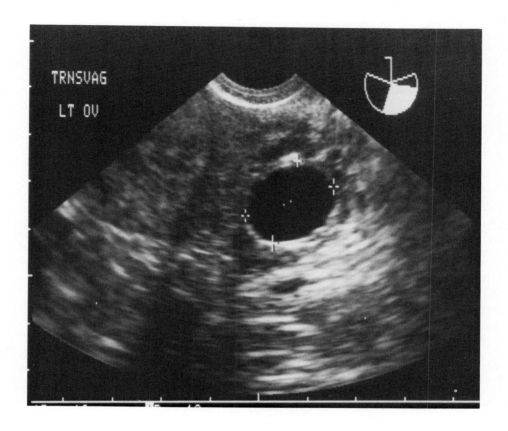

MATURE FOLLICLE

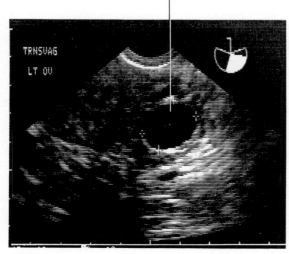

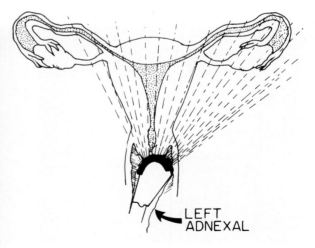

LEFT ADNEXAL

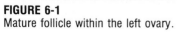

FIGURE 6-1
Mature follicle within the left ovary.

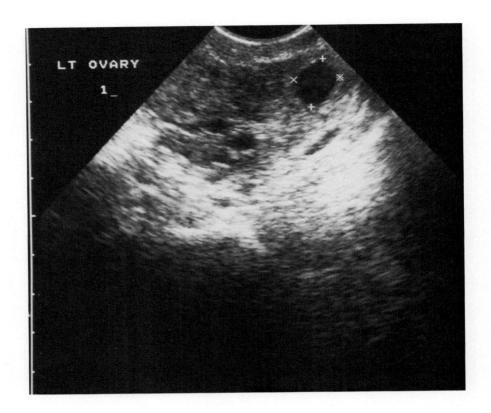

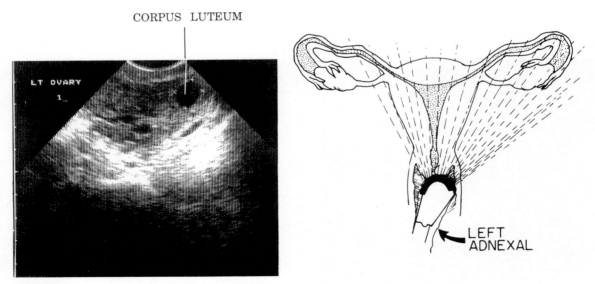

FIGURE 6-2
Postovulatory follicle during a spontaneous cycle with thickened, serrated wall.

FIGURE 6-3
TVS Mimics of a Follicle

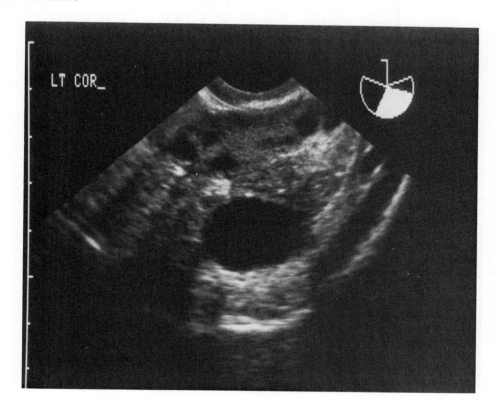

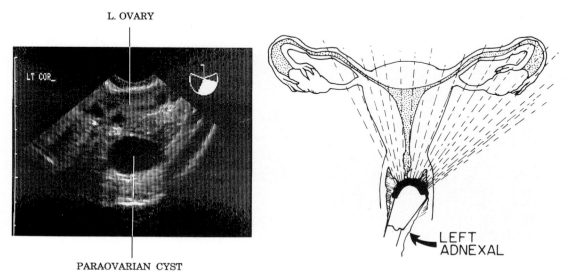

Figure 6-3A. Rounded cystic structure near the left ovary representing a paraovarian cyst.

TVS Mimics of a Follicle *(Continued)*

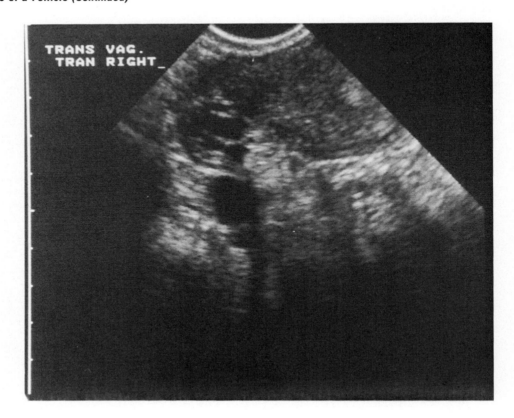

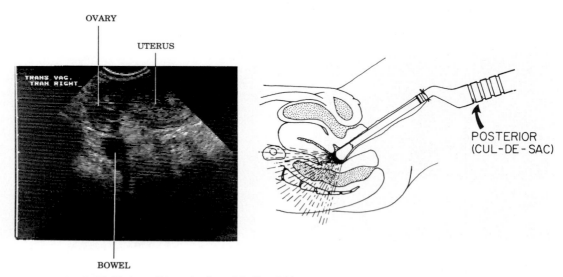

Figure 6-3B. Fluid-filled small bowel adjacent to the right ovary.

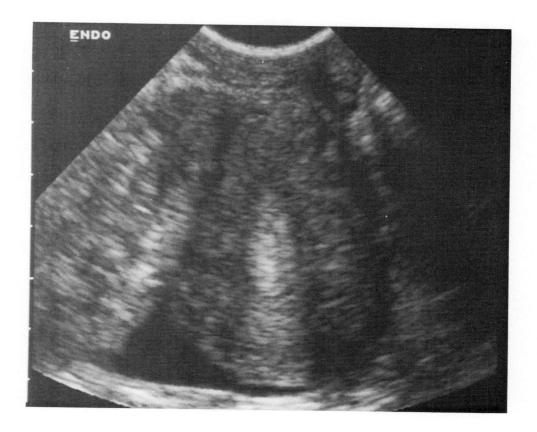

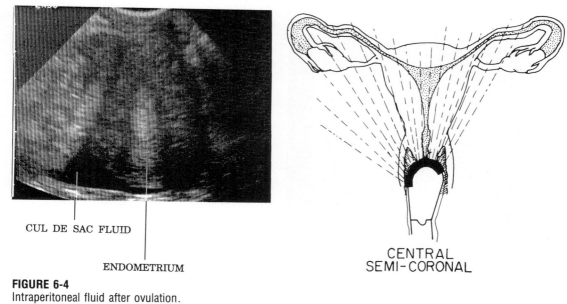

CUL DE SAC FLUID

ENDOMETRIUM

CENTRAL
SEMI-CORONAL

FIGURE 6-4
Intraperitoneal fluid after ovulation.

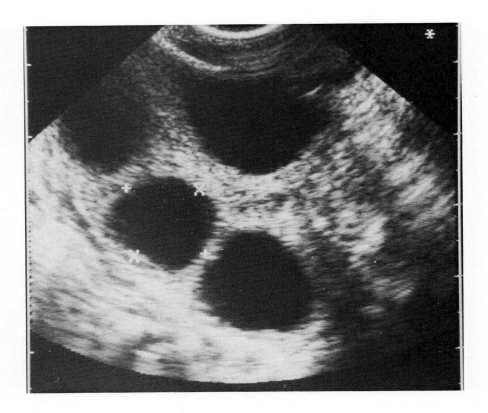

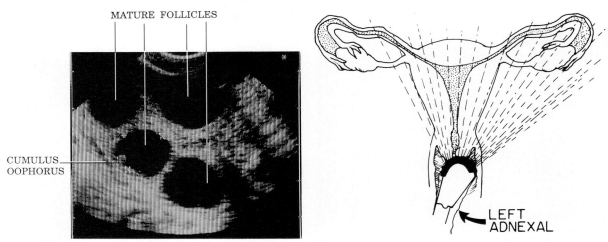

FIGURE 6-5
Multiple mature follicles resulting from CC ovulation induction. A cumulus is seen in the measured
follicle.

FIGURE 6-6
Multiple Follicles at Various Stages of Development

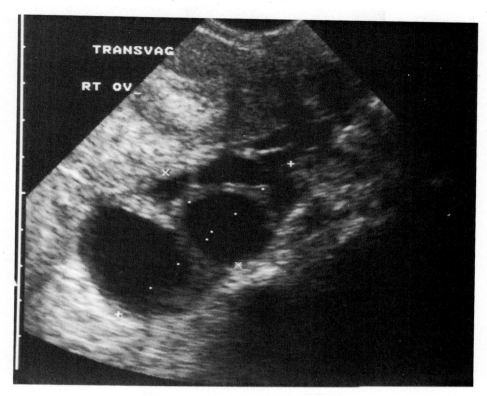

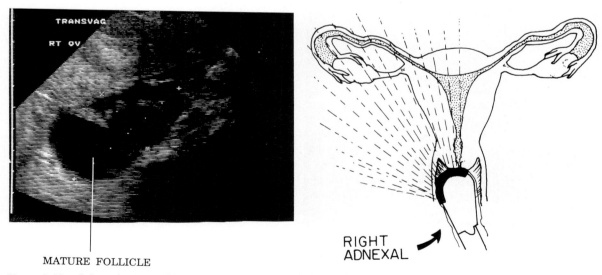

MATURE FOLLICLE

RIGHT
ADNEXAL

Figure 6-6A. Polycystic ovary with development of a single dominant follicle.

Multiple Follicles at Various Stages of Development *(Continued)*

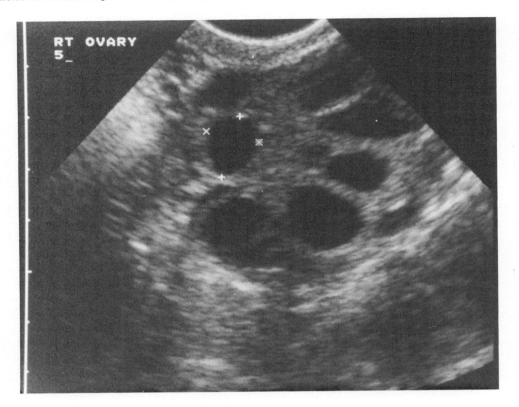

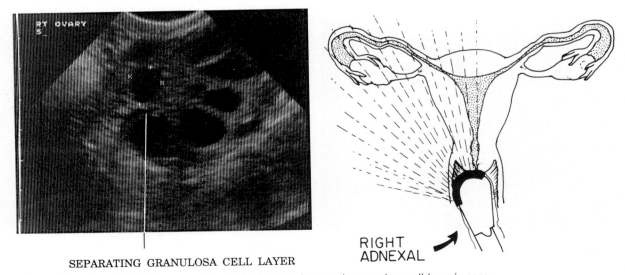

SEPARATING GRANULOSA CELL LAYER

Figure 6-6B. Ovary containing several immature follicles. In one, the granulosa cell layer is separating.

Multiple Follicles at Various Stages of Development *(Continued)*

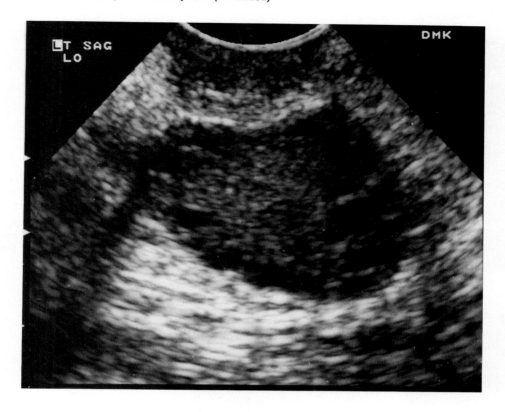

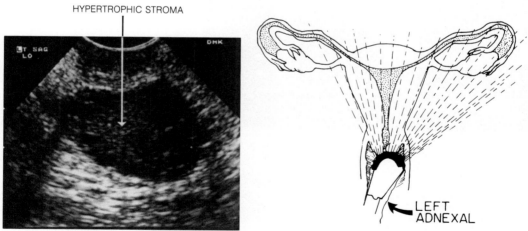

HYPERTROPHIC STROMA

LEFT ADNEXAL

Figure 6-6C. Typical polycystic ovary demonstrating multiple immature follicles along the periphery and increased central echogenicity, probably related to stromal hyperplasia.

FIGURE 6-7
Ovarian Hyperstimulation Syndrome

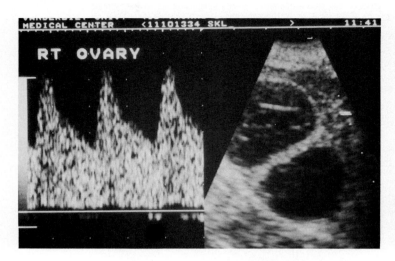

Figure 6-7A. Enlarged right ovary with numerous follicles. Duplex Doppler sonography shows arterial flow within the ovary, thus excluding torsion.

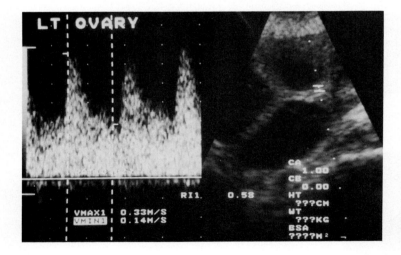

Figure 6-7B. Enlarged left ovary with numerous follicles. Arterial flow is shown as in Figure 6-7A.

Ovarian Hyperstimulation Syndrome *(Continued)*

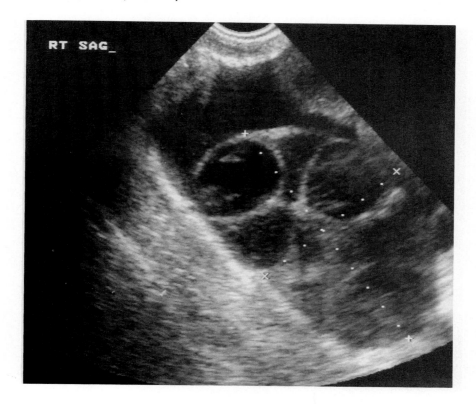

ENLARGED RIGHT OVARY

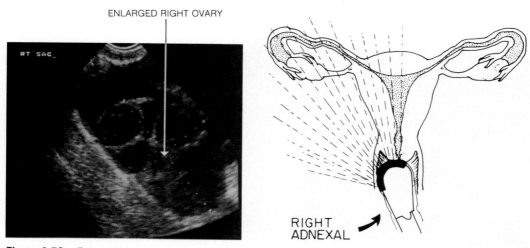

Figure 6-7C. Enlarged right ovary containing several hydropic follicles.

Ovarian Hyperstimulation Syndrome *(Continued)*

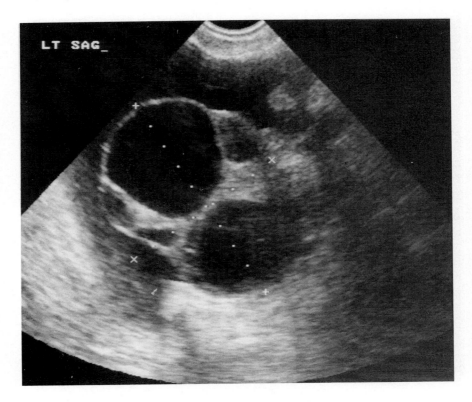

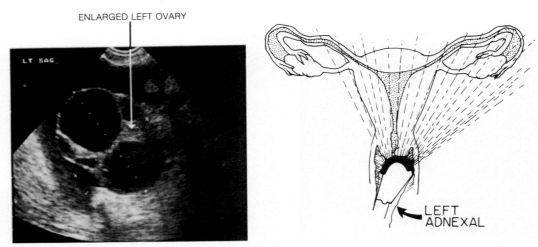

Figure 6-7D. Enlarged left ovary containing several hydropic follicles.

Ovarian Hyperstimulation Syndrome *(Continued)*

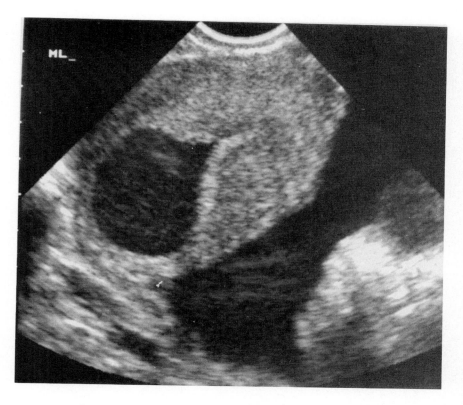

DISTENDED LUMEN

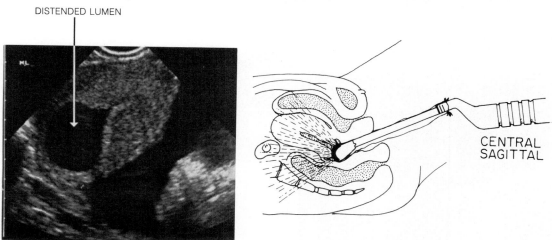

CENTRAL
SAGITTAL

Figure 6-7E. Uterus surrounded by ascites and containing intraluminal fluid.

FIGURE 6-8
Paracervical Vessels

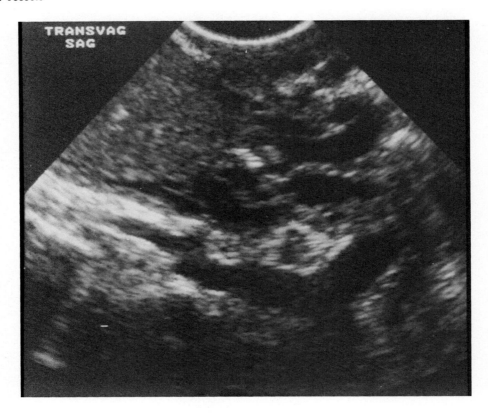

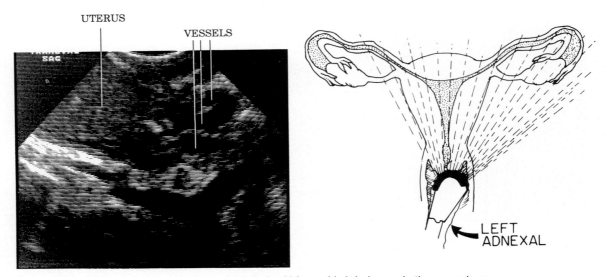

Figure 6-8A. Distended paracervical vessels that should be avoided during aspiration procedures.

Paracervical Vessels *(Continued)*

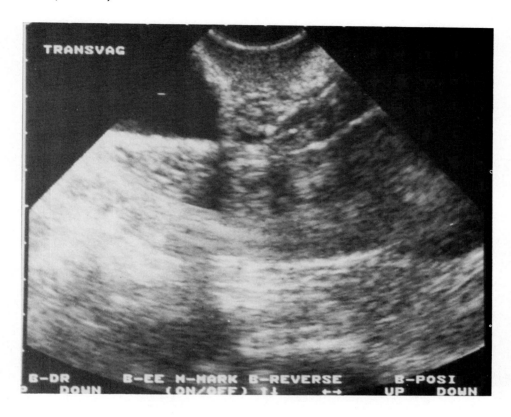

BLADDER

VESSELS

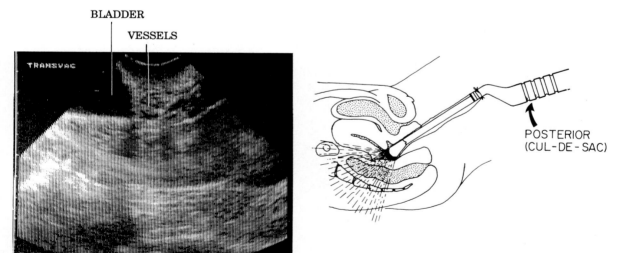

POSTERIOR
(CUL-DE-SAC)

Figure 6-8B. Uterine arteries adjacent to the cervix.

Paracervical Vessels *(Continued)*

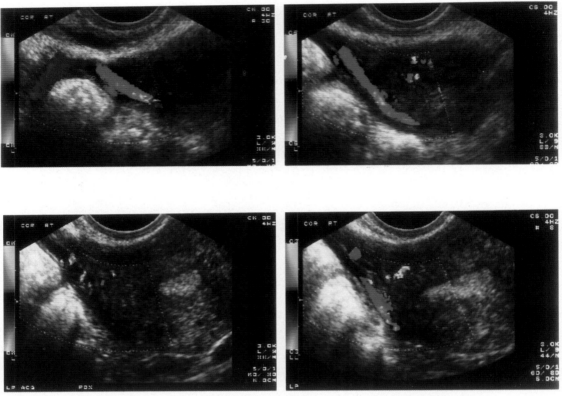

Figure 6-8C. Composite transvaginal color Doppler sonography showing normal vascularity within the uterus and adnexa.

Paracervical Vessels *(Continued)*

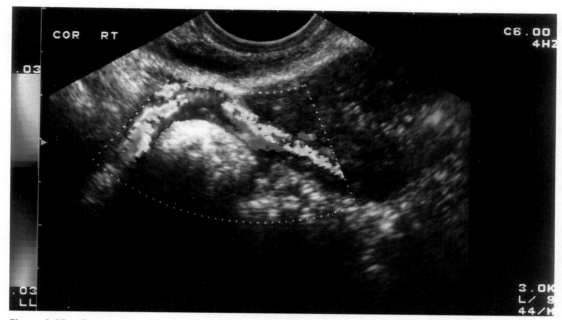

Figure 6-8D. Transvaginal color Doppler sonography showing uterine artery and vein. The uterine vein courses into the myometrium to become the arcuate vein.

Paracervical Vessels *(Continued)*

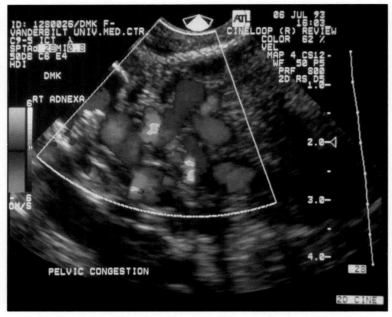

E

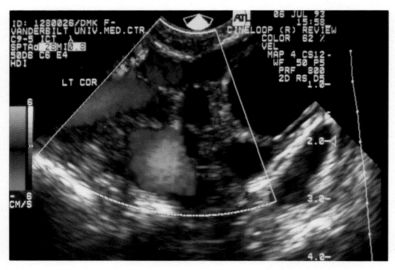

F

Figure 6-8E. Right (**E**) and left (**F**) adnexal transvaginal color Doppler sonography showing distended periuterine veins.

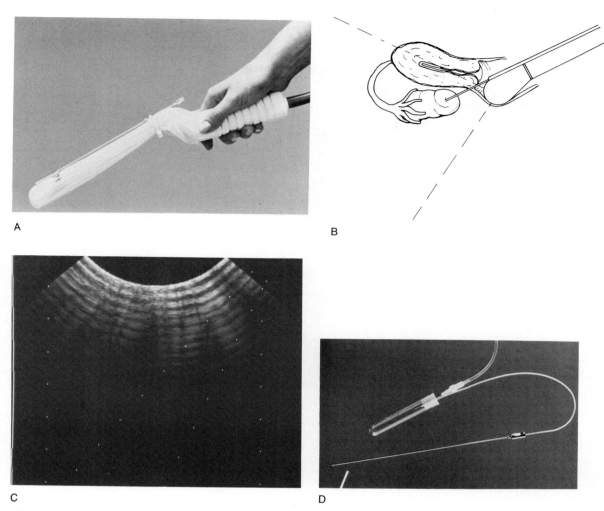

FIGURE 6-9

Guided Procedures. (**A**) Draped probe with needle guide attached. (**B**) Diagram of guided transvaginal follicle aspiration. (**C**) Display on monitor showing path of needle. (**D**) Needle showing scored tip.

FIGURE 6-10
Guided Follicular Aspiration

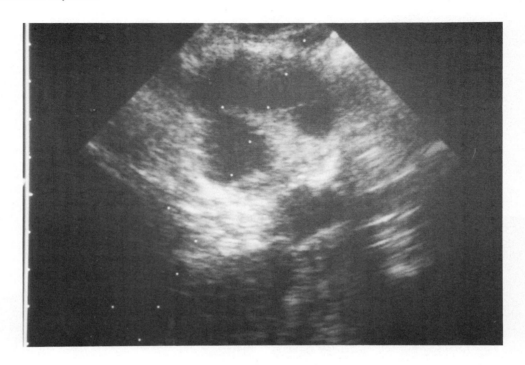

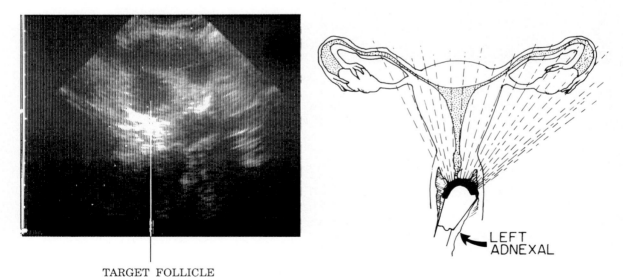

TARGET FOLLICLE

LEFT
ADNEXAL

Figure 6-10A. Before aspiration, the desired follicle aligned within the beam path.

Guided Follicular Aspiration *(Continued)*

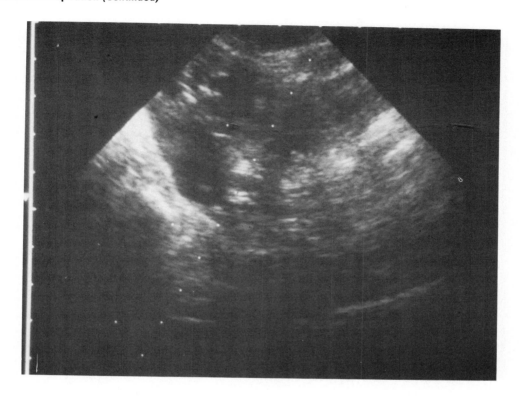

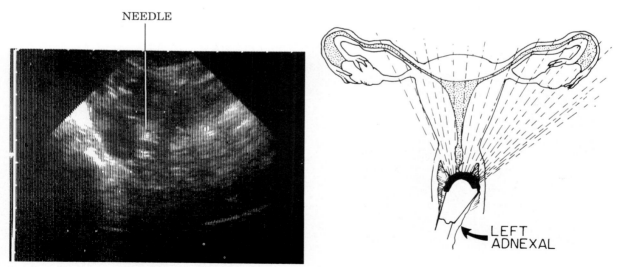

NEEDLE

LEFT
ADNEXAL

Figure 6-10B. After aspiration, the echogenic needle tip seen within the aspirated follicle.

Guided Follicular Aspiration *(Continued)*

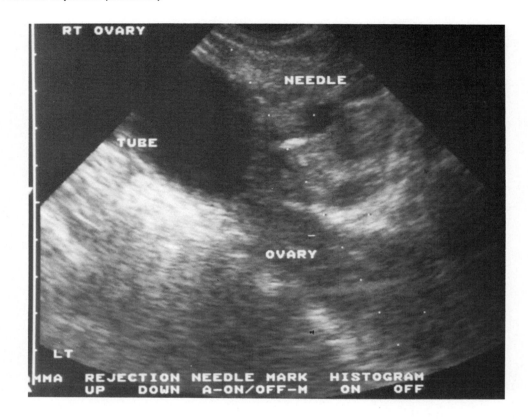

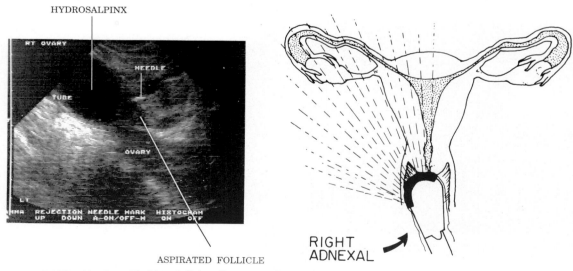

Figure 6-10C. Needle guided into follicle adjacent to a hydrosalpinx.

FIGURE 6-11
Cyst Aspiration Associated With Leuprolide Acetate

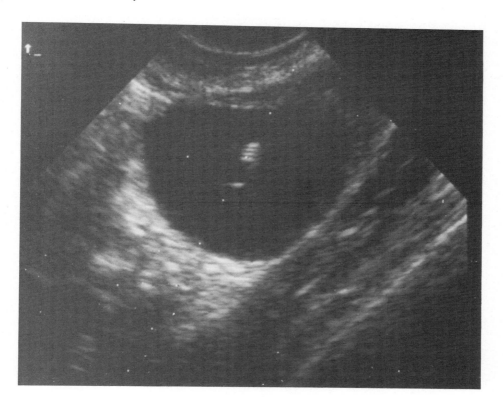

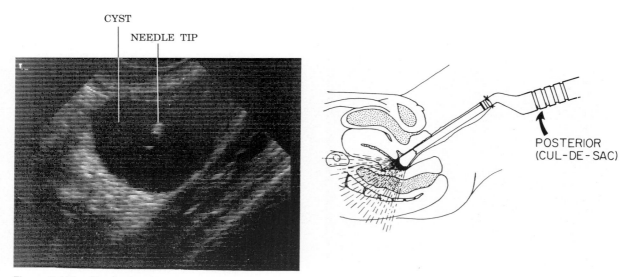

CYST

NEEDLE TIP

POSTERIOR
(CUL-DE-SAC)

Figure 6-11A. Needle tip within cyst.

Cyst Aspiration Associated With Leuprolide Acetate *(Continued)*

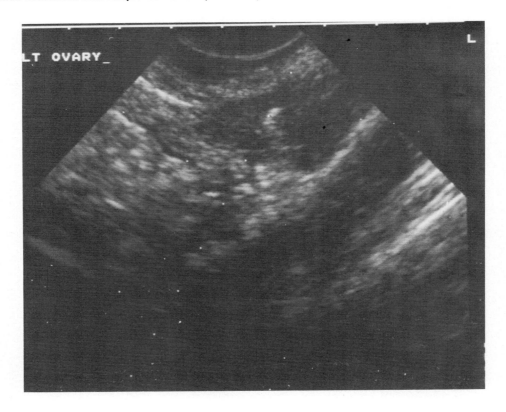

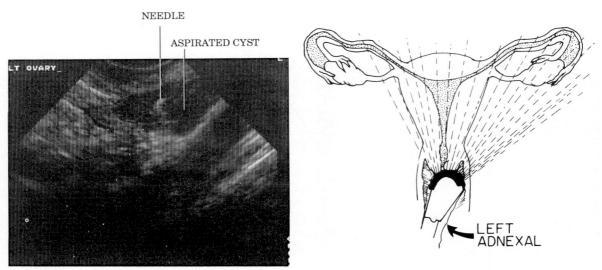

Figure 6-11B. Aspirated cyst.

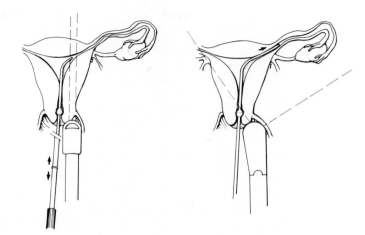

Figure 6-12A. Diagram of TVS guidance.

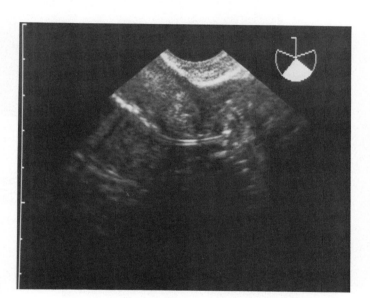

Figure 6-12B. Cannula through ostia.

Tubal Cannulation *(Continued)*

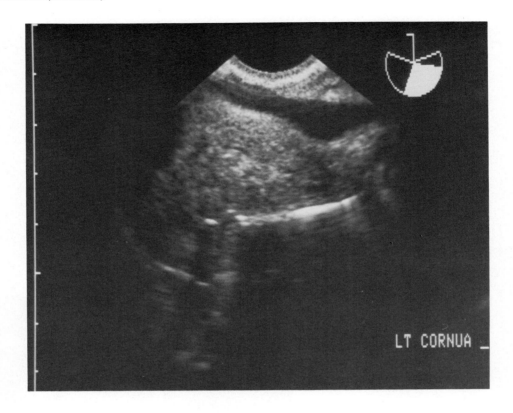

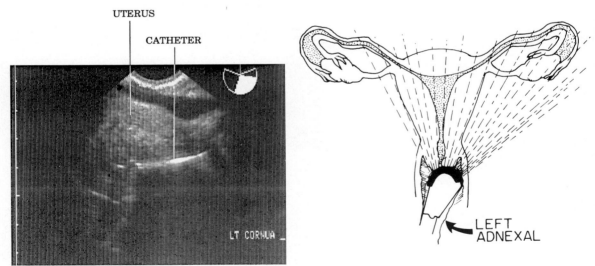

Figure 6-12C. Inner catheter advanced into the isthmic portion of the tube.

Tubal Cannulation *(Continued)*

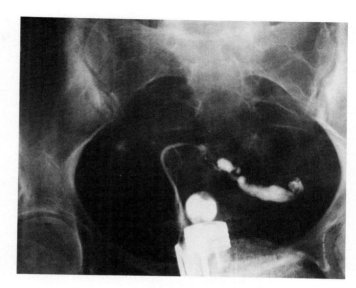

Figure 6-12D. Radiograph of the opened tube after dilation.

Tubal Cannulation *(Continued)*

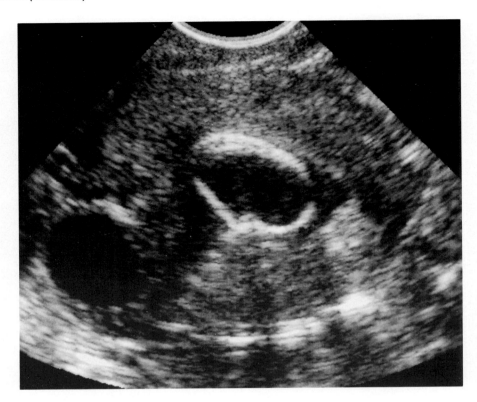

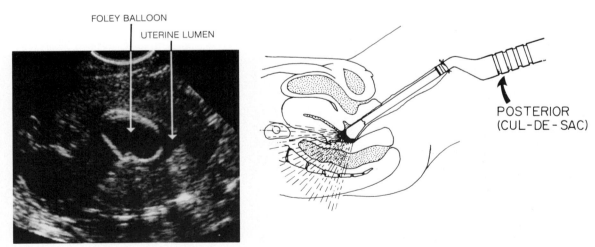

Figure 6-12E. Obstructed tubes after fluid instillation. A Foley catheter balloon occupies the lumen. The right ovary contains a mature follicle. There is no intraperitoneal "spill."

FIGURE 6-13
Endometrial Development. The uterus is shown in sagittal plane, long-axis view

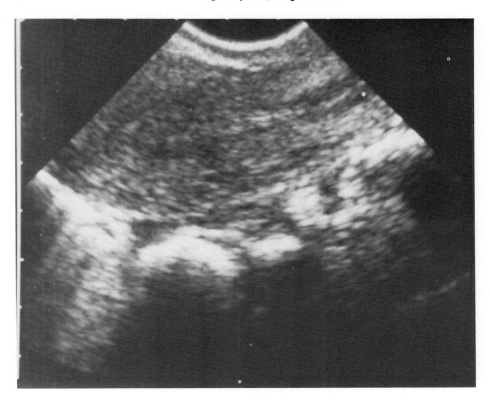

ENDOMETRIUM

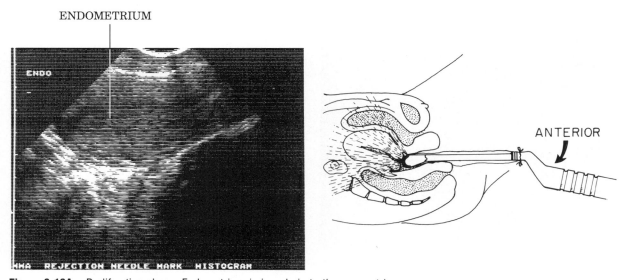

Figure 6-13A. Proliferative phase. Endometrium is isoechoic to the myometrium.

Endometrial Development. The uterus is shown in sagittal plane, long-axis view *(Continued)*

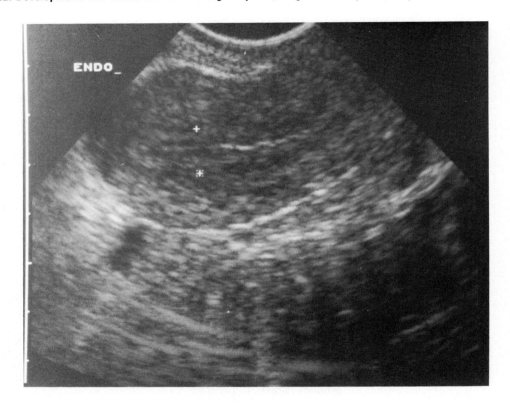

ENDOMETRIUM

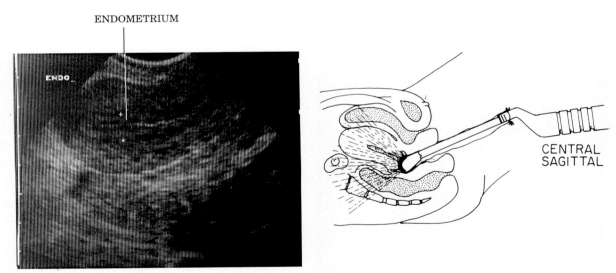

Figure 6-13B. Late proliferative, periovulatory phase showing multilayers.

Endometrial Development. The uterus is shown in sagittal plane, long-axis view *(Continued)*

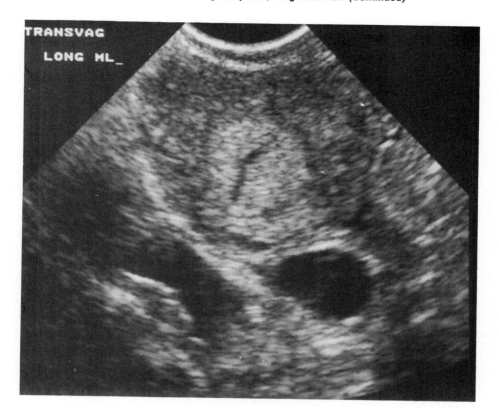

SECRETORY ENDOMETRIUM

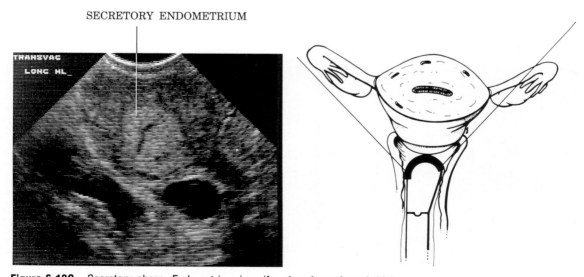

Figure 6-13C. Secretory phase. Endometrium is uniformly echogenic and thick.

FIGURE 6-14
Miscellaneous Applications

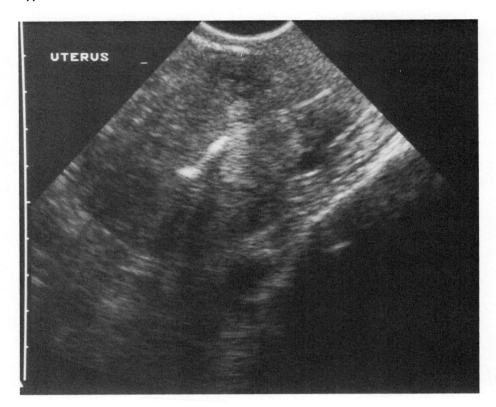

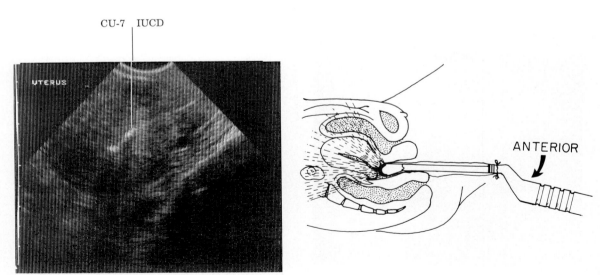

Figure 6-14A. CU-7 IUCD within the upper uterine lumen.

Miscellaneous Applications *(Continued)*

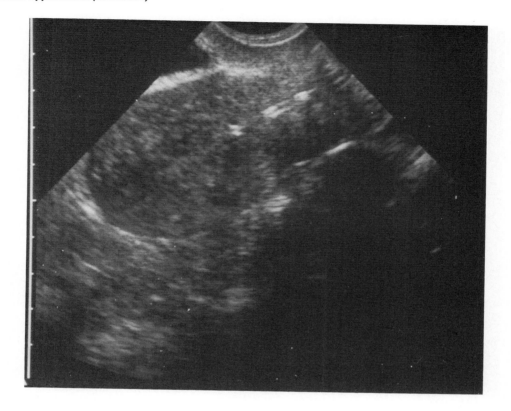

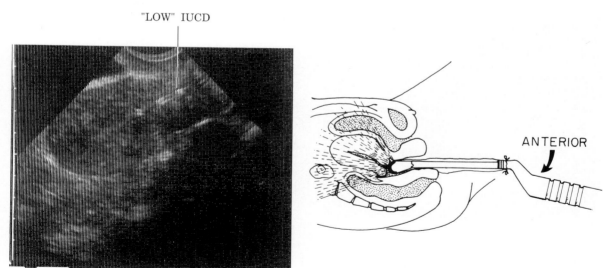

"LOW" IUCD

Figure 6-14B. CU-7 IUCD in the lower corpus, upper cervix.

ANTERIOR

Miscellaneous Applications *(Continued)*

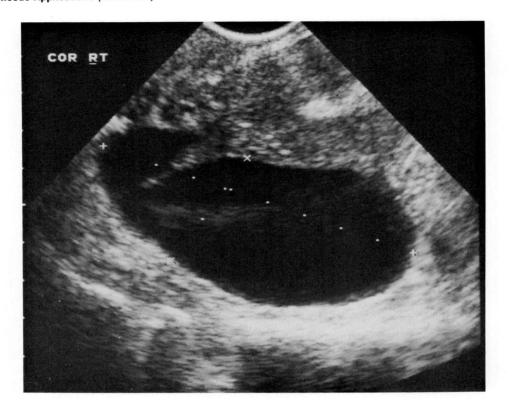

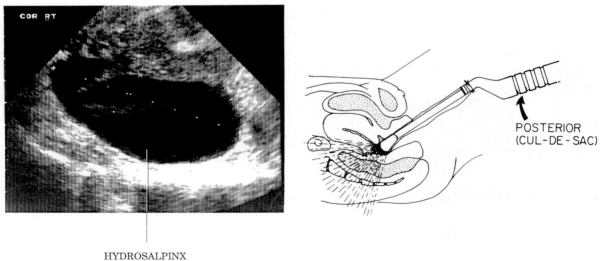

HYDROSALPINX

Figure 6-14C. Hydrosalpinx (between cursors) of the right fallopian tube.

Miscellaneous Applications *(Continued)*

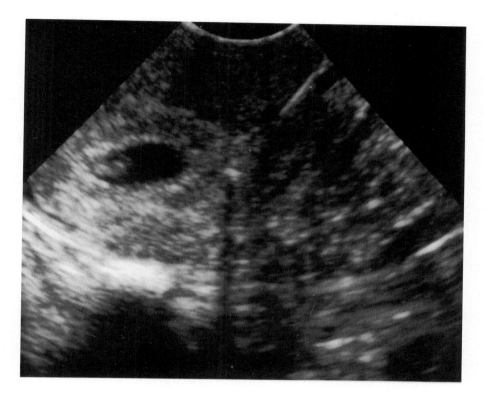

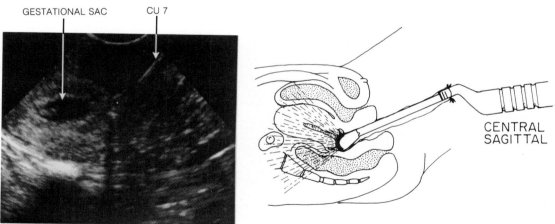

Figure 6-14D. Cu-7 IUCD inferior to an intact gestational sac of 6 weeks.

Transvaginal Sonography: A Clinical Atlas, Second Edition,
edited by Arthur C. Fleischer and Donna M. Kepple.
J.B. Lippincott Company, Philadelphia, © 1995.

CHAPTER 7

Normal Early Pregnancy

Arthur C. Fleischer, MD
Donna M. Kepple, RDMS

INTRODUCTION

Transvaginal sonography (TVS) affords detailed delineation of the anatomic changes that occur in the first trimester of pregnancy. In general, definitive sonographic findings such as the presence of a gestational sac and the presence of an embryo/fetus with or without heart motion can be established 1 week before confirmation by conventional transabdominal scanning techniques (Pennell and coworkers, 1987, 1991; Jain, 1988). Certain anatomic "milestones" can predictably be seen with TVS (Table 7-1).

Transvaginal sonography provides a glimpse at the dynamics of embryonic development, including some transient features. Transient findings may be present for only a few days and are detectable when they are present. A transient finding such as a "double bleb," which represents the developing yolk sac, embryo, and amnion, can be observed.

MILESTONES

One of the earliest sonographic findings in intrauterine pregnancy is the thickening of the decidua that occurs at approximately 3 to 4 weeks (Fig. 7-1). After 4 weeks, a small (3 to 5 mm) hypoechoic area surrounded by an echogenic rim can be seen within the choriodecidual tissue. This is the chorionic sac (Fig. 7-2). The sac usually enlarges from 3 to 10 mm in average dimension and grows at a rate of 1 to 1.1 mm/d or 3.5 cm/wk. At approximately 5 to 6 weeks, a yolk sac/embryo complex can be seen within the chorionic sac (Fig. 7-3). A transient finding of a "double bleb," which represents the yolk sac, embryo, and amnion, is occasionally seen. The embryo can be identified as an echogenic focus immediately adjacent to a pole of the yolk sac. When the embryo measures 5 mm or more, heart motion can consistently be identified, but only if scanners with a high frame rate (more than 30 frames/sec) are used (Fig. 7-4). A recent study shows that normal embryos less than 4 mm may not demonstrate heart motion or may demonstrate a very slow (less than 60 beats per minute) rate, and follow-up examination of these embryos is warranted (Levi and coworkers, 1988, 1990). Measurement of the crown-rump length of the embryo with TVS provides an accurate determination of gestational age (Table 7-2) (Degenhardt and coworkers, 1988).

TABLE 7-1
TVS "Landmarks"

Gestational Age	Sign
4 wks	Choriodecidual thickening; chorionic sac
5 wks	Chorionic sac (5 to 15 mm); yolk sac
6 wks	Yolk sac/embryo; detectable heart motion
7 wks	Embryonic/fetal movement; prominent rhombencephalon
8 wks	Physiologic bowel herniation; arms, legs

SONOGRAPHIC FEATURES

The chorionic sac can be seen in most intrauterine pregnancies when the β-human chorionic gonadotropin (β-hCG) level is higher than 1500 mIU/mL (Table 7-3) (Bree and coworkers, 1989). This is particularly important when examining a patient in whom there is a clinical suspicion of ectopic pregnancy (Fleischer and coworkers, 1990).

Punctate hypoechoic areas representing blood pools or vascular lacunae can be seen surrounding the developing chorion (Fig. 7-5). When these are large (approximating the size of the gestational sac)

and hypoechoic, they are called "retrochorionic hemorrhage" (Fig. 7-6). As documented in one study, these hemorrhages are usually associated with a good prognosis for completion of pregnancy (Stabile and coworkers, 1989). If they are more than one fourth of the volume of the gestational sac size or associated with dissection from the choriodecidua, they may be associated with spontaneous abortion (Pedersen and Mantoni, 1990). Follow-up sonography is recommended in these patients.

The embryo is seen consistently when it measures more than 5 mm, which corresponds to approximately 5 to 6 weerks of gestational age. Heart contractions begin at this time and usually can be estimated to be more than 80 to 90 beats per minute (DuBose and coworkers, 1988; Levi and coworkers, 1990; Rempen, 1990; de Crespigny, 1988). This rate occurs when the heart is forming; there is a slow increase in heart rate up to approximately 10 weeks when the heart rate is usually between 140 and 180 beats per minute (Hertzberg and coworkers, 1988).

If there is slow heart rate after 8 weeks (less than 90 beats per minute), the pregnancy may be compromised. At early development, slow heart rates are seen (less than 85 beats per minute) but after 8 weeks, the heart rate should be between 120 and 160 beats per minute. Although low heart rate can be taken as a sign predictive of poor prognosis,

TABLE 7-2
Crown-Rump Length Versus Gestational Age (wks)

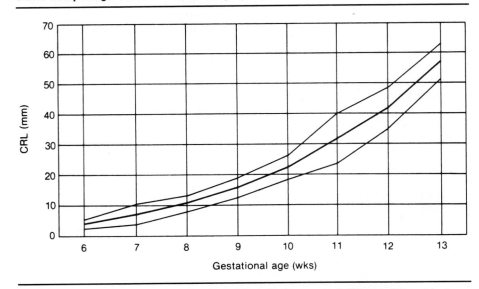

From Degenhardt F, Böhmer S, Behrens O, Mühlhaus K. Transvaginale Ultraschallbiometrie der Scheitel-Steiss-Länge im ersten Trimenon. Z Geburtshilfe Perinatol 1988;192:249–252.

TABLE 7-3
TVS "Milestones" Versus β-hCG

	β-hCG	Days	Weeks
Gestational sac	1000 mIU/mL (IRP)	32	4 +
Yolk sac	7200 mIU/mL (IRP)	36 to 40	5 to 6
Embryo with heart motion	10800 mIU/mL (IRP)	<40	6 +

IRP, international reference preparation.

From Bree RL, Edwards M, Bohm-Velez M, Beyler S, Roberts J, Mendelson EB. Transvaginal sonography in the evaluation of normal early pregnancy: Correlation with HCG level. AJR 1989;153: 75–79.

approximately 10% of embryos/fetuses in normal pregnancies have very slow heart rates (less than 85 beats per minute) (Laboda and coworkers, 1989).

Certain anatomic features of the embryo/fetus can be seen in detail with TVS. Similarly, some of the normal developmental features delineated by TVS may be mistaken for abnormal. For example, an extra yolk sac or allantoic cysts of the developing umbilical cord may be seen in early fetal development and require follow-up scans (Fig. 7-7) (Barzilai and coworkers, 1989; Skibo and coworkers, 1992). The rhombencephalon appears as a hypoechoic area within the posterior aspect of the fetal head corresponding to development of the fourth ventricle and posterior fossa structures and should not be confused with yolk sac, which is extra-amniotic (Fig. 7-8) (Cyr, 1988). Physiologic herniation of the bowel into the base of the umbilical cord can be identified at 8 to 9 weeks, but should spontaneously regress by 12 weeks (Fig. 7-9).

From 8 weeks on, several anatomic structures of the developing fetus can be delineated in detail with TVS. These include the arms, hands, legs, fa-

cial structures, ventricular system, choroid plexus, and spine (Fig. 7-10). The amnion is an extrafetal structure that can be seen as a thin membrane surrounding the fetus. It separates the amniotic cavity from the extraembryonic coelom. Fetal body activity can be identified as early as 6 to 8 weeks and usually consists of flexion or extension of the fetal body and movement of the fetal extremities.

The improved resolution of fetal structures by TVS allows the diagnosis of some fetal gross anomalies such as anencephaly in the first trimester. The problem of misdiagnosis as abnormal of an unusual feature during embryonic/fetal development also exists, however.

Tables 7-4 to 7-7 contain data concerning embryonic and fetal biometry during the first trimester (Timor-Tritsch and coworkers, 1990).

TWIN PREGNANCY

Twin pregnancy can accurately be identified as early as 5 to 6 weeks after conception by the presence of

TABLE 7-4
Gestational Age Versus Crown–Rump Length (cm)

Gestational Age (wks)	5th Percentile	50th Percentile	95th Percentile
6	0.15	0.28	0.47
7	0.47	0.70	1.03
8	0.95	1.32	1.82
9	1.61	2.13	2.83
10	2.43	3.14	4.07
11	3.43	4.34	5.52
12	4.60	5.74	7.20
13	5.94	7.33	9.10
14	7.44	9.11	11.22

From Timor-Tritsch I, Lasser D, Peisner D, Vollebergh J. Embryonic and fetal biometry in the first trimester as depicted with TVS. J Ultrasound Med 1990;9(suppl):41.

TABLE 7-5
Gestational Age Versus Biparietal Diameter (cm)

Gestational Age (wks)	5th Percentile	50th Percentile	95th Percentile
7	0.46	0.47	0.48
8	0.62	0.63	0.64
9	0.82	0.86	0.91
10	1.07	1.16	1.28
11	1.40	1.56	1.82
12	1.83	2.11	2.57
13	2.37	2.85	3.64
14	3.08	3.85	5.15

From Timor-Tritsch I, Lasser D, Peisner D, Vollebergh J. Embryonic and fetal biometry in the first trimester as depicted with TVS. J Ultrasound Med 1990;9(suppl):41.

TABLE 7-6
Gestational Age Versus Head Circumference (cm)

Gestational Age (wks)	5th Percentile	50th Percentile	95th Percentile
9	2.05	3.20	4.78
10	3.23	4.57	6.35
11	4.42	5.91	7.92
12	5.59	7.26	9.49
13	6.78	8.61	11.06
14	7.96	9.95	12.63

From Timor-Tritsch I, Lasser D, Peisner D, Vollebergh J. Embryonic and fetal biometry in the first trimester as depicted with TVS. J Ultrasound Med 1990;9(suppl):41.

TABLE 7-7
Gestational Age Versus Abdominal Circumference (cm)

Gestational Age (wks)	5th Percentile	50th Percentile	95th Percentile
9	1.89	2.85	3.16
10	2.32	3.62	6.95
11	2.85	4.62	9.36
12	3.49	5.88	12.61
13	4.28	7.59	16.98

From Timor-Tritsch I, Lasser D, Peisner D, Vollebergh J. Embryonic and fetal biometry in the first trimester as depicted with TVS. J Ultrasound Med 1990;9(suppl):41.

more than one chorionic sac. Dichorionic placental development can be predicted if the two sacs are separate from each other (Fig. 7-11). Similarly, the amnionicity of twin pregnancies can be seen during the first trimester by establishment of the continuity of the amnion surrounding each fetus (Fig. 7-12). Triplet pregnancies may vary in amnionicity and chorionicity (Fig. 7-13).

SUMMARY

The role of TVS in early pregnancy is to confirm the presence of an intrauterine pregnancy or to provide definitive diagnosis of an ectopic pregnancy by demonstration of an adnexal mass and no intrauterine gestational sac (Fleischer and coworkers, 1990). TVS should be carefully applied, and misdiagnosis should be avoided by adopting a conservative approach.

REFERENCES

Barzilai M, Lyons EA, Levi CS, Lindsay DJ. Vitelline duct cyst or double yolk sac. J Ultrasound Med 1989;8:523.

Bree RL, Edwards M, Bohm-Velez M, Beyler S, Roberts J, Mendelson EB. Transvaginal sonography in the evaluation of normal early pregnancy: Correlation with HCG level. AJR 1989;153:75.

Cyr DR, Mack LA, Nyberg DA, Shepard TH, Shuman WP. Fetal rhombencephalon: Normal US findings. Radiology 1988;166:691.

de Crespigny L, Cooper D, McKenna M. Early detection of intrauterine pregnancy with ultrasound. J Ultrasound Med 1988;7:7.

Degenhardt F, Böhmer S, Behrens O, Mühlhaus K. Transvaginale Ultraschallbiometrie der Scheitel-Steiss-Länge im ersten Trimenon. Z Geburtshilfe Perinatol 1988;192:249.

DuBose TJ, Dickey D, Butschek CM, Porter L, Hill LW, Poole EK. The opinion that the fetal heart rate (FHR) is an indicator of the baby's sex (letter). J Ultrasound Med 1988;7:237.

Fleischer AC, Pennell RG, McKee MS, et al. Sonographic features of ectopic pregnancies as depicted by transvaginal scanning. Radiology 1990;174:375.

Hertzberg BS, Mahony BS, Bowie JD. First trimester fetal cardiac activity: Sonographic documentation of a progressive early rise in heart rate. J Ultrasound Med 1988;7:573.

Jain KA, Hamper UM, Sanders RC. Comparison of transvaginal and transabdominal sonography in the detection of early pregnancy and its complications. AJR 1988;151:1139.

Laboda L, Estroff J, Benacerrat B. First trimester bradycardia: a sign of impending fetal loss. J Ultra Med 1989;8:561.

Levi CS, Lyons EA, Lindsay DJ. Early diagnosis of nonviable pregnancy with endovaginal US. Radiology 1988;167:383.

Levi CS, Lyons EA, Zheng XH, Lindsay DJ, Holt SC. Endovaginal US demonstration of cardiac activity in embryos of less than 5.0 mm in crown-rump length. Radiology 1990;176:71.

Pedersen JF, Mantoni M. Prevalence and significance of subchorionic hemorrhage in threatened abortion: A sonographic study. AJR 1990;154:535.

Pennell RG, Baltarowich OH, Kurtz AB, et al. Complicated first-trimester pregnancies: Evaluation with endovaginal US versus transabdominal technique. Radiology 1987;165:79.

Pennell RG, Needleman L, Pajak T, et al. Prospective comparison of vaginal and abdominal sonography in normal early pregnancy. J Ultrasound Med 1991;10:63.

Rempen A. Diagnosis of viability in early pregnancy with vaginal sonography. J Ultrasound Med 1990;9:711.

Skibo LK, Lyons EA, Levi CS. First-trimester umbilical cord cysts. Radiology 1990;182:719.

Stabile I, Campbell S, Grudzinskas JG. Threatened miscarriage and intrauterine hematomas: Sonographic and biochemical studies. J Ultrasound Med 1989;8:289.

Timor-Tritsch IE, Lasser D, Peisner D, Vollebergh J. Embryonic and fetal biometry in the first trimester as depicted with TVS. J Ultrasound Med 1990;9 (suppl):41.

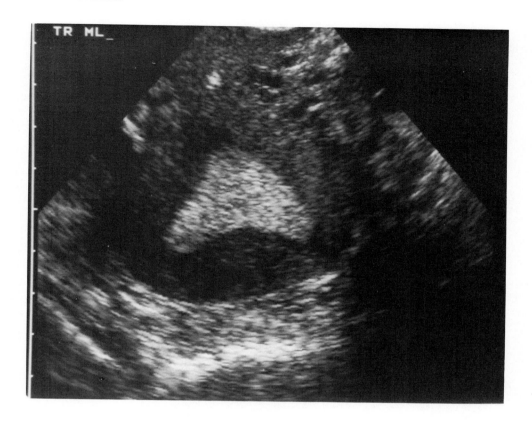

DECIDUALIZED   ENDOMETRIUM

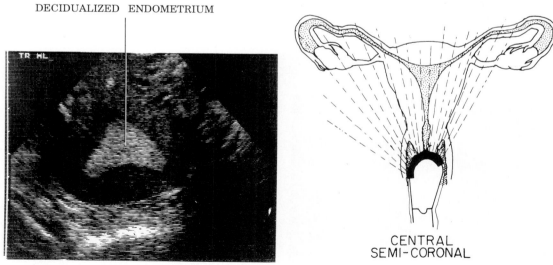

CENTRAL
SEMI-CORONAL

FIGURE 7-1
Thickened Decidua at 2 5/7 Weeks After a Successful IVF-ER Procedure.

FIGURE 7-2
Chorionic Sac Within Thickened Choriodecidua of a 4- to 5-Week Intrauterine Pregnancy

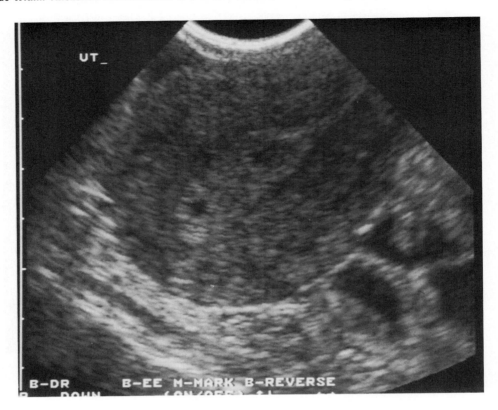

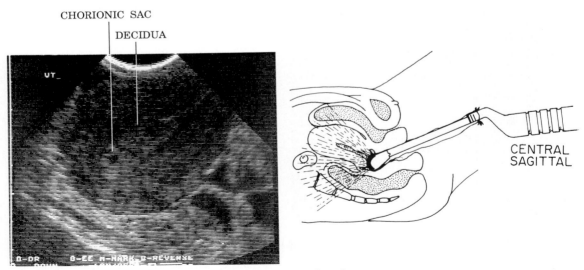

Figure 7-2A. Chorionic sac with decidualized endometrium at 4 weeks.

Chorionic Sac Within Thickened Choriodecidua of a 4- to 5-Week Intrauterine Pregnancy
(Continued)

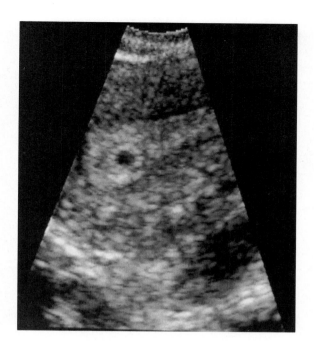

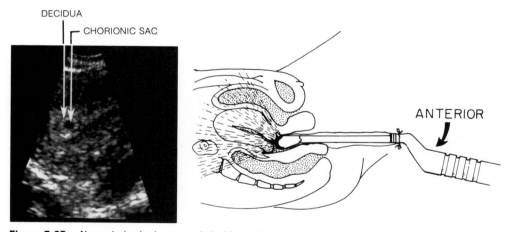

Figure 7-2B. Normal chorionic sac and decidua at 5 weeks.

Chorionic Sac Within Thickened Choriodecidua of a 4- to 5-Week Intrauterine Pregnancy
(Continued)

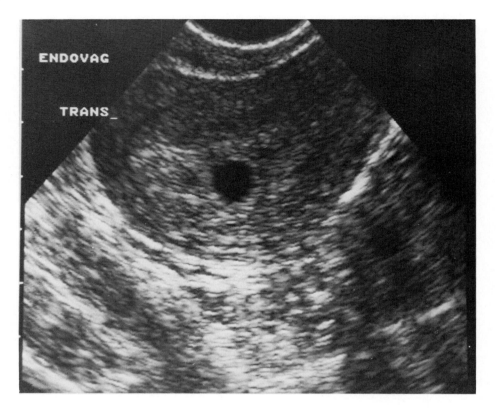

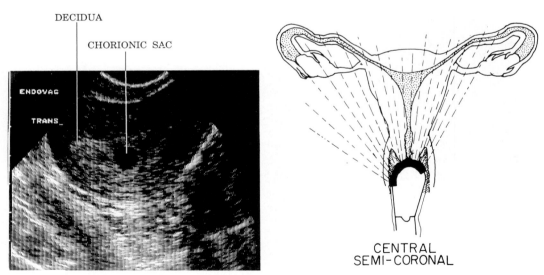

Figure 7-2C. Chorionic sac within thickened choriodecidua at 5 weeks. β-hCG = 1500 mIU/mL (2nd Int. St.).

FIGURE 7-3
Five- to Six-Week Intrauterine Pregnancy

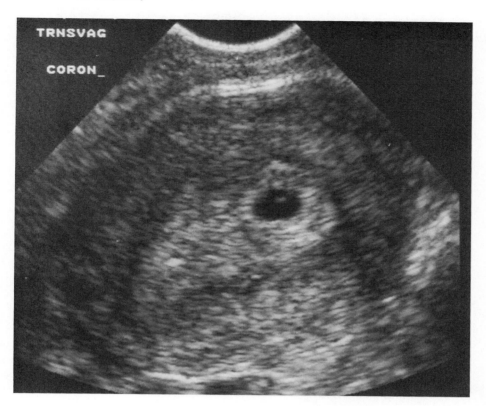

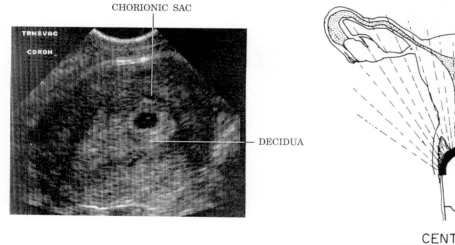

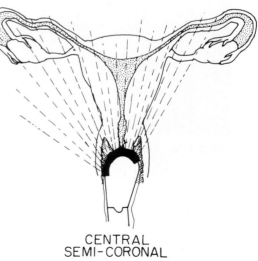

CENTRAL
SEMI-CORONAL

Figure 7-3A. Chorionic sac with developing yolk sac.

Five- to Six-Week Intrauterine Pregnancy *(Continued)*

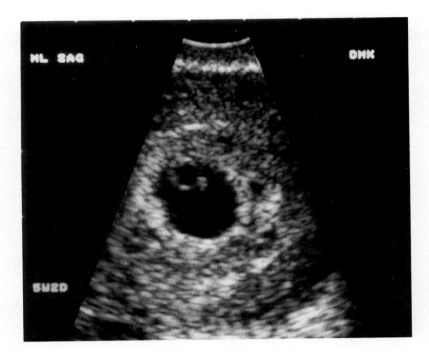

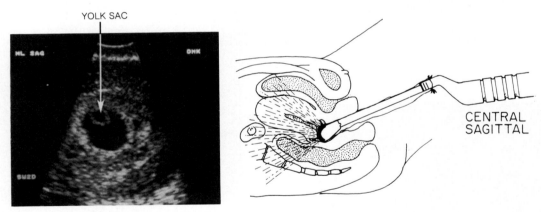

Figure 7-3B. Yolk sac within gestational sac.

Five- to Six-Week Intrauterine Pregnancy *(Continued)*

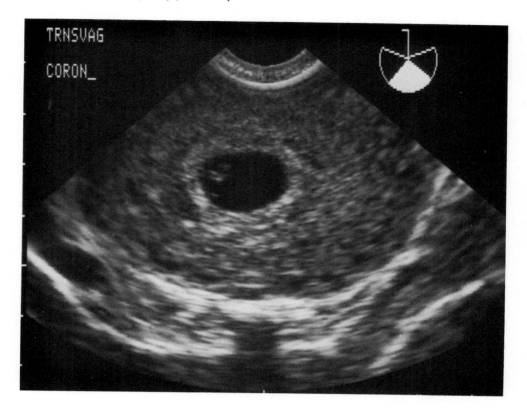

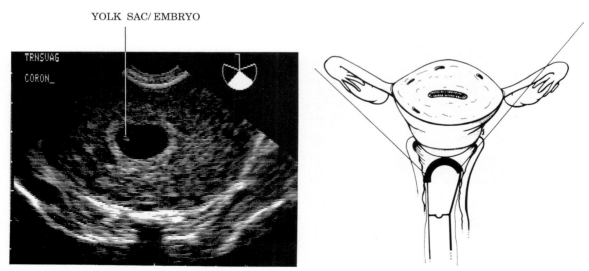

YOLK SAC/ EMBRYO

Figure 7-3C. Chorionic sac with developing yolk sac/embryo.

Five- to Six-Week Intrauterine Pregnancy *(Continued)*

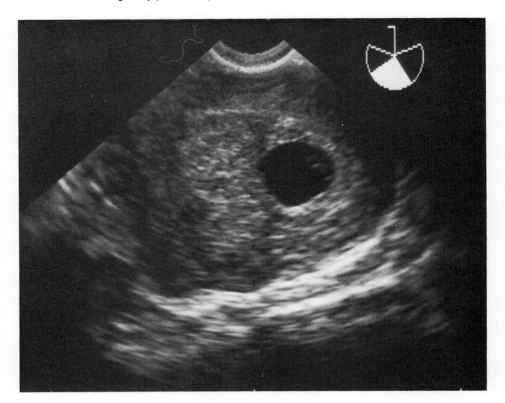

YOLK SAC/ EMBRYO

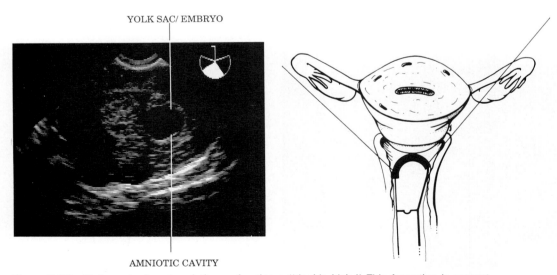

AMNIOTIC CAVITY

Figure 7-3D. Yolk sac/embryo/amniotic sac forming a "double bleb." This formation is present for 1 or 2 days only.

Five- to Six-Week Intrauterine Pregnancy *(Continued)*

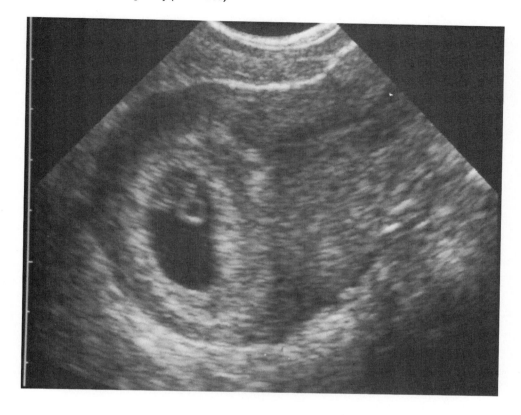

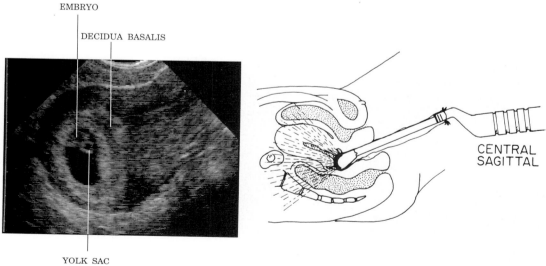

EMBRYO

DECIDUA BASALIS

YOLK SAC

CENTRAL
SAGITTAL

Figure 7-3E. Yolk sac/embryo within the gestational sac.

FIGURE 7-4
Six- to Seven-Week Intrauterine Pregnancy

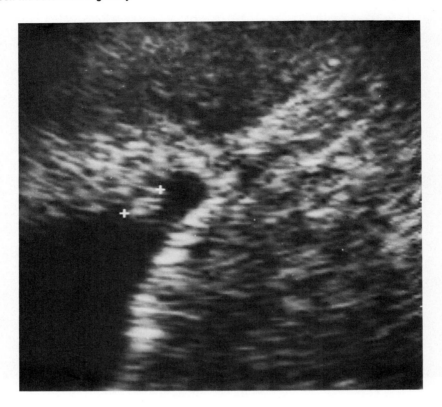

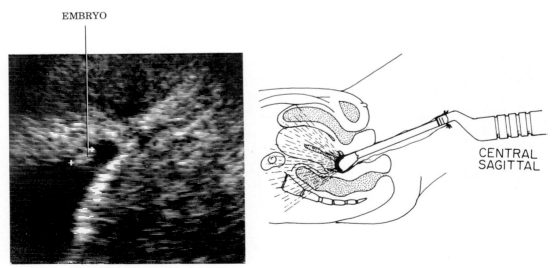

Figure 7-4A. Magnified scan of 4-mm embryo within the inferior aspect of the gestational sac.

Six- to Seven-Week Intrauterine Pregnancy (Continued)

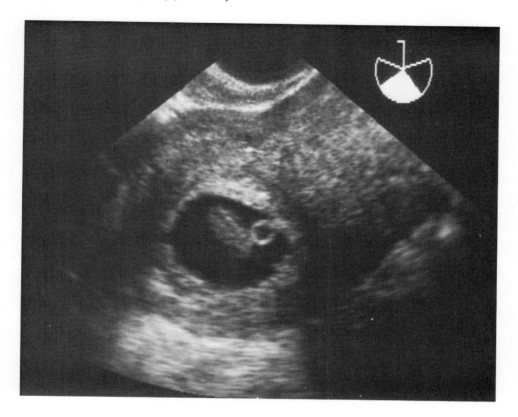

DEVELOPING SPINE

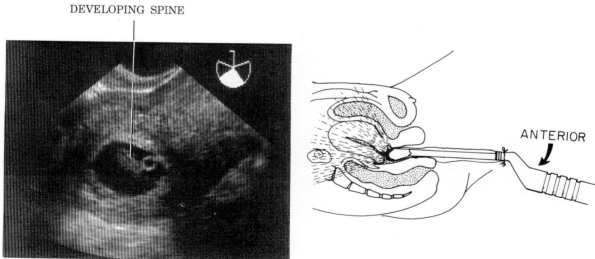

ANTERIOR

Figure 7-4B. Developing spine and spinal cord in 6-week embryo. The yolk sac is adjacent to the embryo.

Six- to Seven-Week Intrauterine Pregnancy *(Continued)*

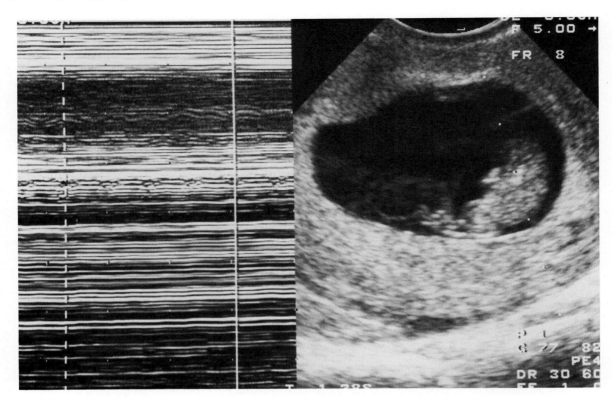

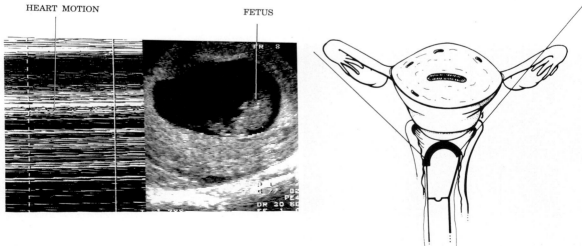

Figure 7-4C. Heart motion depicted in M-mode of a 7-week embryo.

Six- to Seven-Week Intrauterine Pregnancy *(Continued)*

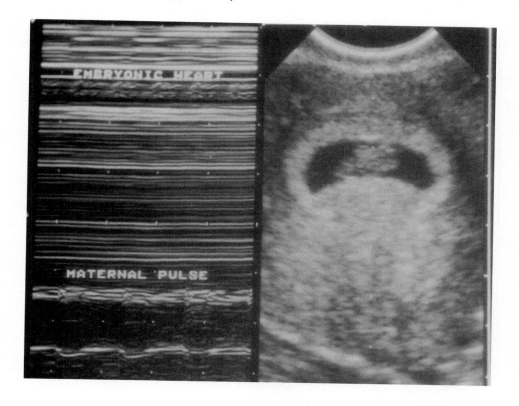

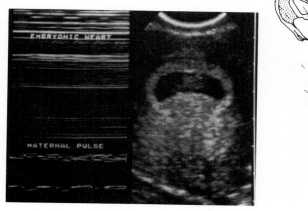

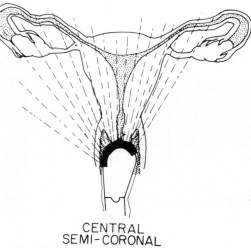

CENTRAL
SEMI-CORONAL

Figure 7-4D. Embryonic heart and maternal M-mode showing that the embryonic heart rate is approximately double the maternal heart rate.

FIGURE 7-5
Normal Variants

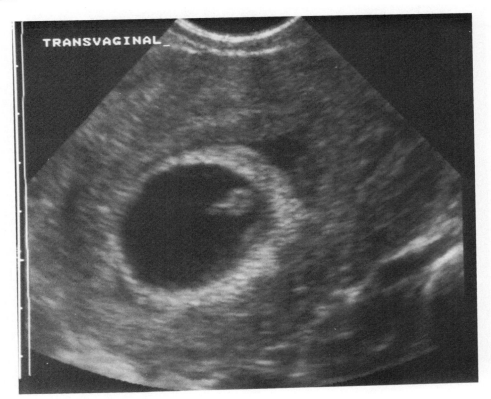

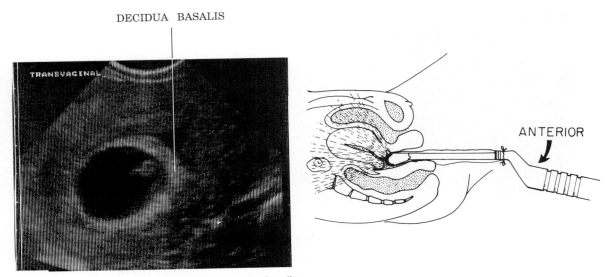

DECIDUA BASALIS

ANTERIOR

Figure 7-5A. Vascular lacunae behind the decidua basalis.

Normal Variants *(Continued)*

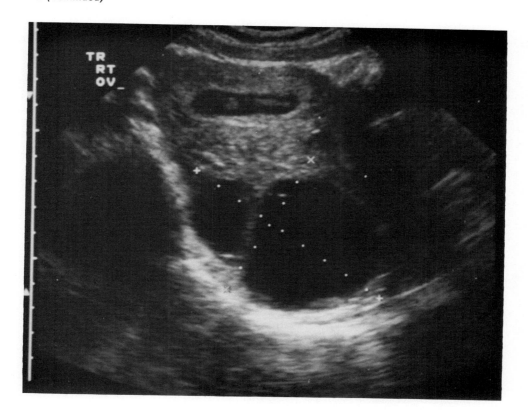

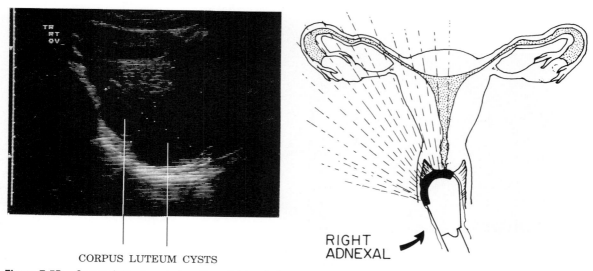

CORPUS LUTEUM CYSTS

RIGHT ADNEXAL

Figure 7-5B. Corpus luteum cysts in a 6-week intrauterine pregnancy.

Normal Variants *(Continued)*

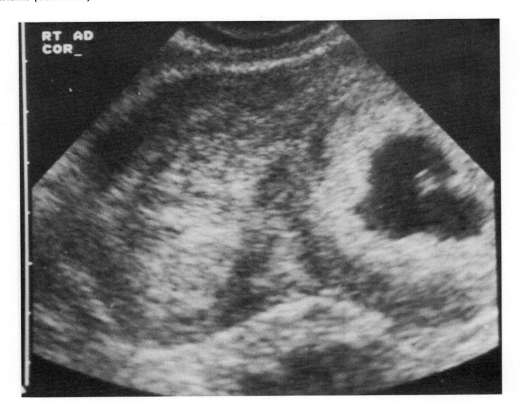

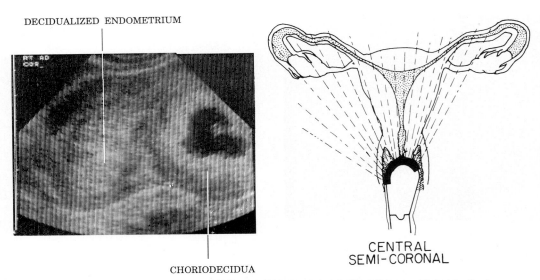

Figure 7-5C. Bicornuate uterus with 7-week intrauterine pregnancy in the left horn and decidualized endometrium in the right horn.

Normal Variants *(Continued)*

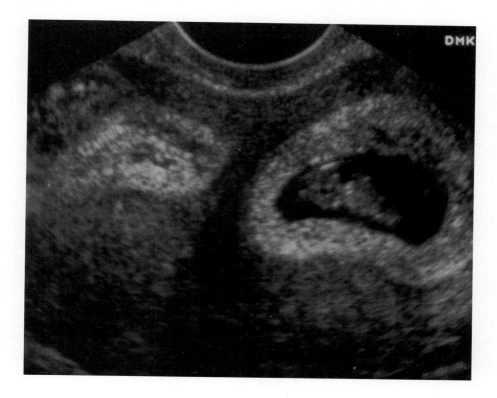

NON-GRAVID HORN

DECIDUALIZED ENDOMETRIUM

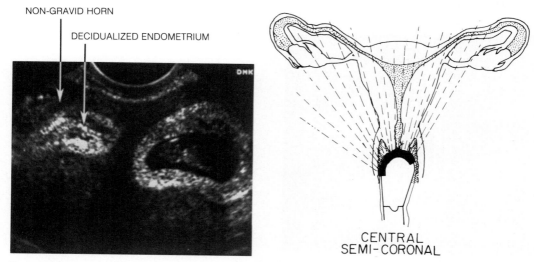

CENTRAL
SEMI-CORONAL

Figure 7-5D. Bicornuate uterus with one gravid horn and one nongravid horn with decidualized endometrium.

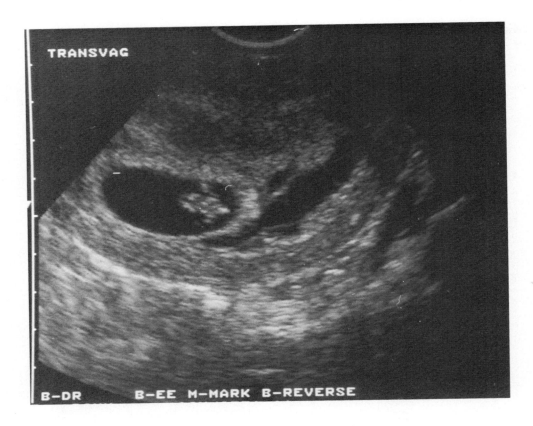

RETROCHORIONIC HEMORRHAGE

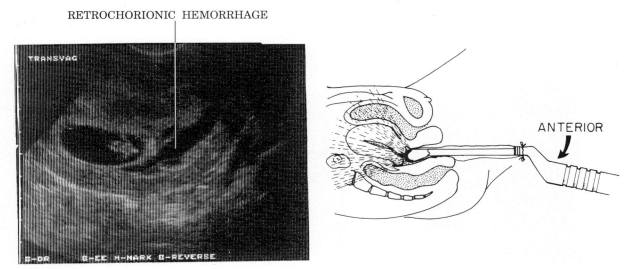

FIGURE 7-6
Retrochorionic hemorrhage appearing as hypoechoic area adjacent to the gestational sac.

FIGURE 7-7
Eight-Week Fetus

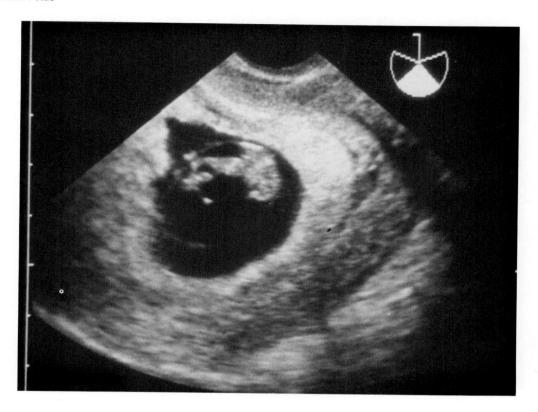

PHYSIOLOGICAL BOWEL HERNIATION

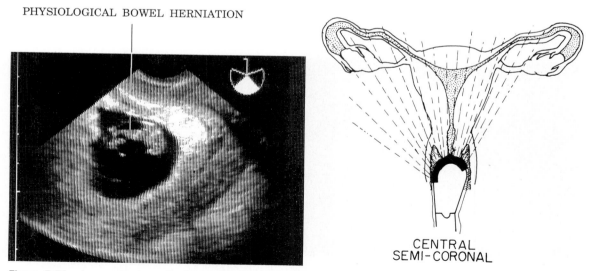

CENTRAL
SEMI-CORONAL

Figure 7-7A. Long-axis view of a fetus with physiologic bowel herniation and an allantoic cyst contiguous within the developing umbilical cord.

Eight-Week Fetus *(Continued)*

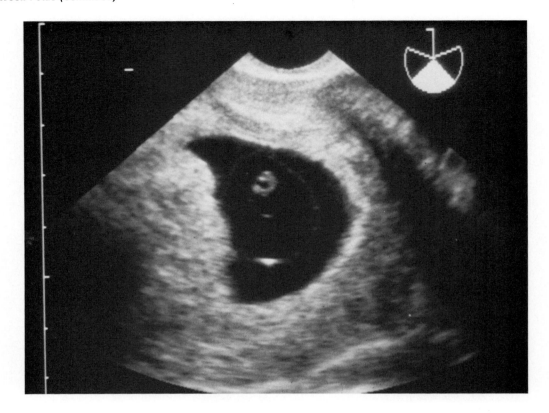

UMBILICAL CORD

ALLANTOIC CYST

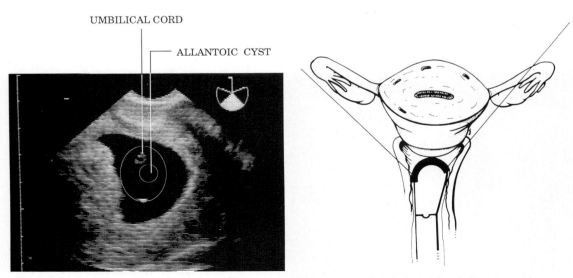

Figure 7-7B. Short-axis view of the same fetus as in Fig. 7-7A with physiologic bowel herniation and an allantoic cyst contiguous within the developing umbilical cord.

FIGURE 7-8
Rhombencephalon

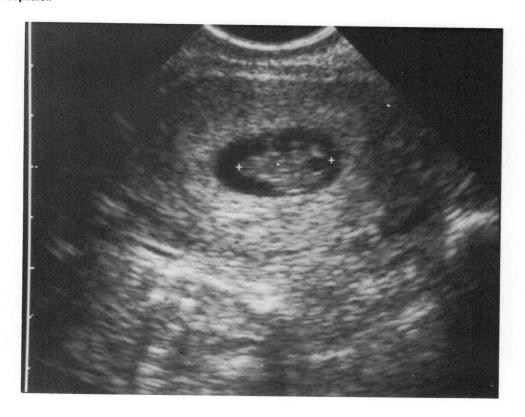

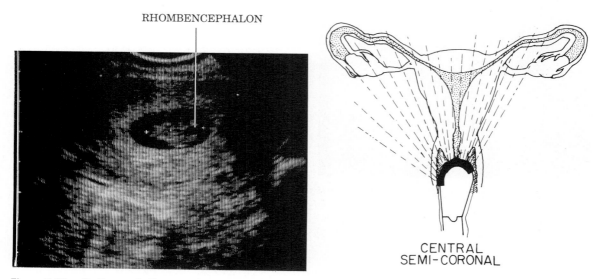

RHOMBENCEPHALON

CENTRAL
SEMI-CORONAL

Figure 7-8A. Cystic area in the posterior portion of the cranium in a 7-week embryo, representing the rhombencephalon.

Rhombencephalon *(Continued)*

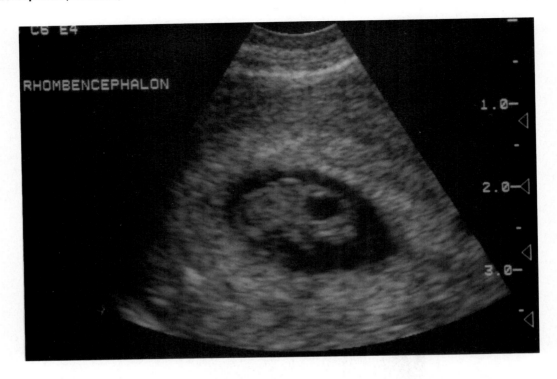

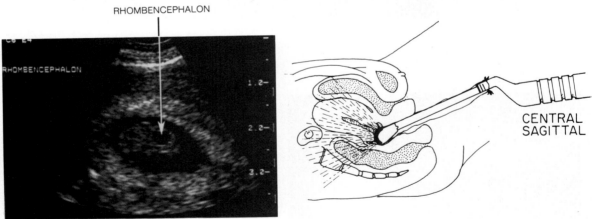

Figure 7-8B. Prominent rhombencephalon in an 8-week embryo.

Rhombencephalon *(Continued)*

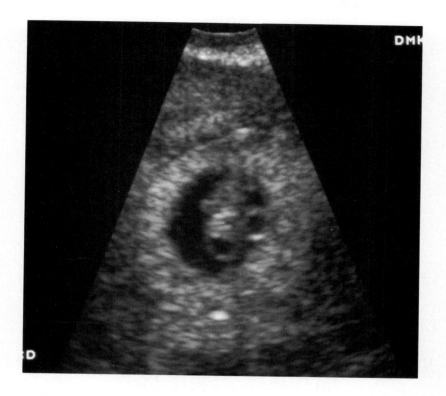

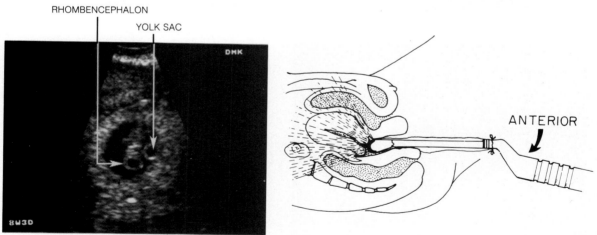

Figure 7-8C. Rhombencephalon adjacent to the yolk sac in an 8-week, 3-day pregnancy.

FIGURE 7-9
Physiologic Bowel Herniation

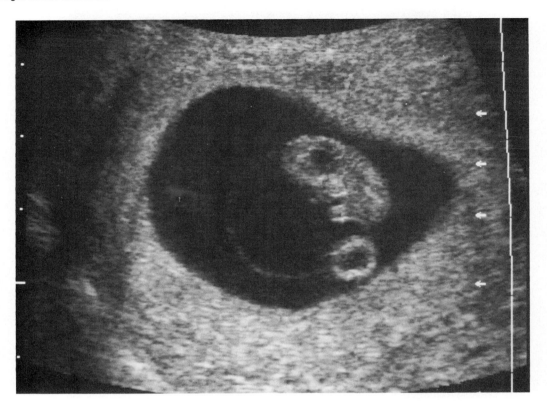

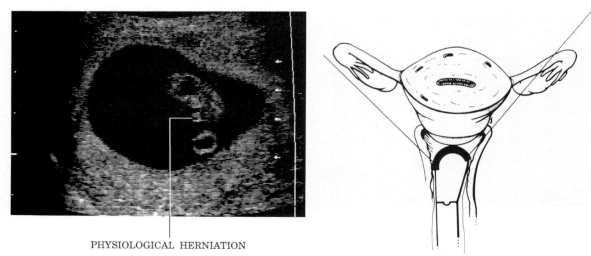

PHYSIOLOGICAL HERNIATION

Figure 7-9A. Physiologic bowel herniation into the base of the umbilical cord at 9 weeks of pregnancy.

Physiologic Bowel Herniation *(Continued)*

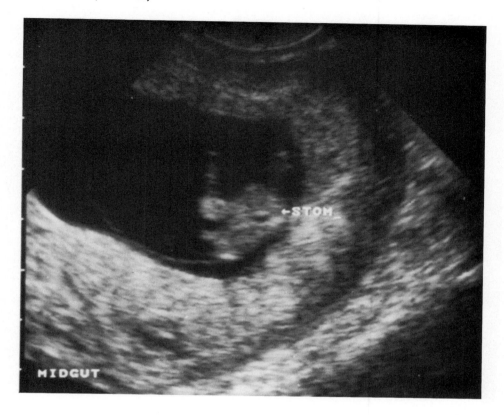

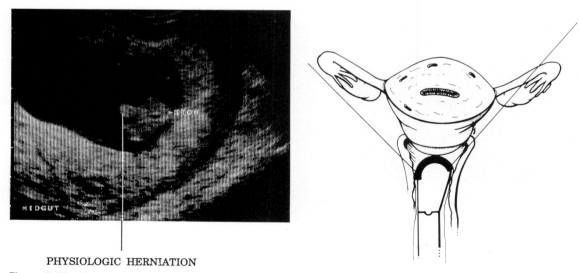

PHYSIOLOGIC HERNIATION

Figure 7-9B. More prominent herniation in a 9-week fetus. This prompted a repeat scan at 12 weeks that showed return of bowel contents into the abdomen.

Physiologic Bowel Herniation *(Continued)*

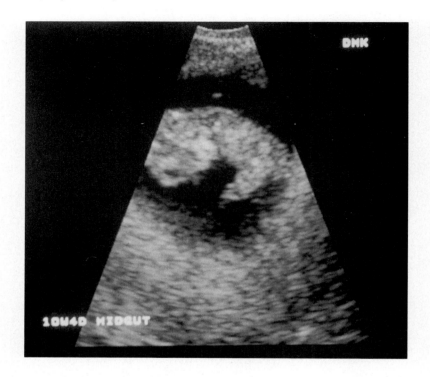

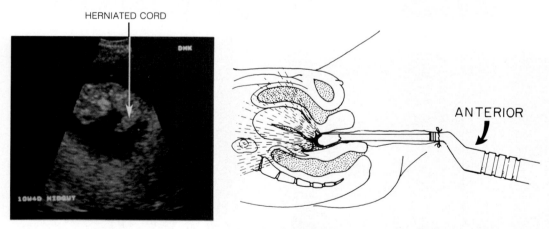

Figure 7-9C. Physiologic midgut herniation of a 10-week, 1-day fetus. This should completely regress by 11 to 12 weeks.

FIGURE 7-10
Normal 9- to 12-Week Fetus and Membranes

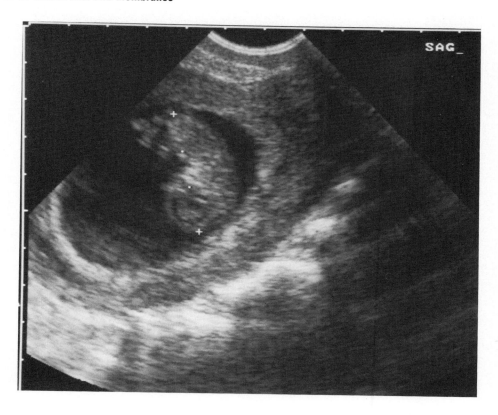

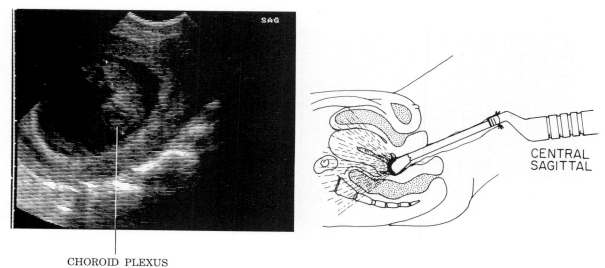

CHOROID PLEXUS

CENTRAL
SAGITTAL

Figure 7-10A. Normal lateral ventricles and choroid plexus in a 10-week fetus.

Normal 9- to 12-Week Fetus and Membranes *(Continued)*

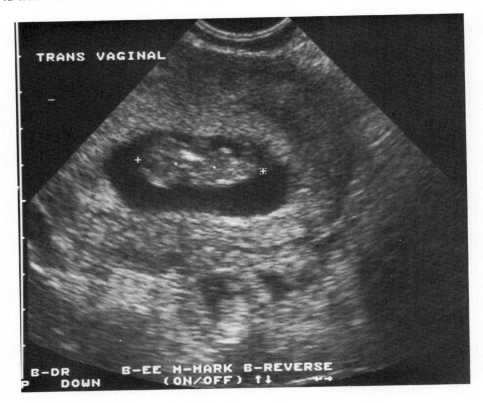

FETUS

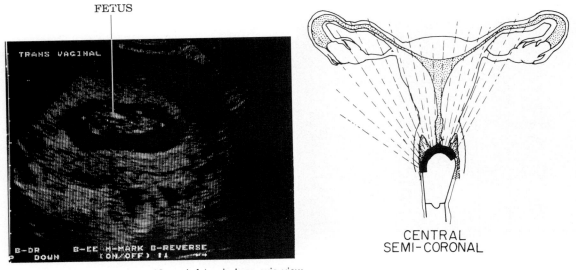

Figure 7-10B. Normal 9- to 12-week fetus in long-axis view.

Normal 9- to 12-Week Fetus and Membranes *(Continued)*

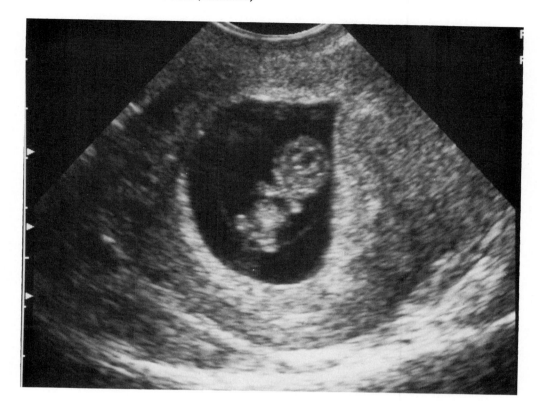

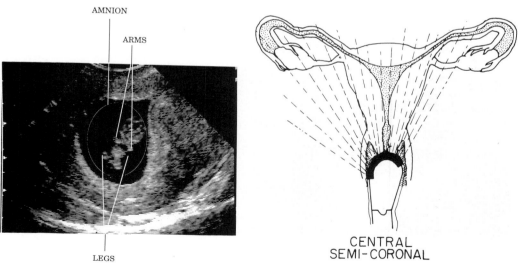

Figure 7-10C. Normal arms and legs of a 9- to 12-week fetus. The amnion is seen as a thin interface surrounding the fetus.

Normal 9- to 12-Week Fetus and Membranes *(Continued)*

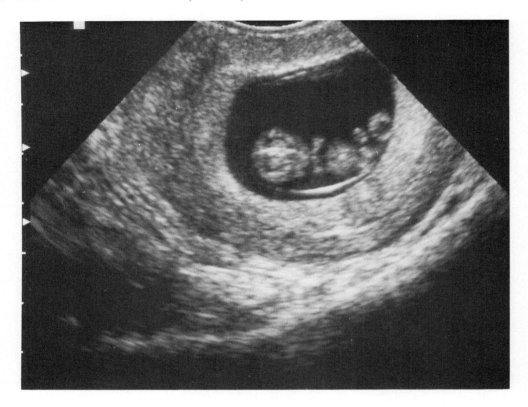

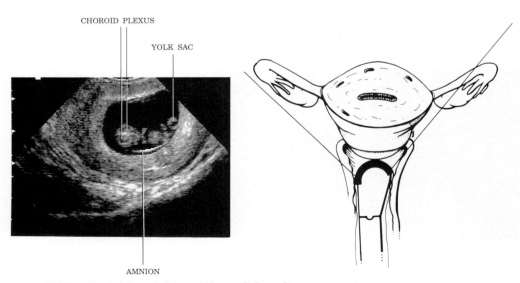

Figure 7-10D. Normal 9-week fetus within amniotic cavity.

Normal 9- to 12-Week Fetus and Membranes *(Continued)*

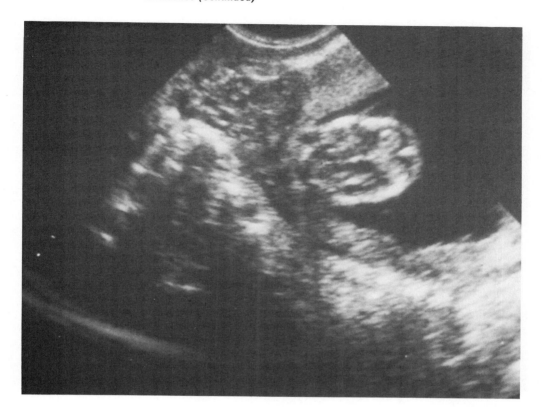

CEREBELLUM

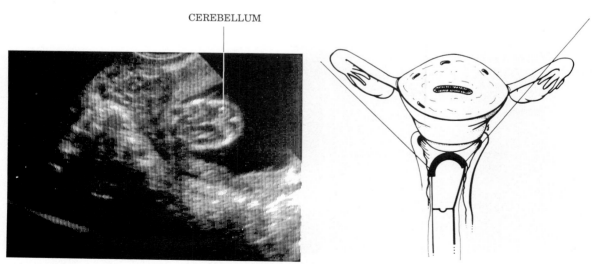

Figure 7-10E. Normal cerebellum in an 11-week fetus.

Normal 9- to 12-Week Fetus and Membranes *(Continued)*

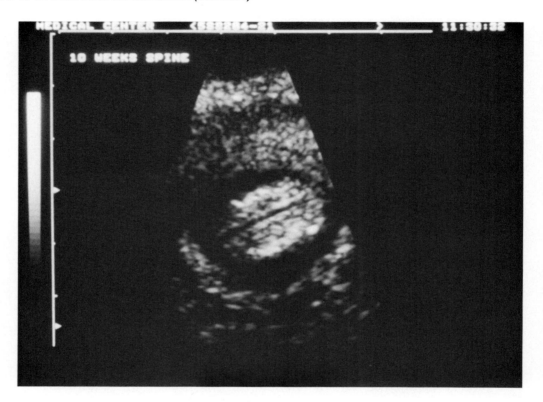

SPINE

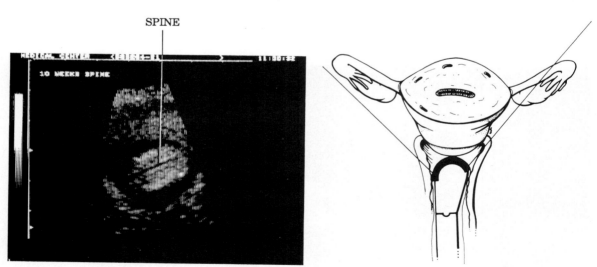

Figure 7-10F. Normal developing spine of a 10-week fetus.

Normal 9- to 12-Week Fetus and Membranes *(Continued)*

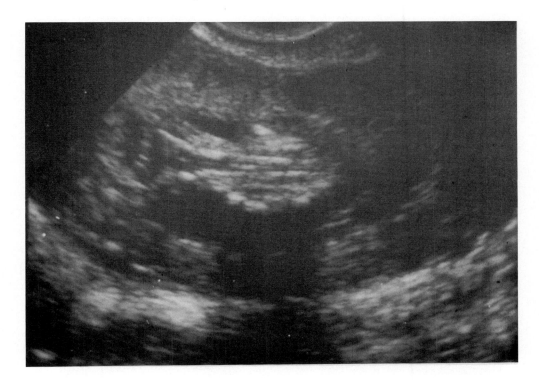

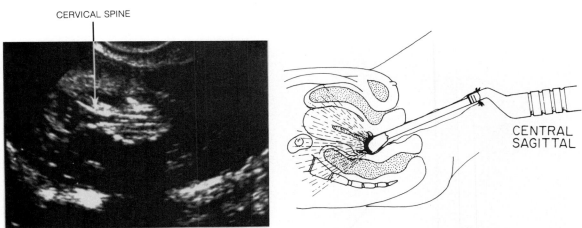

Figure 7-10G. Normal flaring of the pedicles of the cervical spine of a 12-week fetus.

Normal 9- to 12-Week Fetus and Membranes *(Continued)*

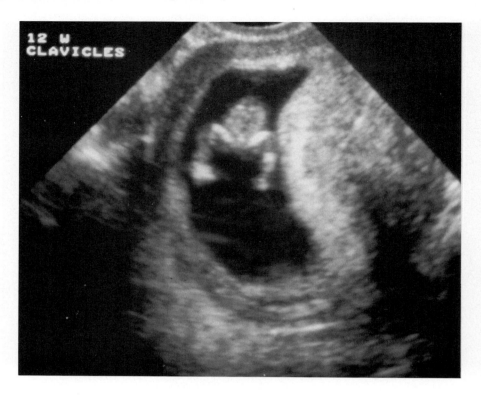

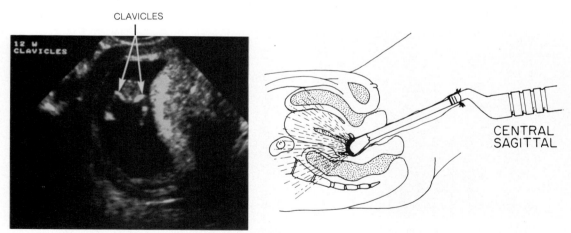

Figure 7-10H. Clavicles in a 12-week fetus. These are among the first bones to ossify.

Normal 9- to 12-Week Fetus and Membranes *(Continued)*

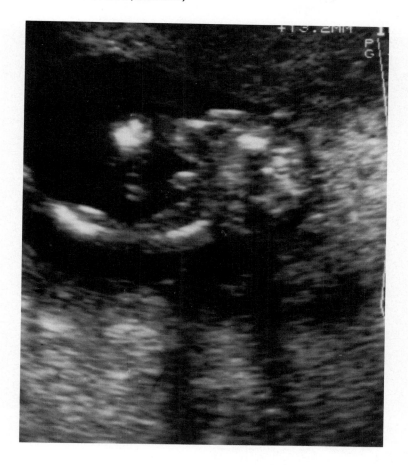

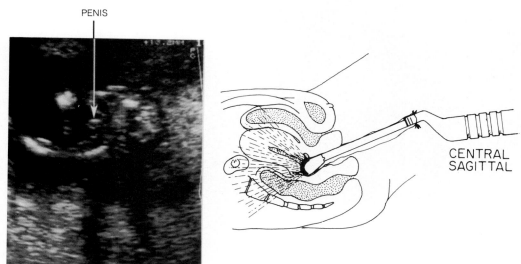

Figure 7-10I. Penis in a 12-week fetus.

FIGURE 7-11
Normal Diamniotic Twin Intrauterine Pregnancy

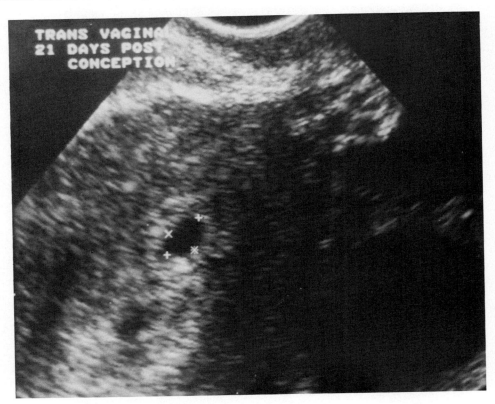

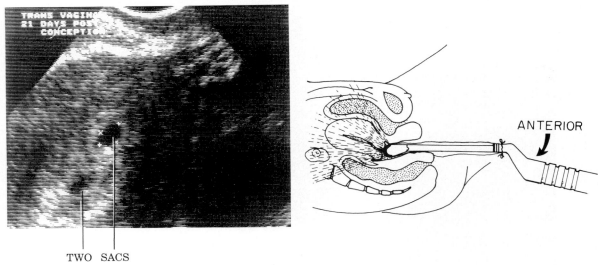

TWO SACS

Figure 7-11A. Twin separate (dizygotic) sacs at 5 weeks.

Normal Diamniotic Twin Intrauterine Pregnancy *(Continued)*

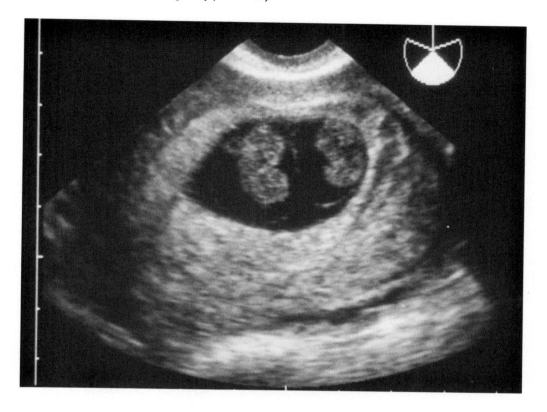

DIAMNIOTIC TWINS

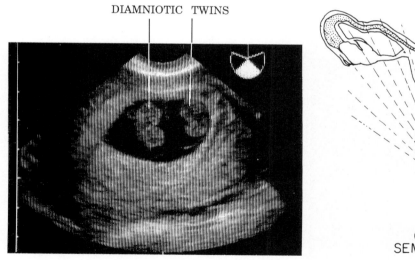

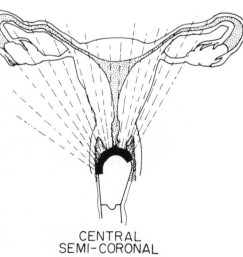

CENTRAL
SEMI-CORONAL

Figure 7-11B. Diamniotic twin intrauterine pregnancy at 7 weeks.

FIGURE 7-12
Monoamniotic Twin Intrauterine Pregnancy

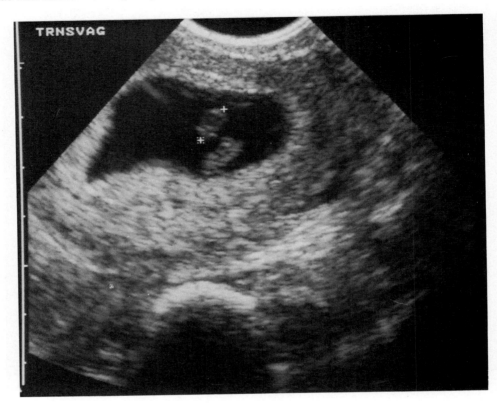

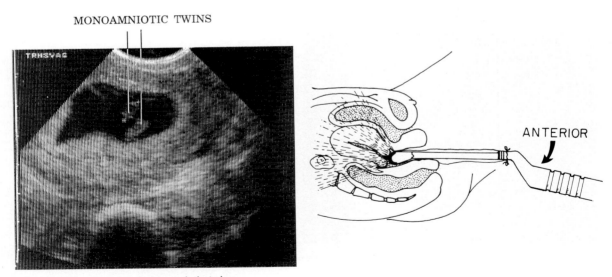

Figure 7-12A. Six-week monoamniotic twins.

Monoamniotic Twin Intrauterine Pregnancy *(Continued)*

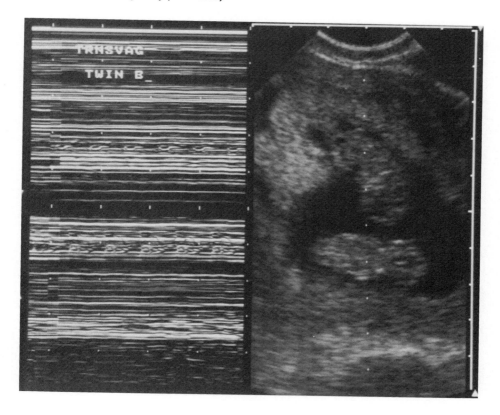

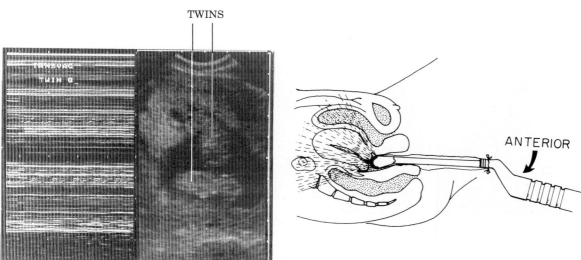

Figure 7-12B. M-mode showing viability of twins.

FIGURE 7-13
Triplets

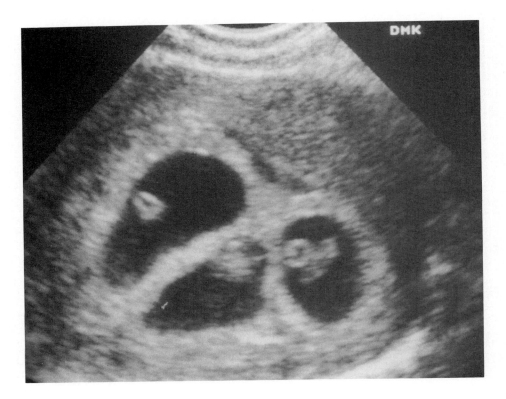

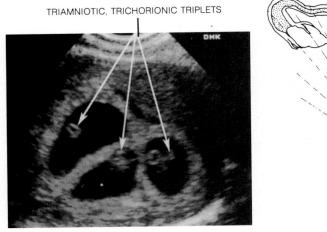

TRIAMNIOTIC, TRICHORIONIC TRIPLETS

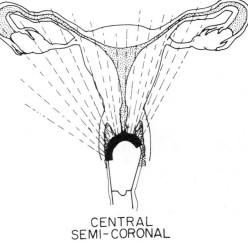

CENTRAL
SEMI-CORONAL

Figure 7-13A. Triamniotic, trichorionic triplets at 7 weeks.

Triplets *(Continued)*

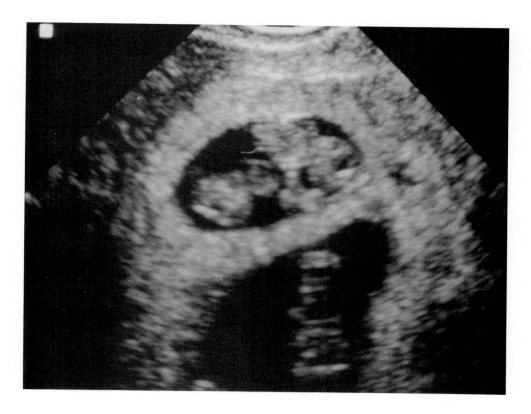

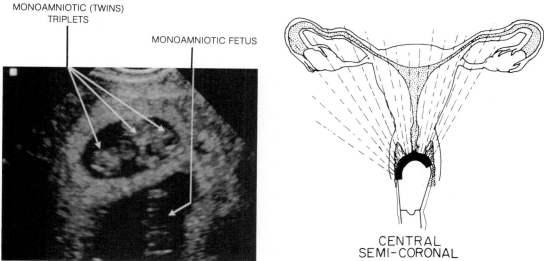

Figure 7-13B. Diamniotic, dichorionic triplet pregnancy at 8 weeks. One fetus is monoamniotic, monochorionic. The other two are monoamniotic, monochorionic.

Transvaginal Sonography: A Clinical Atlas, Second Edition,
edited by Arthur C. Fleischer and Donna M. Kepple.
J.B. Lippincott Company, Philadelphia, © 1995.

CHAPTER **8**

Complicated Early Pregnancy

Arthur C. Fleischer, MD
Donna M. Kepple, RDMS

INTRODUCTION

Transvaginal sonography (TVS) depicts detailed anatomic structures and reveals some functional aspects of early pregnancies, such as heart and body motion. TVS provides important clinical assessment of complicated pregnancies for optimal management of patients. Specifically, TVS can be used to determine the presence of an embryo/fetus, the presence of heart motion, the intactness of the choriodecidua, and the location (intrauterine or extrauterine) of the gestation. (Pennell, 1987).

EMBRYONIC/FETAL DEMISE

In a normal pregnancy, heart motion should be demonstrated by TVS in embryos that are larger than 5 mm or are 5 to 6 weeks of gestation. The heart rate is relatively slow during early heart development (70 to 90 beats per minute) but increases at approximately 8 weeks to approximately 120 beats per minute (DuBose, 1989; Hertzberg and coworkers, 1988). Some researchers have observed that embryos between 6 and 9 weeks of gestation with slow heart rates (less than 85 beats per minute) have a tendency to spontaneously abort (Laboda and coworkers, 1989). The embryo with a slow heart rate

should be reexamined in 3 to 5 days for signs of reversion to a normal heart rate.

Early embryonic demise has a variety of appearances, ranging from a gestational sac devoid of a yolk sac or embryo to a yolk sac/embryo complex without embryonic heart motion (Fig. 8-1). Embryonic demise should be suspected when there is a lack of enlargement of the embryo on serial scans coupled with deflation of the sac or yolk sac. In some cases of embryonic demise, there is deflation of the yolk sac coupled with an increase in its internal echogenicity (Fig. 8-2E). The yolk sac can become enlarged and hydropic in embryonic demise (see Fig. 8-2F).

Some have reported that the amnion is either too small or too large for the embryo, resulting in imminent fetal demise. In one study, if crown-rump length (CRL) minus amnion measures less than 0.5 mm, then the result is an indication that the amnion is too small (Bromley and coworkers, 1991). Conversely, the amnion may be too large for a compromised embryo or fetus if the amnion minus CRL is greater than 0.8 mm (Horrow, 1992).

Pregnancy should not be terminated based on a single sonographic examination that demonstrates a lack of heart motion during the embryonic stage (3 to 5 mm CRL) of development. A follow-up scan is usually indicated to confirm the lack of embryonic or fetal viability. In general, an embryo should be seen in a sac larger than 6 to 9 mm; embryonic heart motion should be seen when the sac is 10 to 14 mm in size (Bree and coworkers, 1989).

Embryonic loss is believed to occur in approximately 20% to 30% of all developing early pregnancies (Biggers, 1982). It is more likely in the patient with a history of abortion (habitual aborter) or who has had a previous fetus with chromosomal abnormality.

ABORTION

Incomplete spontaneous abortion demonstrates echogenic tissue within the uterine lumen arising from retained choriodecidua (see Fig. 8-2A through 2D). Completed abortion may be diagnosed occasionally when there is no echogenic tissue (decidualized endometrium or blood) within the uterine lumen and when the cervical os is closed (see Fig. 8-2D). The relative amount of remaining choriodecidua can be estimated using a prolate ellipsoid formula:

$$\text{vol in mL} = \text{length [cm]} \times \text{height [cm]} \\ \times \text{width [cm]} \times 0.5$$

Early trophoblastic disease demonstrates a pattern similar to retained choriodecidua, and hydropic villi are usually not present before 14 weeks (Fig. 8-3A) (Dillon and coworkers, 1993).

Patients who experience vaginal bleeding in the first trimester may demonstrate areas of retrochorionic hemorrhage on TVS. Retrochorionic hemorrhage appears as relatively hypoechoic areas behind the chorionic layer. If the hemorrhage is small and remote to the decidua basalis, the chance for pregnancy completion is better than if the hemorrhage extends behind the decidua basalis or is more than 25% of the size of the gestational sac (see Fig. 8-3B) (Sauerbrei and Pham, 1986).

ECTOPIC PREGNANCY

Transvaginal sonography is an accurate means of diagnosing an ectopic pregnancy (Nyberg and coworkers, 1987; Dashefsky and coworkers, 1988; Fleischer and coworkers, 1990). First, an intrauterine gestational sac can be excluded 1 to 2 weeks earlier with TVS than with transabdominal scanning. Second, the ability to detect the adnexal mass that represents an ectopic pregnancy is significantly enhanced with TVS.

The role of TVS in the detection of ectopic pregnancy has been elevated since the enhancement of medical treatment for ectopic pregnancies (Kurjak and coworkers, 1991; Pellerito and Taylor, 1993; Jaffe and Warsof, 1992). For example, ectopic pregnancies that demonstrate a live embryo may be treated differently than those that do not. Some ectopic pregnancies with a living embryo may be treated with direct instillation of potassium chloride, whereas pregnancies without a living embryo may be treated with methotrexate. It is possible that failure of methotrexate treatment may be predicted based on the changes in vascularity in ectopic pregnancies treated this way (Atri, 1993).

When an ectopic pregnancy is suspected but is not apparent on TVS, transvaginal color Doppler sonography can be used for further evaluation (Emerson and coworkers, 1992; Atri and coworkers, 1993; Brown, 1993). In positive cases, a vascular ring can be identified (see Chap 12).

Intraluminal fluid or blood surrounding the thin decidua reaction in an ectopic pregnancy occasionally stimulates the appearance of a malformed gestational sac. The thickened decidual reaction that surrounds intraluminal fluid or blood (pseudosac) seen in some advanced ectopic pregnancies can be distinguished from a normal gestational sac because the choriodecidual thickening at the decidua basalis is not present (Fig. 8-4). Rarely, cystic spaces can be observed within the thickened decidua, which represents decidual "cysts" (Ackerman and coworkers, 1993).

In the adnexa, TVS demonstrates the presence of a "tubal ring" consisting of an echogenic rim and a hypoechoic center (Fig. 8-5). This structure is typically seen in the adnexal regions adjacent to but separate from the uterus and ovary. An embryo may or may not be seen within the gestational sac because a large number of ectopic gestations have chromosomal abnormalities with resultant embryonic demise and they fail to develop a sonographically detectable embryo. One can usually distinguish the tubal ring from a corpus luteum because the corpus luteum is located within the displaced rim of ovarian tissue. In some patients with a centrally located corpus luteum, the TVS appearance of a tubal ring is mimicked. Some corpora lutea appear as hypoechoic masses that have broken linear interfaces within, probably representing synechiae. Most hematomas associated with ectopic pregnancy appear as solid rounded masses that displace the uterus and bowel out of the cul-de-sac. In unruptured tubal ectopic pregnancies, the tubal ring is distinct. The distended tube surrounding the tubal mass may be identified.

If rupture has occurred, the fallopian tube is enlarged, fusiform, and contains irregularly echogenic material. Intraperitoneal blood may be the result of blood oozing from the fimbriated end of the fallopian tube because of detachment of the chorionic tissue from the tubal wall (Fig. 8-6). It may also result from attempts at tubal abortion, in which the gestational sac is passed out through the fimbriated end of the tube. The intraperitoneal fluid associated with a ruptured ectopic pregnancy usually has echoes within it, reflecting a predominance of clotted blood rather than serous fluid. The low-level echoes arising from blood elements suspended within intraperitoneal fluid move in a swirling pattern with the peristaltic motion of the bowel.

Unusual types of ectopic pregnancy can be recognized with TVS. These include cornual, cervical, and ovarian ectopic pregnancies. Cornual ectopic pregnancies form eccentric to the endometrial lumen and extend to within 3 to 5 mm of the uterine serosa. Hypoechoic blood lacunae may be seen surrounding the gestation. Cervical ectopic pregnancies form proximal to the endometrial tissue and distend the cervix. They can be distinguished from cervical inclusion cysts by the relatively thick choriodecidual layer that surrounds the hypoechoic lumen (Fig. 8-7). This appearance is similar to that of choriodecidua in the process of being aborted, except cervical ectopic pregnancies are usually better defined and remote from the endometrial lumen. Ovarian ectopic pregnancies are rare. The examples that have been seen appear as hypoechoic areas within the ovary when a solid component of an embryo is present.

Abnormal multifetal pregnancies can be detected by TVS (Fig. 8-8). The number of amniotic and chorionic membranes can be assessed.

SUMMARY

Transvaginal sonography has an important role in the evaluation of a complicated early pregnancy. Specifically, incomplete abortion, embryonic demise, and ectopic pregnancy are readily diagnosed.

REFERENCES

Ackerman T, Levi C, Lyons E. Decidual cysts: Endovaginal sonographic sign of ectopic pregnancy. Radiology 1993;189:727.
Atri M. Ectopic pregnancy: Evaluation with endovaginal color Doppler flow imaging. Radiology 1993a;187:19.
Atri M, Bret PM, Tulandi T. Spontaneous resolution of ectopic pregnancy: Initial appearance and evolution at transvaginal US. Radiology 1993b;186:83.

Biggers S. In vitro fertilization and embryo transfer in human beings. N Engl J Med 1982;304:336.
Bree RL, Edwards M, Bohm-Velez M, Beyler S, Roberts J, Mendelson EB. Transvaginal sonography in the evaluation of normal early pregnancy: Correlation with hCG level. AJR 1989;153:75.
Bromley B, Harlow BL, Laboda LA, Benacerraf BR. Small sac size in the first trimester: A predictor of poor fetal outcome. Radiology 1991;178:375.
Brown DL. Diagnosis of ectopic pregnancy with endovaginal color Doppler US. Radiology 1993;4:20.
Dashefsky SM, Lyons EA, Levi CS, Lindsay DJ. Suspected ectopic pregnancy: Endovaginal and transvesical US. Radiology 1988;169:181.
Dillon EH, Case CQ, Ramos IM, Holland CK, Taylor KJW. Endovaginal US and Doppler findings after first-trimester abortion. Radiology 1993;186:87.
DuBose T. Fetal heart rates. J Ultrasound Med 1989;8:407. Letter to the Editor.
Emerson D, Cartier M, Alteri L. Diagnostic efficacy of endovaginal color Doppler flow imaging in an ectopic pregnancy screening program. Radiology 1992;183:413.
Fleischer AC, Pennell RG, McKee MS, et al. Sonographic features of ectopic pregnancies as depicted by transvaginal scanning. Radiology 1990;174:375.
Hertzberg BS, Mahony BS, Bowie JD. First trimester fetal cardiac activity: Sonographic documentation of a progressive early rise in heart rate. J Ultrasound Med 1988;7:573.
Horrow MM. Enlarged amniotic cavity: A new sonographic sign of early embryonic death. AJR 1992;158:359.
Jaffe R, Warsof SL. Color Doppler imaging in the assessment of uteroplacental blood flow in abnormal first trimester intrauterine pregnancies: An attempt to define etiologic mechanisms. J Ultrasound Med 1992;11:41.
Kurjak A, Zalud I, Schulman H. Ectopic pregnancy: Transvaginal color Doppler of trophoblastic flow in questionable adnexa. J Ultrasound Med 1991;10:685.
Laboda LA, Estroff JA, Benacerraf BR. First trimester bradycardia. J Ultrasound Med 1989;8:561.
Levi CS, Lyons EA, Lindsay DJ. Early diagnosis of nonviable pregnancy with endovaginal US. Radiology 1988;167:383.
Nyberg DA, Mack LA, Jeffrey RB, Laing FC. Endovaginal sonographic evaluation of ectopic pregnancy: A prospective study. AJR 1987;149:1181.
Pellerito JS, Taylor KJW. Ectopic pregnancy: Evaluation with endovaginal color Doppler flow imaging-response. Radiology 1993;187:21.
Pennell RG, Baltarowich OH, Kurtz AB, et al. Complicated first-trimester pregnancies: Evaluation with endovaginal US versus transabdominal technique. Radiology 1987;165:79.
Sauerbrei EE, Pham DH. Placental abruption and subchorionic hemorrhage in the first half of pregnancy: US appearance and clinical outcome. Radiology 1986;160:109.

FIGURE 8-1
Embryonic Demise

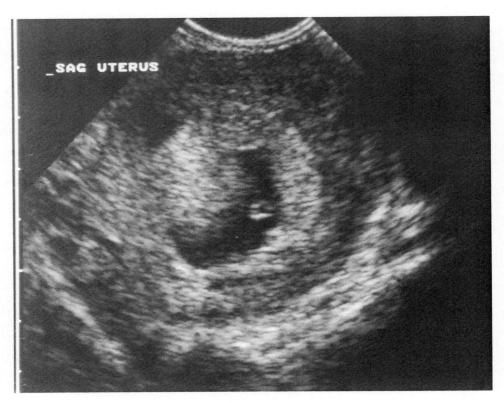

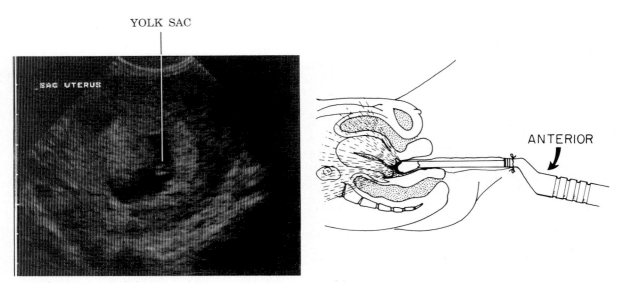

Figure 8-1A.   Initial TVS showing yolk sac within the gestational sac.

Embryonic Demise *(Continued)*

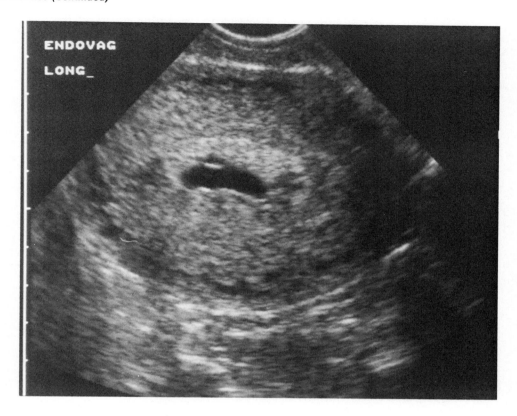

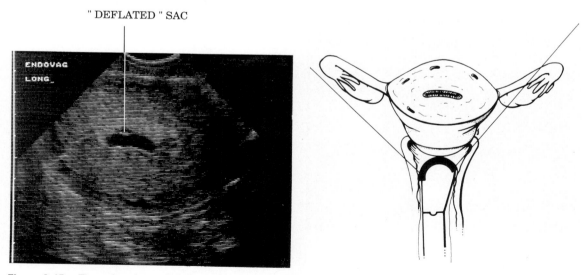

Figure 8-1B. Three days later, deflation of the gestational sac.

Embryonic Demise *(Continued)*

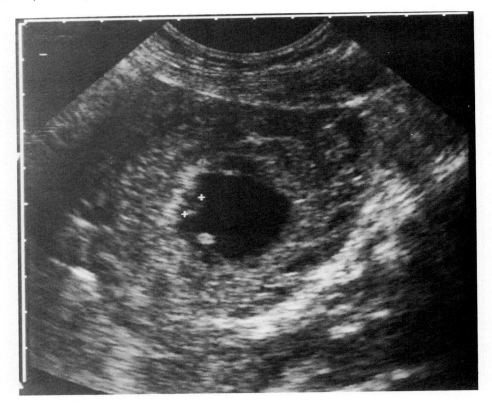

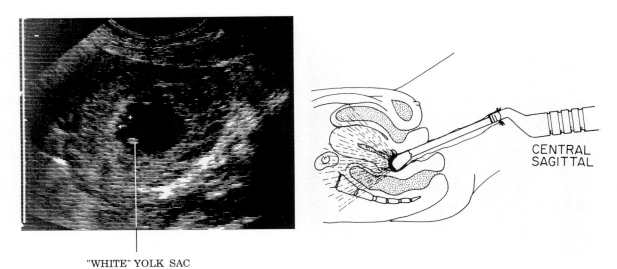

"WHITE" YOLK SAC

Figure 8-1C. Echogenic or "white" yolk sac associated with embryonic demise.

Embryonic Demise *(Continued)*

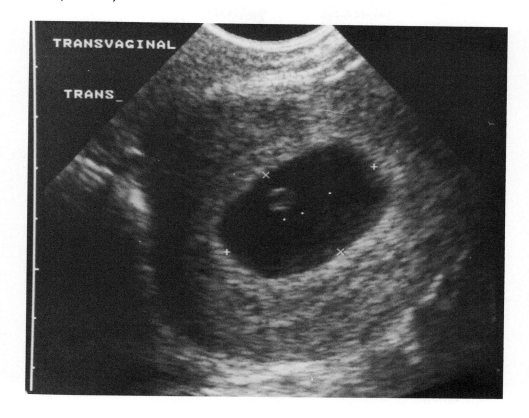

YOLK SAC

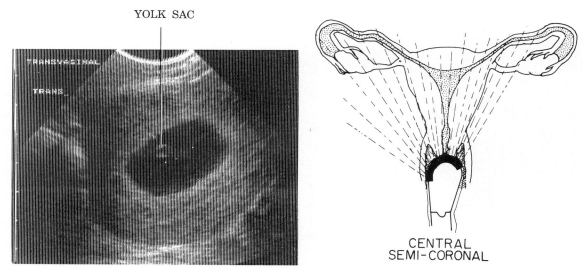

CENTRAL
SEMI-CORONAL

Figure 8-1D. Relatively large gestational sac with deflated yolk sac.

Embryonic Demise *(Continued)*

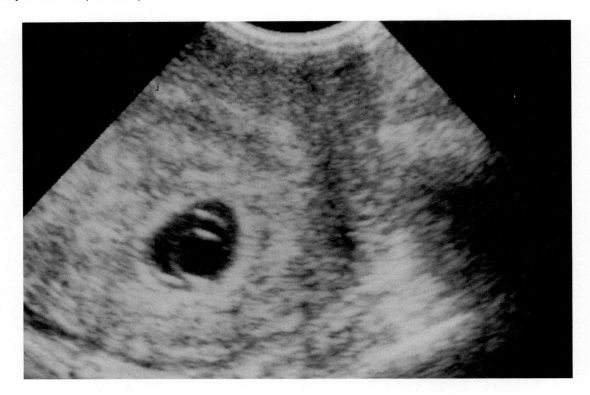

ENLARGED YOLK SAC

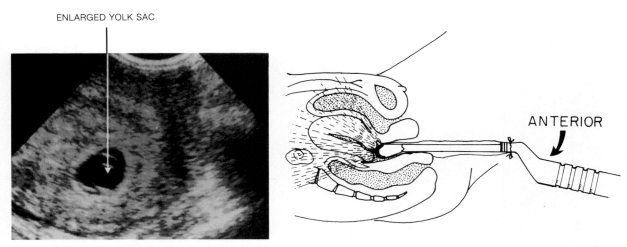

ANTERIOR

Figure 8-1E. Enlarged hydropic yolk sac, probably associated with embryonic demise.

FIGURE 8-2
Abortion

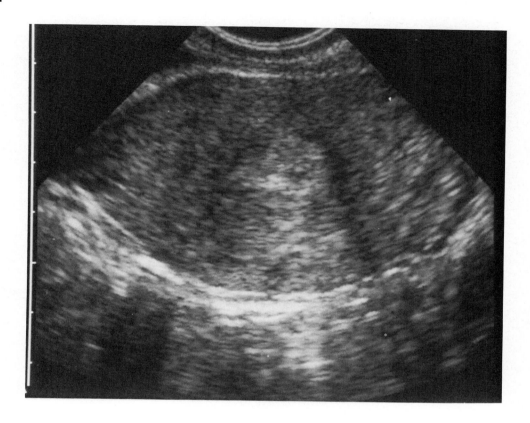

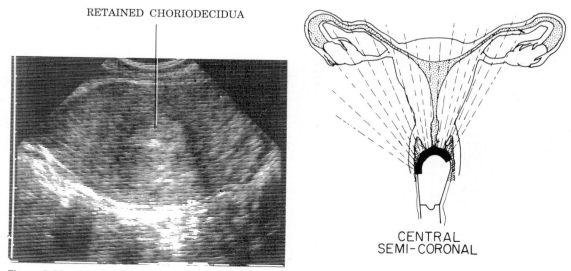

RETAINED CHORIODECIDUA

CENTRAL
SEMI-CORONAL

Figure 8-2A. Incomplete abortion appearing as echogenic tissue within the uterus.

Abortion *(Continued)*

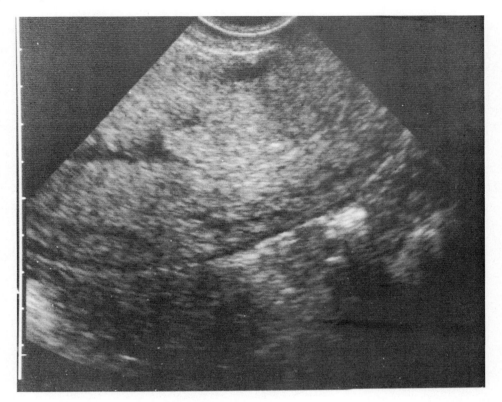

RETAINED CHORIODECIDUA

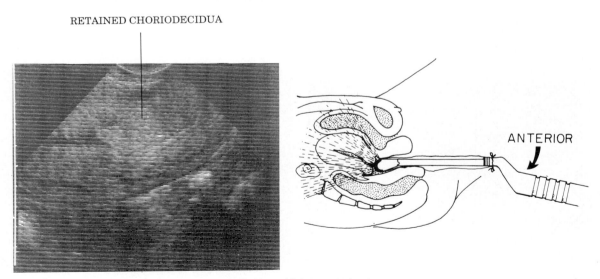

Figure 8-2B. Incomplete abortion with choriodecidua with lower uterine lumen.

Abortion *(Continued)*

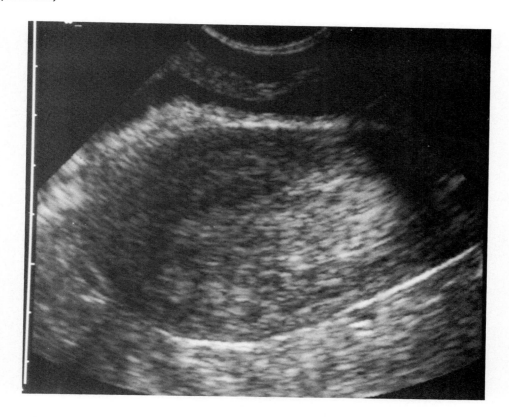

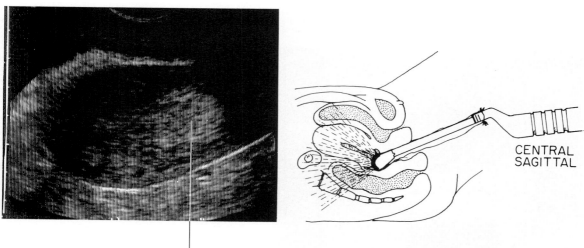

CHORIODECIDUA

Figure 8-2C. Abortion-in-progress showing choriodecidua within the lower uterine lumen.

Abortion *(Continued)*

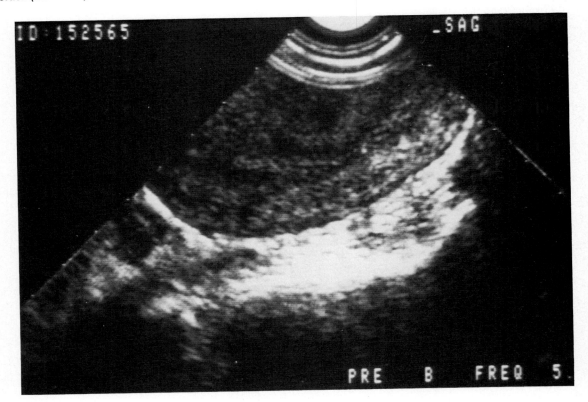

ENDOMETRIUM

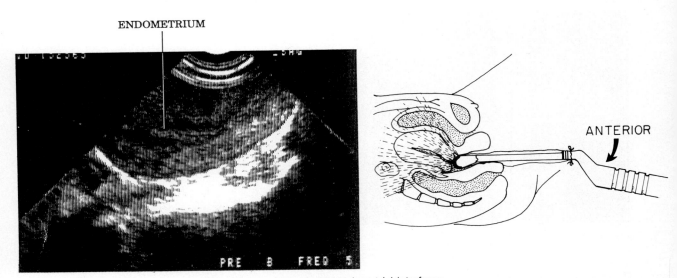

Figure 8-2D. Completed abortion showing closely opposed, thin endometrial interfaces.

Abortion *(Continued)*

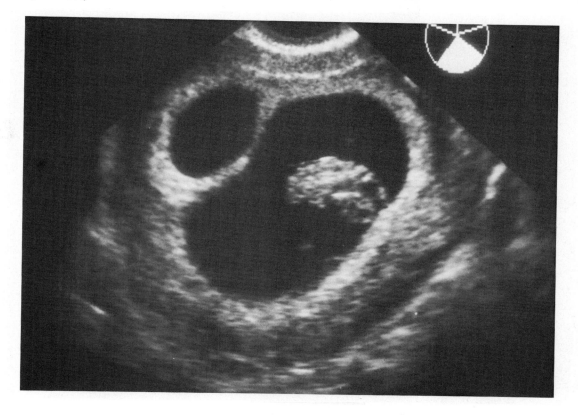

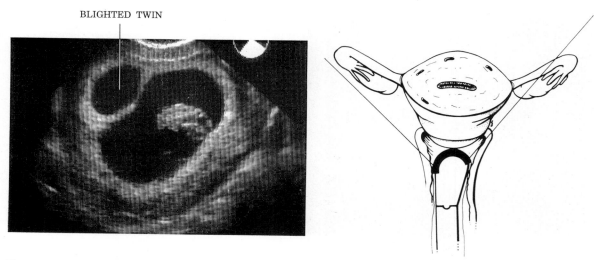

Figure 8-2E. Blighted twin in an empty sac adjacent to a living embryo within an intact gestational sac.

Abortion *(Continued)*

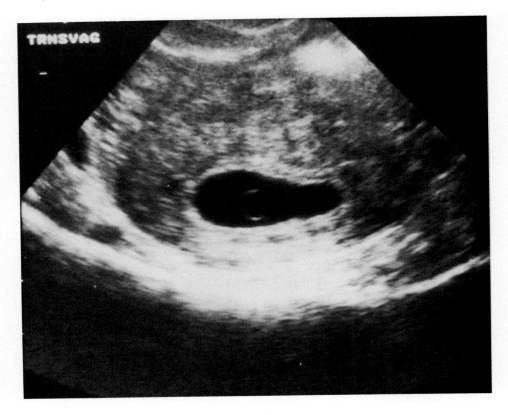

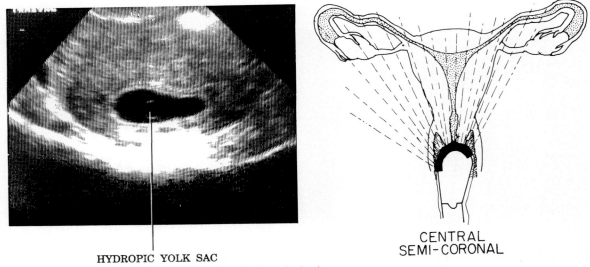

HYDROPIC YOLK SAC

CENTRAL
SEMI-CORONAL

Figure 8-2F. Hydropic yolk sac associated wtih embryonic demise.

FIGURE 8-3
Other Conditions Associated With Bleeding

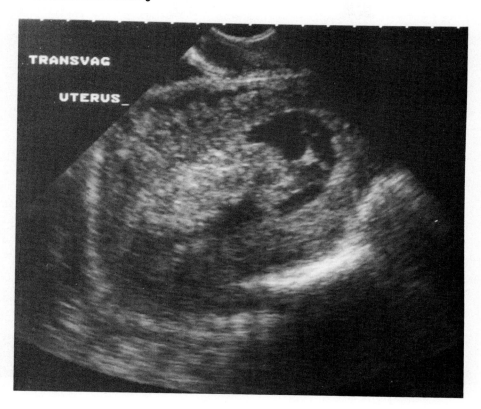

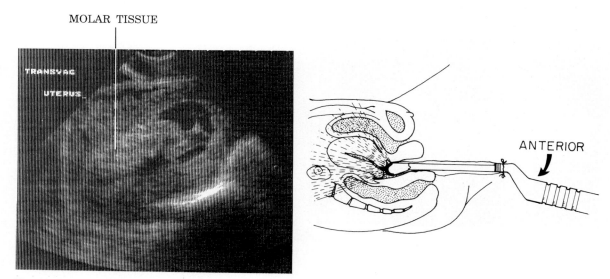

Figure 8-3A. Early molar pregnancy (gestational trophoblastic disease) simulating the appearance of an incomplete abortion.

Other Conditions Associated With Bleeding *(Continued)*

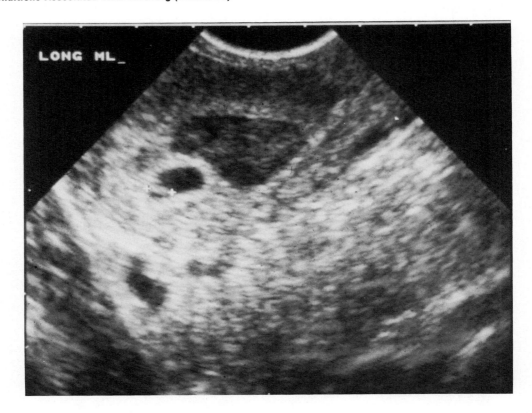

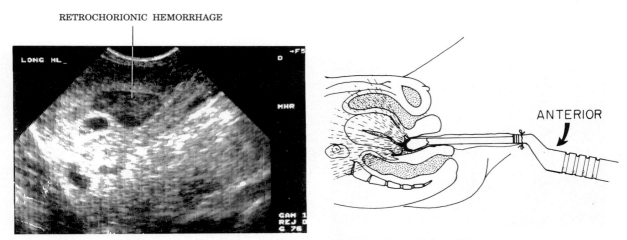

Figure 8-3B. Retrochorionic hemorrhage surrounding a gestational sac containing a living embryo.

Other Conditions Associated With Bleeding *(Continued)*

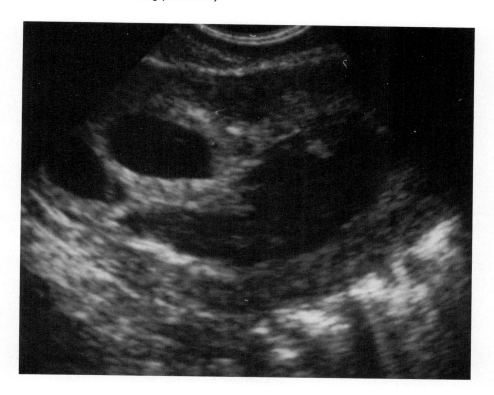

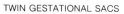
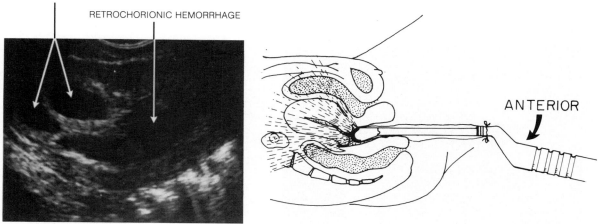

Figure 8-3C. Retrochorionic hemorrhage adjacent to two gestational sacs of a twin diamniotic, dichorionic pregnancy.

Other Conditions Associated With Bleeding *(Continued)*

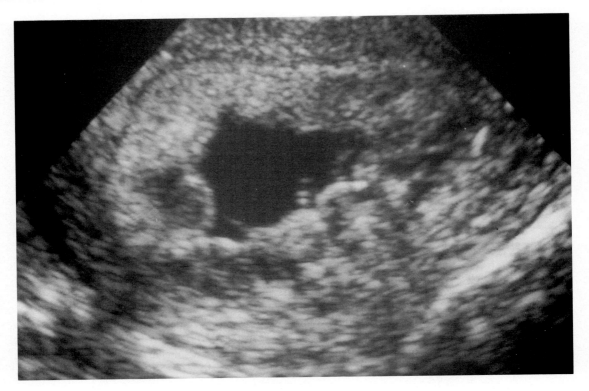

CHORIODECIDUA

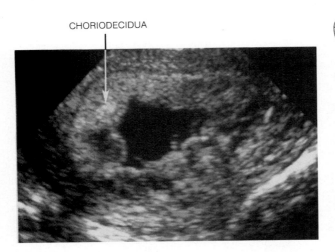

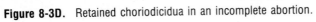

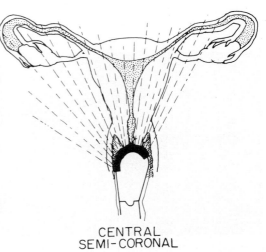

CENTRAL
SEMI-CORONAL

Figure 8-3D. Retained choriodicidua in an incomplete abortion.

FIGURE 8-4
Ectopic Pregnancy—Uterine Findings

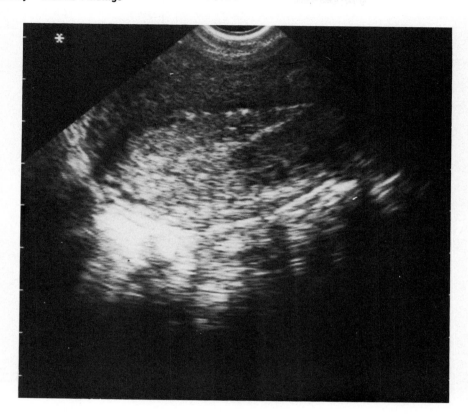

DECIDUALIZED ENDOMETRIUM

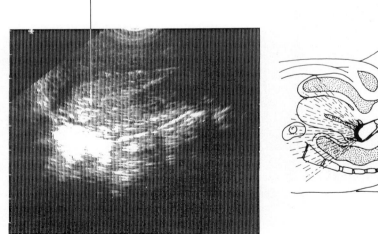

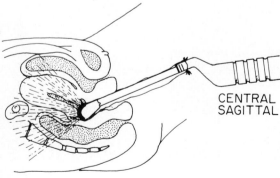

CENTRAL
SAGITTAL

Figure 8-4A. Decidual thickening.

Ectopic Pregnancy—Uterine Findings *(Continued)*

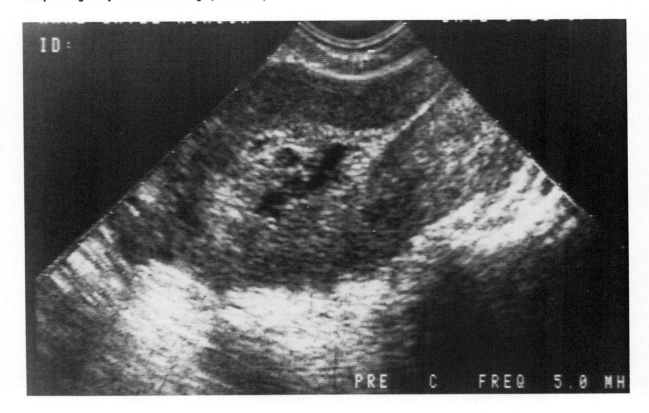

NECROTIC DECIDUA

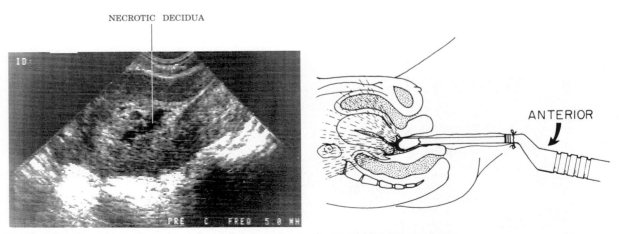

ANTERIOR

Figure 8-4B.   Necrotic decidua with several hypoechoic areas. (Courtesy of R. Pennell, M.D.)

Ectopic Pregnancy—Uterine Findings *(Continued)*

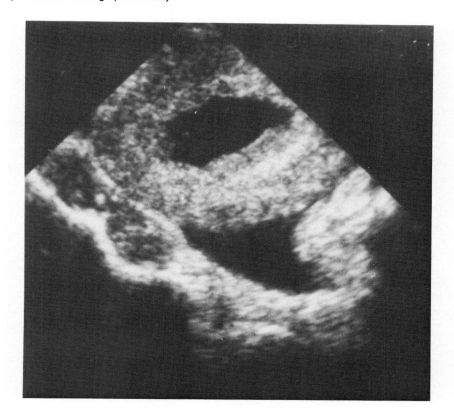

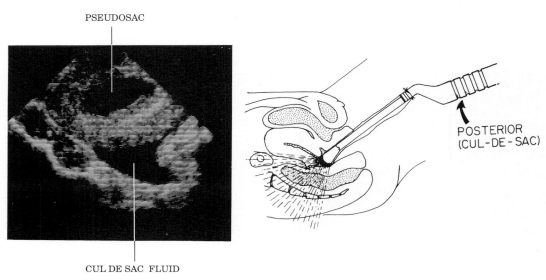

PSEUDOSAC

CUL DE SAC FLUID

POSTERIOR
(CUL-DE-SAC)

Figure 8-4C. Pseudosac showing irregular decidual thickening. There is fluid in the cul-de-sac.

Ectopic Pregnancy—Uterine Findings *(Continued)*

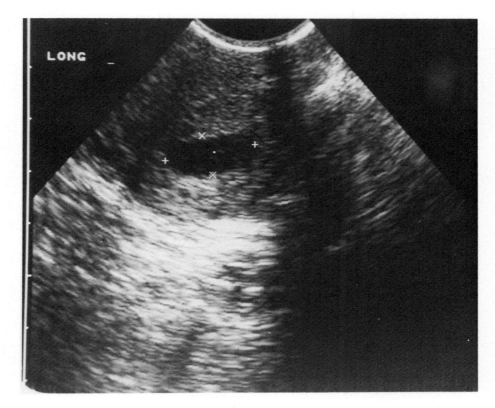

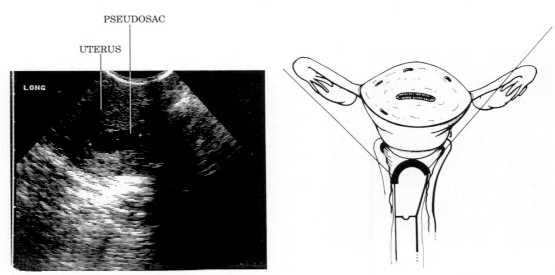

Figure 8-4D. Pseudosac resulting from fluid accumulation within the uterine lumen.

Ectopic Pregnancy—Uterine Findings *(Continued)*

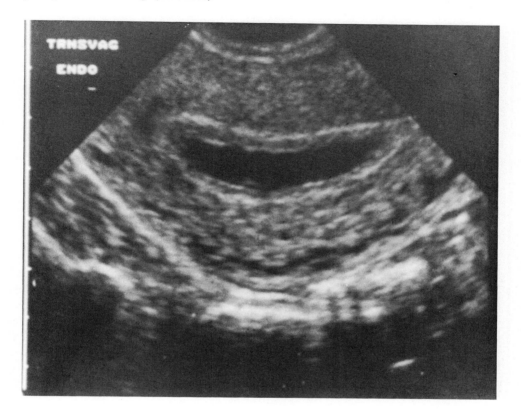

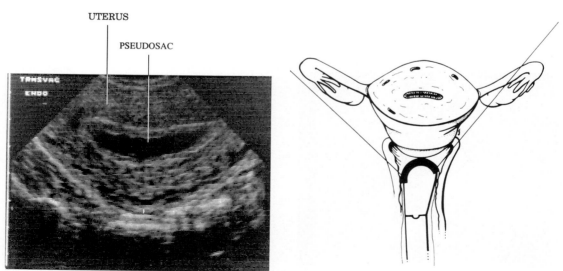

Figure 8-4E. Pseudosac with concentric and thin decidual thickening.

Ectopic Pregnancy—Uterine Findings *(Continued)*

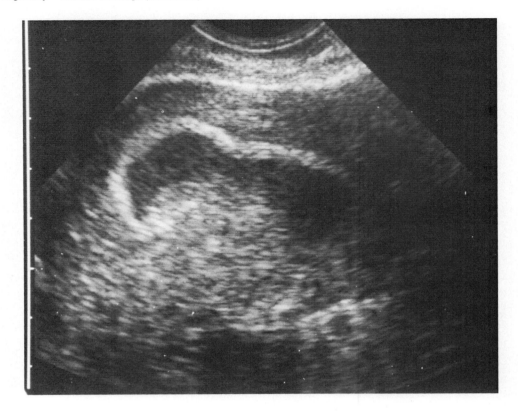

HEMORRHAGIC PSEUDOSAC

UTERUS

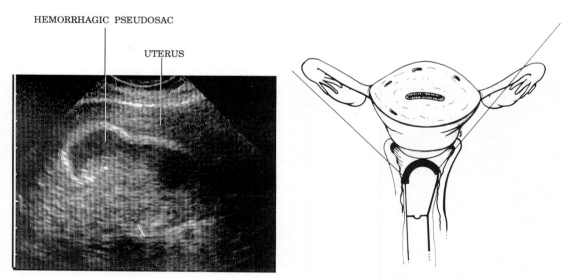

Figure 8-4F. Hemorrhage within the pseudosac of an advanced ectopic pregnancy.

FIGURE 8-5
Ectopic Pregnancy—Adnexal Findings

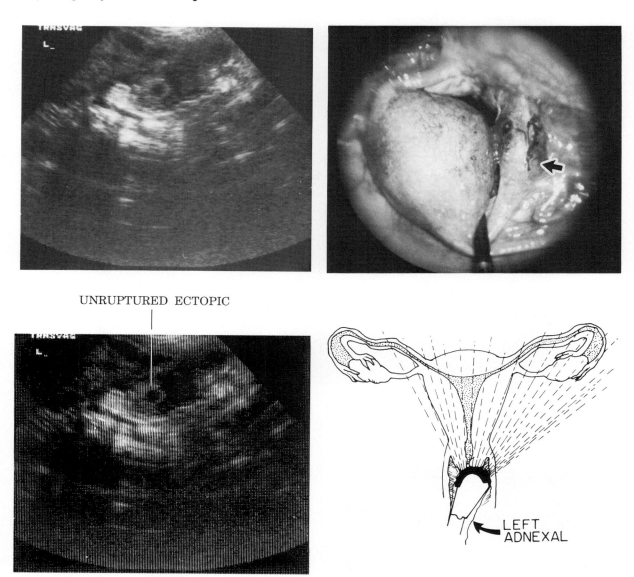

Figure 8-5A. "Tubal ring" representing an unruptured ectopic pregnancy in the left uterine tube. Laparoscopic appearance of the unruptured ectopic pregnancy is a bulge in the left fallopian tube (*arrow*). (Courtesy of C. Herbert, M.D.)

Ectopic Pregnancy—Adnexal Findings *(Continued)*

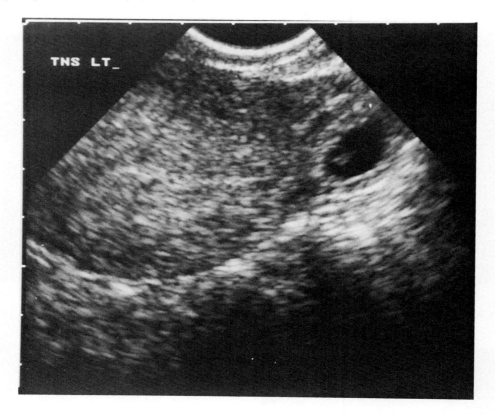

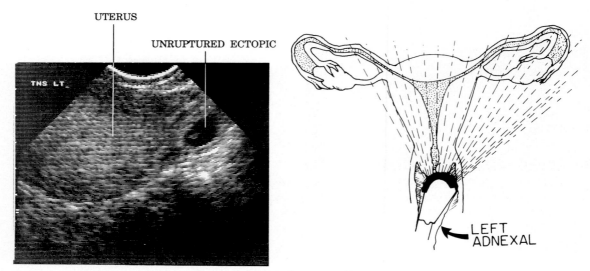

Figure 8-5B. Unruptured ectopic pregnancy adjacent to the nongravid uterus.

Ectopic Pregnancy—Adnexal Findings *(Continued)*

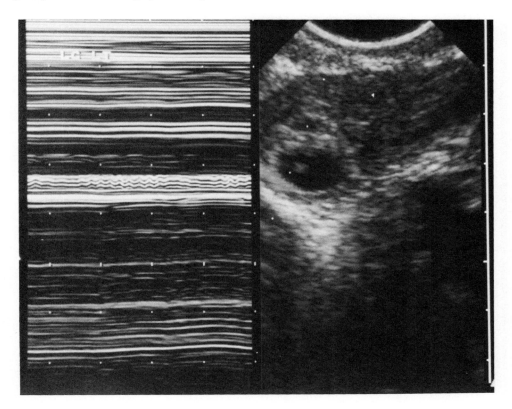

UNRUPTURED ECTOPIC

POSTERIOR
(CUL-DE-SAC)

Figure 8-5C. Unruptured ectopic pregnancy seen in Figure 8-5*B* containing embryo with heart motion as shown on M-mode.

Ectopic Pregnancy—Adnexal Findings *(Continued)*

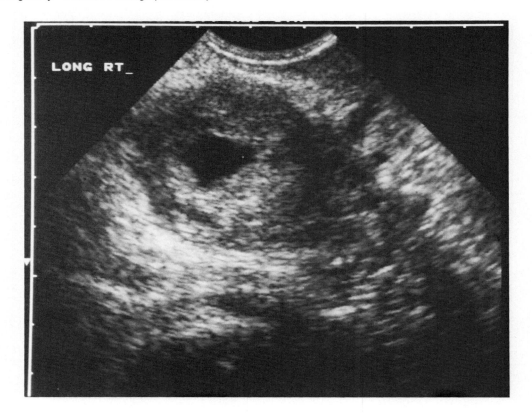

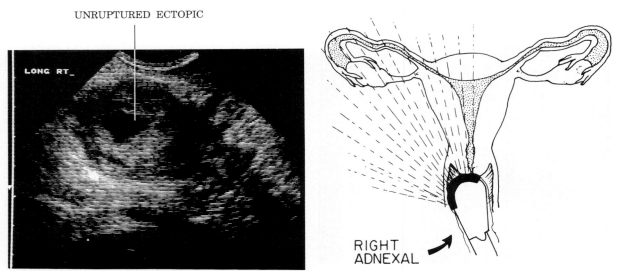

Figure 8-5D. Unruptured ectopic pregnancy surrounded by a thickened tubal wall.

Ectopic Pregnancy—Adnexal Findings *(Continued)*

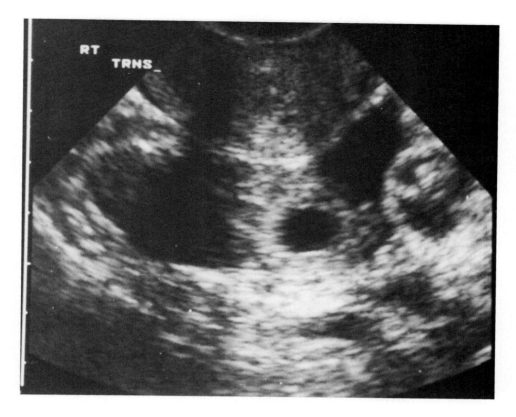

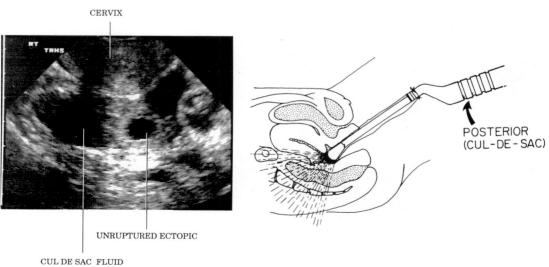

CERVIX

UNRUPTURED ECTOPIC

CUL DE SAC FLUID

POSTERIOR
(CUL-DE-SAC)

Figure 8-5E. Unruptured ectopic pregnancy appearing as a tubal mass. Cul-de-sac fluid resulted from blood oozing from the fimbriated end of the tube.

Ectopic Pregnancy—Adnexal Findings *(Continued)*

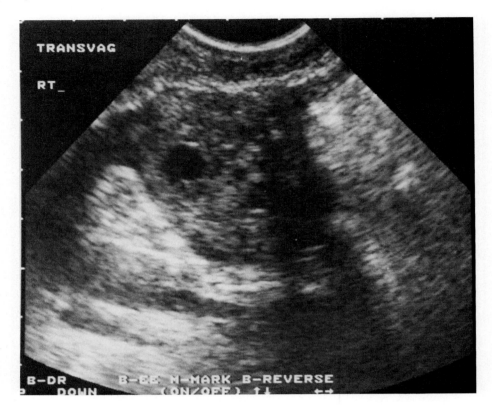

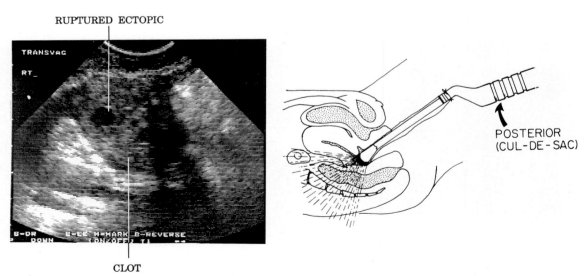

Figure 8-5F. Ruptured ectopic pregnancy resulting in hematosalpinx.

Ectopic Pregnancy—Adnexal Findings *(Continued)*

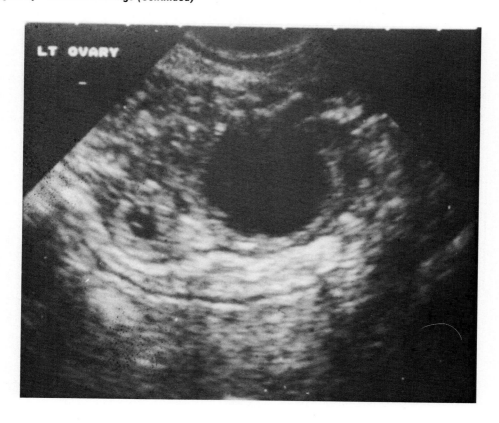

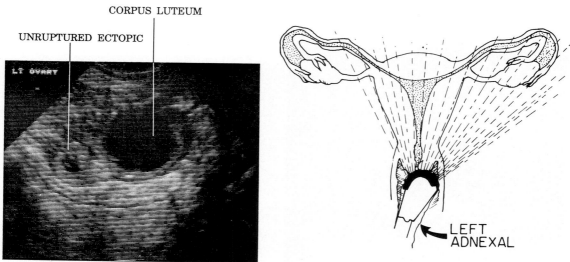

Figure 8-5G. Corpus luteum adjacent to an unruptured ectopic pregnancy.

Ectopic Pregnancy—Adnexal Findings *(Continued)*

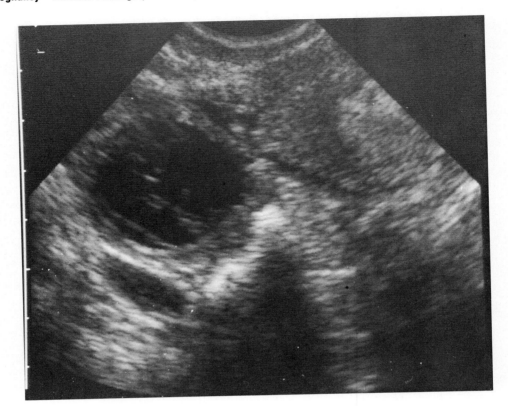

HEMORRHAGIC CORPUS LUTEUM CYST

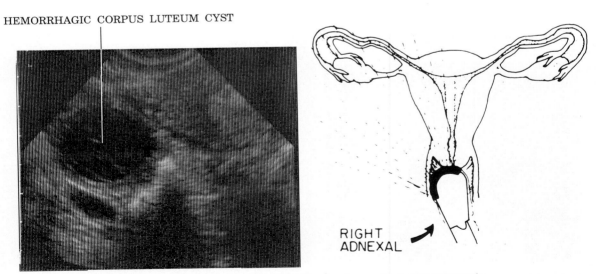

RIGHT
ADNEXAL

Figure 8-5H. Hemorrhagic corpus luteum with fine internal septae in a patient with an ectopic pregnancy.

Ectopic Pregnancy—Adnexal Findings *(Continued)*

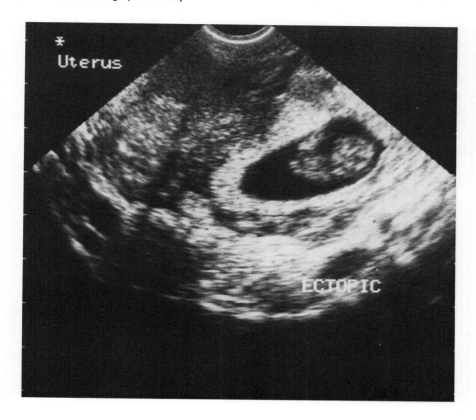

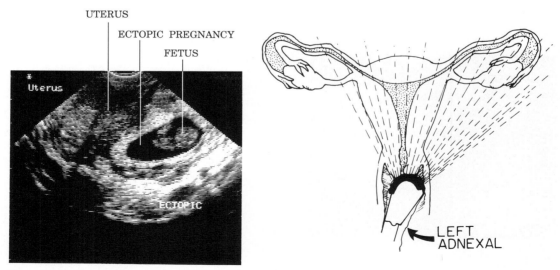

Figure 8-5I. Unruptured ectopic pregnancy with a living 8-week-old fetus.

Ectopic Pregnancy—Adnexal Findings *(Continued)*

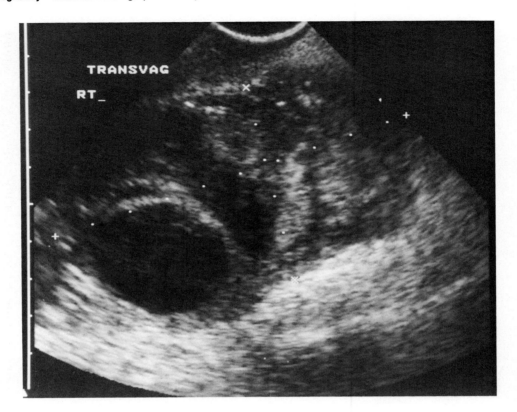

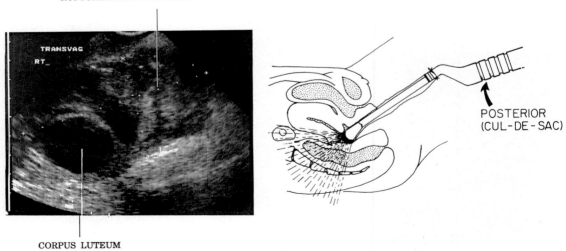

Figure 8-5J. Hematosalpinx and hematoperitoneum adjacent to a corpus luteum cyst.

FIGURE 8-6
Ectopic Pregnancy—Cul-De-Sac Findings

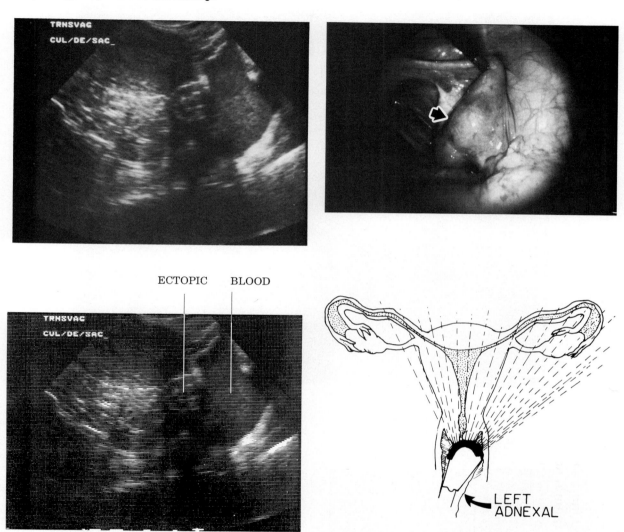

Figure 8-6A. Echogenic or "particulate" intraperitoneal fluid surrounding an unruptured ectopic pregnancy due to bleeding into the peritoneum from the fallopian tube. At laparoscopy, an unruptured ectopic pregnancy (*arrow*) was apparent within the intact left tube. (Courtesy of C. Herbert, M.D.)

Ectopic Pregnancy—Cul-De-Sac Findings *(Continued)*

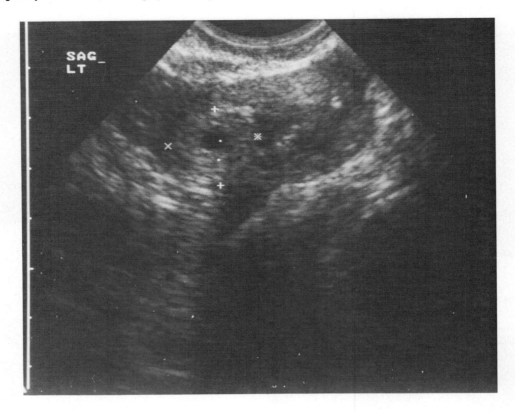

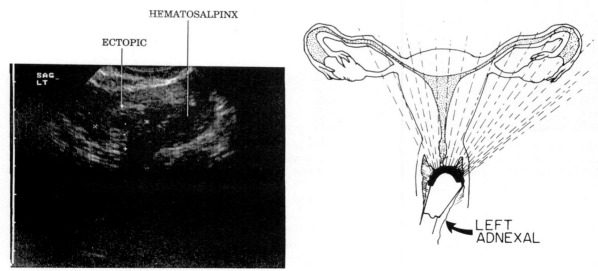

Figure 8-6B. Unruptured ectopic pregnancy within a hematosalpinx.

FIGURE 8-7
Unusual Ectopic Pregnancies

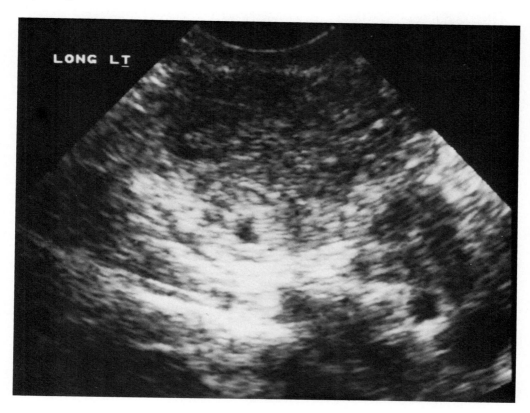

CORNUAL PREGNANCY

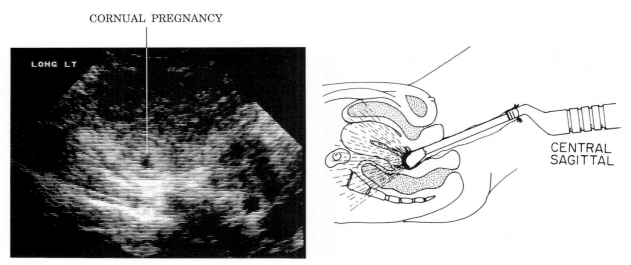

Figure 8-7A. Cornual ectopic pregnancy eccentric to the endometrial lumen and within 5 mm of the uterine serosa.

Unusual Ectopic Pregnancies *(Continued)*

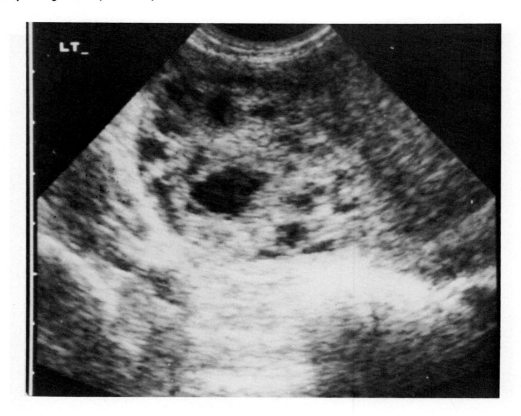

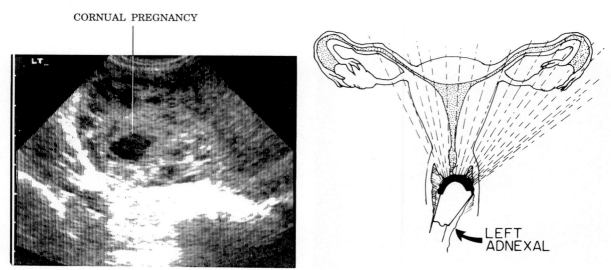

Figure 8-7B. Cornual ectopic pregnancy with thick choriodecidual ring and lacunae.

Unusual Ectopic Pregnancies *(Continued)*

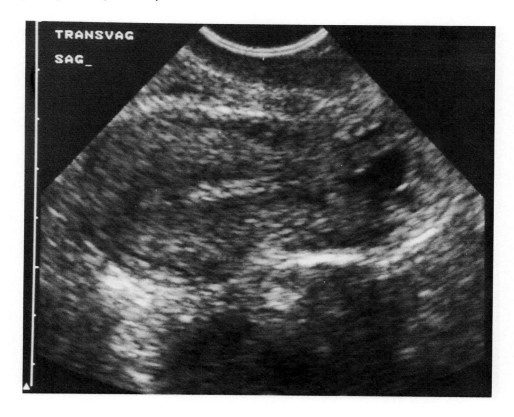

CERVICAL ECTOPIC

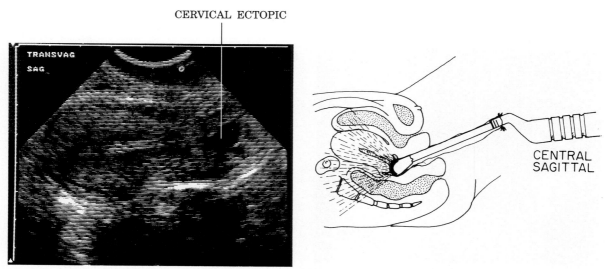

CENTRAL
SAGITTAL

Figure 8-7C. Cervical ectopic pregnancy in a patient with previous diethylstilbesterol exposure (see Figs. 12-3*A* through 12-3*D*).

Unusual Ectopic Pregnancies *(Continued)*

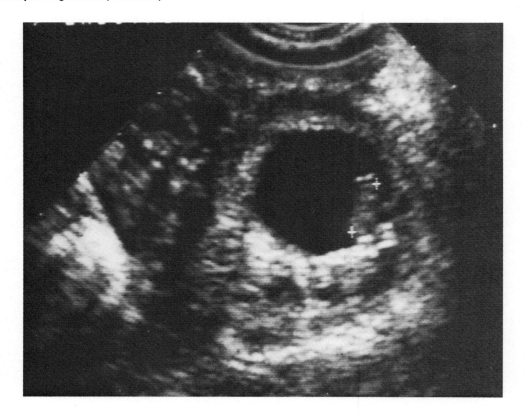

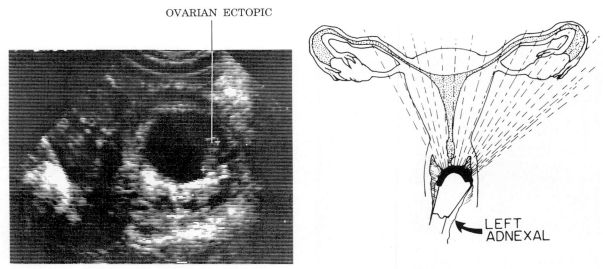

OVARIAN ECTOPIC

LEFT ADNEXAL

Figure 8-7D. Ovarian ectopic pregnancy with a dead embryo within the gestational sac. (Courtesy of L. Needleman, M.D.)

Unusual Ectopic Pregnancies *(Continued)*

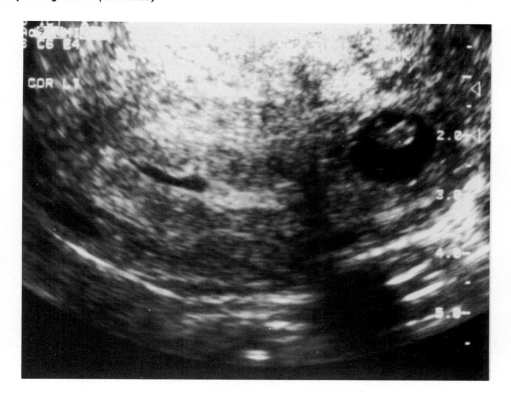

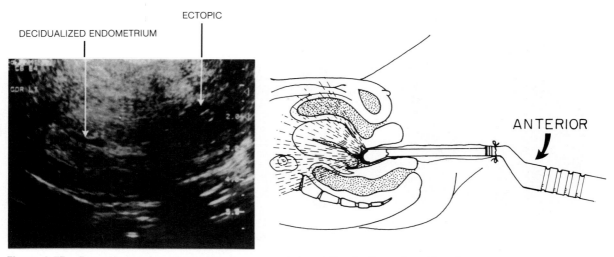

Figure 8-7E. Eccentric location of the ectopic pregnancy in relation to the endometrium in an isthmic ectopic pregnancy.

Unusual Ectopic Pregnancies *(Continued)*

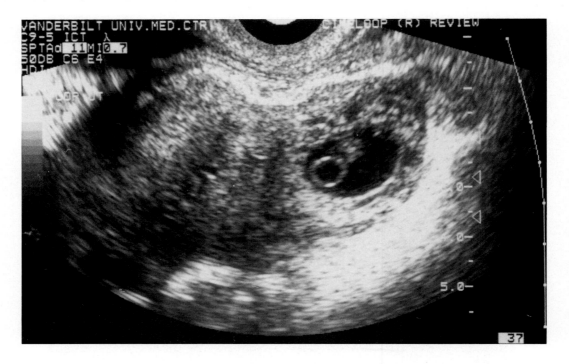

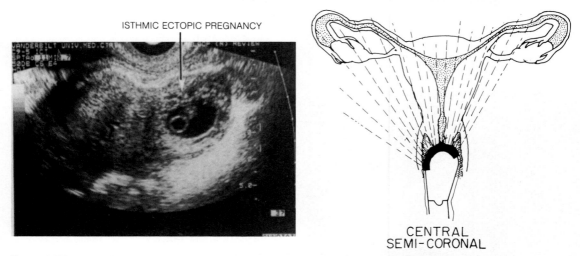

Figure 8-7F. Bulge between the isthmic ectopic pregnancy and the uterus suggests the possibility of a cornual ectopic pregnancy.

FIGURE 8-8
Multiple Pregnancies

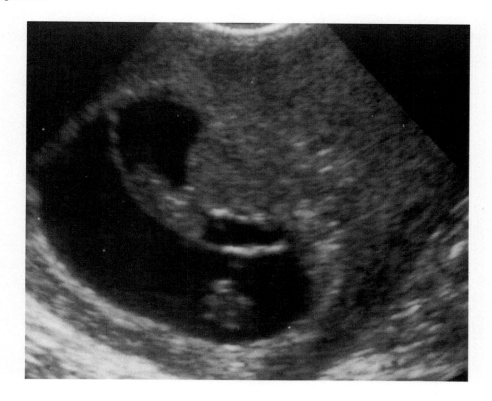

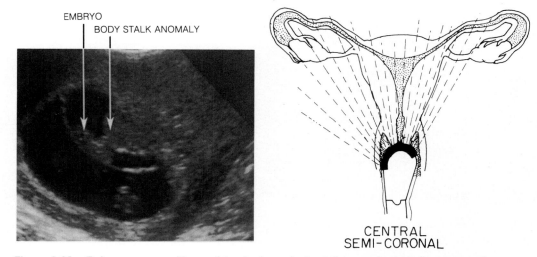

Figure 8-8A. Twin pregnancy with one fetus having a body stalk anomaly, including a severely shortened cord.

Multiple Pregnancies *(Continued)*

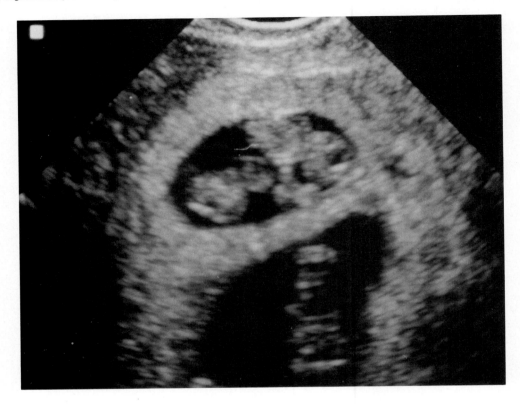

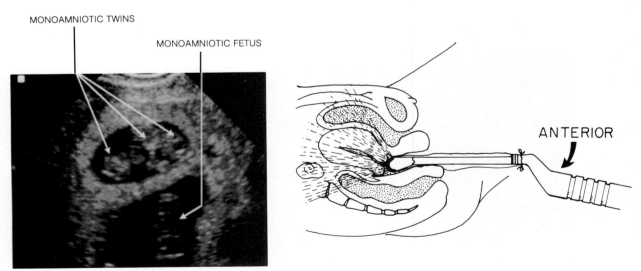

Figure 8-8B. Triplet pregnancy with two embryos contained within one amnion, and the third within its own sac.

Transvaginal Sonography: A Clinical Atlas, Second Edition,
edited by Arthur C. Fleischer and Donna M. Kepple.
J.B. Lippincott Company, Philadelphia, © 1995.

CHAPTER **9**

Lower Urinary Tract

Martin J. Quinn, MD, MRCOG

INTRODUCTION

Transvaginal sonography (TVS) is a simple, noninvasive technique for the assessment of the lower urinary tract in women with urinary incontinence (Quinn and coworkers, 1988). High-frequency endoprobes with reduced external dimensions permit objective assessment of the bladder outlet at rest and during provocative maneuvers. Women without urinary symptoms have a well-supported bladder neck that remains closed during a cough. Opening of the bladder neck with concurrent urinary leakage during a cough, establishes a diagnosis of genuine stress incontinence (Quinn and coworkers, 1989).

Symptoms and signs may not establish the underlying cause of the lower urinary tract symptoms. Urodynamic investigations have been developed to determine their cause (Enhorning, 1961; Bates and coworkers, 1970; Hilton and Stanton, 1981). Twin-channel subtraction cystometry defines detrusor instability, whereas synchronous videocystourethrography remains the reference standard for the diagnosis of genuine stress incontinence (Versi and Cardozo, 1986). These investigations are invasive and require facilities and established staff to per-

form and interpret them (Stanton, 1983). Limited sensitivity and specificity of some aspects of urodynamic testing have been demonstrated and their reproducibility has not been established because most women are unwilling to undergo repetitive testing (Richardson, 1986). For these reasons, urodynamic testing is not universally accepted, and there is divergence of opinion as to which patients may benefit from such investigations (Shah, 1984; Jarvis and coworkers, 1980; Benness, 1989; Stanton and coworkers, 1988).

Radiologic techniques, notably bead-chain cystourethrography, provide indirect images of anatomic relationships, although dynamic assessment is limited to the displacement of the bladder neck during provocative maneuvers (Green, 1962). Specific anatomic configurations have not proven to be specific for a diagnosis of genuine stress incontinence, although some typical patterns exist (Hodgkinson, 1970). Videocystourethrography includes direct imaging the bladder neck and taking synchronous pressure measurements but requires urethral catheterization and radiologic facilities (Bates and coworkers, 1970). Ultrasound has been proposed as a suitable alternative technique and abdominal, perineal, and rectal routes have been investigated (Brown and coworkers, 1985; Gordon and coworkers, 1989; Richmond and coworkers, 1986). Lack of image resolution, distortion of the anatomic field, and limited patient acceptance have restricted their development. The vaginal route ensures that the endoprobe is adjacent to the important landmarks without discomfort to the patient (Quinn and coworkers, 1988). An offset field, high operating frequency, and reduced external dimensions ensure enhanced resolution of the image without distortion of the anatomic features. In contrast to bead-chain cystourethrography, the effect of an increase in intraabdominal pressure on the continence mechanism and the presence of urinary leakage are directly visible. Each scan may be completed in 5 minutes with urethral catheterization, contrast medium, and radiologic facilities (Quinn and coworkers, 1988).

The primary requirement of a new technique is to differentiate genuine stress incontinence from detrusor instability because these are the most common urinary complaints and their treatment differs markedly (Hilton, 1987). Some researchers suggest that determining the presence or absence of genuine stress incontinence is most important because, in most cases, an accurate suprapubic operation cures both conditions (McGuire and Savastano, 1985). Comparison of the anatomic consequences of different suprapubic operations is an additional benefit of the technique because the position of the bladder neck relative to the inferior border of the symphysis pubis may be objectively assessed (Quinn and coworkers, 1989). Despite the improved success rate of suprapubic surgery, a proportion of patients have persistent or recurrent postoperative symptoms, the cause of which have not been elucidated (Hertogs and Stanton, 1985). Controlled studies will determine the precise role of transvaginal ultrasound in the management of patients with lower urinary tract symptoms.

TECHNIQUE

Successful imaging of the lower urinary tract requires equipment capable of static and dynamic assessment in both recumbent and sitting positions. A 7-MHz mechanical sector scanner with an offset field (45°), wide field angle (112°), high frame rate (20 Hz), and reduced external dimensions (maximum diameter 22 mm) is important (Bruel & Kjaer A/S, Naerum, Denmark; Fig. 9-1). These specifications ensure imaging of a sagittal section of the anterior pelvis in the plane of the symphysis pubis. The high frame ensures imaging of the continence

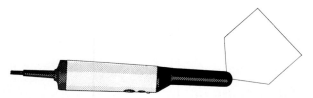

FIGURE 9-1
Endoprobe. The operating characteristics of the endoprobe are critical for imaging the lower urinary tract. The endoprobe has an operating frequency of 7 MH$_2$ and scans through an arc of 112° over a focal range of 1 to 6 cm. The field is offset and the crystal has a frame rate of 20 frames per second so that the dynamic effects of a cough on the continence mechanism may be visualized.

mechanism during a cough, and the reduced external dimensions avoid any distortion of the anatomic features. Linear array systems may provide appropriate images of the lower urinary tract, although they are most often available at frequencies of 5 MHz with a convex array and limited aperture that may prevent satisfactory resolution of the anatomic features.

Complete assessment of the patient includes history, examination, and ultrasound scanning in both supine and sitting positions. The patient should have a full bladder. After explanation of the procedure, the patient assumes a supine position on a flat couch. The endoprobe is placed in the finger of a sterile disposable glove and liberally covered with coupling gel. The first structures to be visualized are the symphysis pubis and the pubic ramus with the bladder and urethra immediately posterior to the symphysis (Figs. 9-2 and 9-3). Examination in the recumbent position permits accurate assessment of the relative positions of the bladder neck and the inferior border of the symphysis pubis in the sagittal plane. Examination in the sitting position during provocative maneuvers is a sensitive technique for the diagnosis of genuine stress incontinence (Quinn and coworkers, 1989). The patient sits on a commode with a sheet over the lower half of her body; places the endoprobe at the introitus, where it is held in the correct plane by the examiner so that the patient may sit erect to carry out a series of provocative maneuvers. Opening of the bladder neck with urinary leakage concurrent with a cough establishes a diagnosis of genuine stress incontinence (Quinn and coworkers, 1987).

Limiting features of the technique include inadequate bladder filling, moderate or severe prolapse of the anterior vaginal wall, and distortion of the

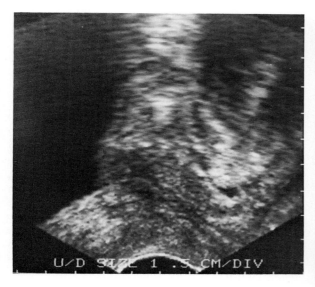
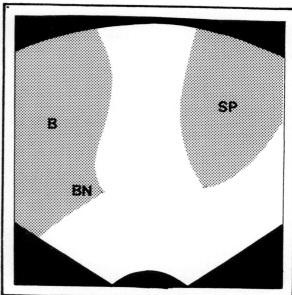

FIGURE 9-2
Bladder appearing as a hypoechoic structure because of stored urine. The course of the urethra is indicated by the acoustic characteristics of the adjacent tissues. In the midline sagittal plane, the symphysis pubis appears as a dense, uniform, hyperechoic feature. In all scans, the longitudinal axis of the patient extends from the top, left corner of the scan (head) to the bottom right corner (feet). *B*, bladder; *BN*, bladder neck; *SP*, symphysis pubis.

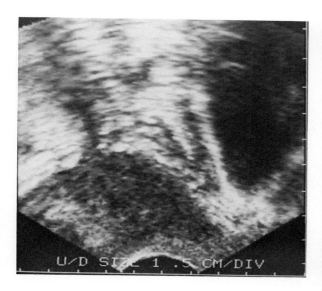
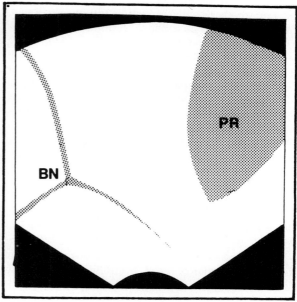

FIGURE 9-3
The same patient as in Figure 9-2 shown with the bladder emptied and the pubic bone scanned in an oblique plane. The trabecular bone of the body of the pubis appears as a hypoechoic feature in contrast to the hyperechoic, cortical bone of the inferior border. *BN*, bladder neck; *PR*, pubic ramus.

anatomic features. Minor degrees of prolapse do not restrict ultrasound scanning, although moderate or severe prolapse prevents examination with the patient in the sitting position. The precise effect of the endoprobe on adjacent tissues is visible throughout the scan and may be observed in the ultrasound monitor. Reorientation of the endoprobe avoids any perineal distorting effect. Patient acceptance is enhanced by the reduced external dimensions and the offset field that ensures the tip of the endoprobe is placed no more than 1 to 2 cm within the vagina throughout the examination.

SONOGRAPHIC ANATOMY OF THE LOWER URINARY TRACT

Sonographic appearances of the lower urinary tract depend on the differing acoustic impedances of the different structures—urine, cartilage, and trabecular and cortical bone. Additional information may be gained by introducing foreign materials with an independent acoustic pattern, such as catheters or microtransducers.

Symphysis Pubis and Pubic Ramus

The symphysis pubis is a secondary cartilaginous joint with sonographic appearances determined by the pad of cartilage connecting the pubic bones. Cartilage appears as a dense, homogeneous, echogenic pattern differentiated from the surrounding connective tissue by the shape of the inferior half of the pubis and its immobility during a cough or Valsalva maneuver (see Fig. 9-2). The symphysis is a uniform midline structure that provides a fixed reference point from which reproducible measurements may be made. The pubis adjacent to the symphysis is composed of trabecular bone with a dense inferior cortex that appears as a hypoechoic body with a hyperechoic inferior border (see Fig. 9-3).

Bladder and Urethra

The position of the bladder is identified by the hypoechoic appearance of the stored urine (see Fig. 9-2). The course of the urethra is identified by the acoustic properties of the adjacent tissues, including its vascular supply (see Figs. 9-2 and 9-3). The bladder neck may refer to a number of different structures. Radiologically, it is the junction of the bladder and the urethra; histologically, it is the junction of squamous and transitional epithelium; urodynamically, it denotes a gradient in pressure. In this chap-

ter, it represents the junction of the urethra and a comfortably full bladder (holding 200 to 500 mL of urine).

Sonographic Appearances of Urinary Incontinence

In patients without urinary symptoms, dynamic assessment of the bladder neck in the sitting position may be associated with slight posterior or inferior displacement of the bladder neck, but there is no associated leakage of urine (Quinn and coworkers, 1988; Quinn and coworkers, 1989).

Examination in the sitting position establishes the presence of genuine stress incontinence (Quinn and coworkers, 1989). Opening of the bladder neck and proximal urethra, with urinary leakage concurrent with a cough, is the hallmark of genuine stress incontinence (Fig. 9-4). This finding is sensitive and specific for the diagnosis of genuine stress incontinence, differentiating this condition from detrusor instability in a consecutive series of 124 patients (Quinn and coworkers, 1989). Patients with relatively minor symptoms of stress incontinence, for example, urinary leakage during vigorous exercise, may not demonstrate these sonographic findings because the increase in intraabdominal pressure cannot be reproduced in the testing situation. Downward displacement of the bladder neck is ob-

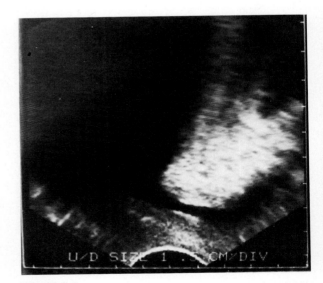

FIGURE 9-4
Genuine stress incontinence. The opening of the bladder neck and proximal urethra shown with urinary leakage concurrent with a cough.

served, although this is not specific to establish a diagnosis of genuine stress incontinence (Hodgkinson, 1970).

Opening of the bladder neck resulting from detrusor instability occurs under different circumstances and in a different fashion from that associated with genuine stress incontinence (Fig. 9-5). Detrusor instability may be provoked by a change in position, hand-washing, coughing, or bladder filling. Much of the justification or objective assessment of patients with urinary incontinence derives from the observation that a cough may provoke urinary leakage in patients with detrusor instability, which may be mistaken for genuine stress incontinence. Cough-induced instability is differentiated from urinary leakage resulting from genuine stress incontinence because there is a clear interval between increase in intraabdominal pressure and subsequent opening of the bladder neck that may be recognized during ultrasound examination.

ANATOMIC EFFECTS OF SUPRAPUBIC OPERATIONS

There are many operations used for the treatment of urinary stress incontinence. Because abdominal operations have more consistent results than vaginal procedures, different forms of suprapubic operations have become increasingly popular (Stanton and Cardozo, 1979). There are three main categories of suprapubic operation:

Retropubic urethropexy, in the form of colposuspension, or Marshall-Marchetti-Krantz procedure (Burch, 1961; Krantz, 1980)
Needle-suspension procedure (Pereyra, 1959; Raz, 1981; Stamey, 1980)
Sling operations (Hohenfellner and Petri, 1980).

All these operations prevent downward displacement of the urethrovesical junction with an increase in intra-abdominal pressure. Despite improved results, a proportion of patients have persistent or recurrent urinary symptoms after these procedures.

After colposuspension, different anatomic configurations are associated with successful and unsuccessful results. Successful outcomes are associated with absence of displacement of the bladder neck so that an increase in intraabdominal pressure does not cause displacement or opening of the bladder neck (Fig. 9-6). Unsuccessful outcomes, including early and late recurrent stress incontinence

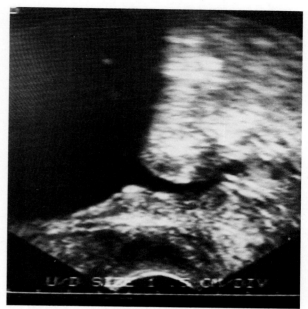

FIGURE 9-5
The opening of the bladder neck and urinary leakage associated with detrusor instability. The timing and appearance are different from those associated with urinary stress incontinence.

(RSI), frequency—urgency syndrome, and persistent urinary incontinence, are associated with four different anatomic configurations. RSI occurs in two situations. Early RSI occurs in the immediate postoperative period and results from primary failure of the supporting sutures. Any increase in intraabdominal pressure leads to downward displacement and opening of the bladder neck with a cough. Late RSI in the early postmenopausal years may occur after an apparently successful operation some years before menopause. Examination of the patient shows that, although the sutures are intact, there is sufficient loss of support to allow urinary leakage with a cough. Inaccurate placement of the supporting sutures relative to the bladder neck may be associated with either persistent incontinence or persistent postoperative frequency–urgency (Figs. 9-7 and 9-8). If the sutures are placed adjacent to the vaginal vault, securing them to the iliopectineal ligament causes indentation of the bladder base by the vaginal shelf (see Fig. 9-7). There is no elevation of the bladder neck, and stress incontinence persists. Placing the sutures between the vaginal vault and the bladder neck leads to indentation of trigone by the vaginal shelf (see Fig. 9-8), persistent symptoms

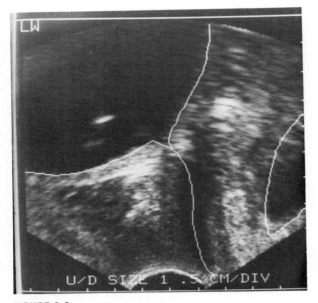

FIGURE 9-6
Successful colposuspension. The bladder neck is elevated to
a new position behind the symphysis pubis. Nonabsorbable
suture material in the vaginal fornices and the iliopectineal
ligament appear as a hyperechoic feature. The symphysis pubis, bladder floor, neck, and urethra are outlined. An increase
in intra-abdominal pressure is not associated with downward
displacement of the urethrovesical junction.

of frequency–urgency, and de novo appearance of
detrusor instability (Jarvis, 1981; Langer and coworkers, 1988). A well-executed suprapubic operation cures most patients with combined symptoms
of stress incontinence and detrusor instability. Inaccurate placement of the supporting sutures raises a

vaginal shelf beneath the trigone that may be associated with the postoperative development of detrusor instability (Quinn and coworkers, 1989; Jarvis,
1981; Langer and coworkers, 1988).

Successful outcomes after needle-suspension
operations are associated with anatomic appearances similar to those of colposuspension in which
the bladder neck is elevated and there is no downward displacement with a cough or Valsalva maneuver (Figs. 9-9 and 9-10). They have been associated with a significant incidence of early RSI in the
immediate postoperative period. This results from
ipsilateral or bilateral failure of the supporting sutures and recurrent stress incontinence.

SUMMARY

Transvaginal sonography is a simple, noninvasive
technique for the objective assessment of the lower
urinary tract in patients with urinary incontinence.
In contrast to other radiologic techniques, TVS produces direct dynamic images of the effects of provocative maneuvers on the continence mechanism
without urethral catheterization and exposure to
x-rays. Equipment specifications are important in
providing high-resolution images without distortion of the anatomic features. These include an operating frequency of 7 MHz, an offset field, reduced
external dimensions, and a high frame rate. Examination in the sitting position is a sensitive and specific technique for the diagnosis of genuine stress
incontinence. Examination in the recumbent position permits accurate determination of the position

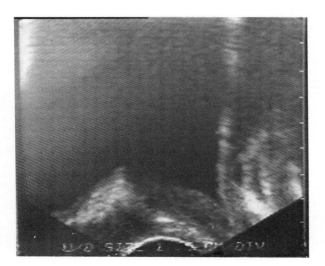

FIGURE 9-7
Persistent stress incontinence after colposuspension. The supporting sutures have been placed closer to the vaginal vault
than the bladder neck, with the result that there is no support
of the bladder neck and the vaginal shelf indents the bladder
base.

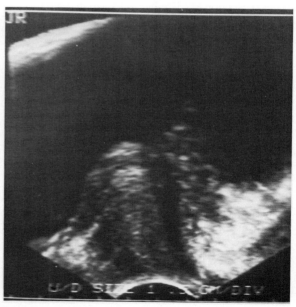

FIGURE 9-8
Frequency–urgency syndrome after colposuspension. The vaginal shelf is beneath the trigone rather than at the level of the bladder neck.

of the bladder neck relative to the inferior border of the symphysis pubis. Persistent or recurrent postoperative symptoms after suprapubic surgery are associated with a variety of anatomic configurations caused by inaccurate surgical technique. Preexisting detrusor instability combined with stress incontinence may be cured by an accurate suprapubic operation, where an inaccurate operation may cause postoperative detrusor instability.

In its present format, TVS will not replace all aspects of traditional urodynamic studies, although it should avoid many time-consuming and invasive investigations in patients who have urinary incontinence.

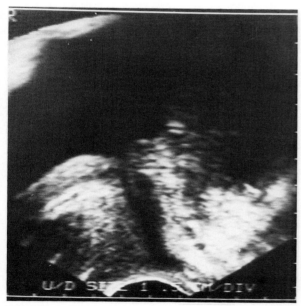

FIGURE 9-9
Successful Stamey needle-suspension. The bladder neck is elevated above the inferior border of the symphysis pubis. There is no displacement of the urethrovesical junction with an increase in ultra-abdominal pressure.

FIGURE 9-10
The same patient as in Figure 9-9 during a Valsalva maneuver. The bladder neck remains in a fixed position although the bladder base is rotated toward the symphysis.

REFERENCES

Bates CP, Whiteside CG, Turner-Warwick R. Synchronous cine/pressure/flow cystourethrography with special reference to stress and urge incontinence. Br J Urol 1970;42:714.

Benness CJ, Barnick CG, Cardozo L. Is there a place for routine videocystourethrography in the assessment of lower urinary tract dysfunction? Neurourology and Urodynamics 1989;8:291.

Brown MC, Sutherst JR, Murray A, Richmond DH. Potential use of ultrasound in place of x-ray fluoroscopy in urodynamics. Br J Urol 1985;57:88.

Burch JC. Urethrovaginal fixation to Cooper's ligament for correction of stress incontinence, cystocele and prolapse. Am J Obstet Gynecol 1961;117:805.

Enhorning G. Simultaneous recording of intravesical and intraurethral pressure. Acta Chir Scand 1961; 125(suppl):276.

Gordon D, Pearce M, Norton P, Stanton SL. Comparison of ultrasound and lateral chain urethrocystography in the determination of bladder neck descent. Am J Obstet Gynecol 1989;160:182.

Green T. Development of a plan for the diagnosis and treatment of urinary stress incontinence. Am J Obstet Gynecol 1962;83:632.

Hertogs K, Stanton SL. Lateral bead-chain urethrocystography after successful and unsuccessful colposuspension. Br J Obstet Gynaecol 1985;92:1179.

Hilton P. Urinary incontinence in women. BMJ 1987; 299:455.

Hilton P, Stanton SL. Urethral pressure measurement by microtransducer. I. An analysis of variance; II. An analysis of rotation variations. In: Sundin T, Mattiasson A, eds. Proceedings 11th Annual Meeting International Continence Society. Lund, Sweden, 1981:69.

Hodgkinson CP. Stress urinary incontinence—1970. Am J Obstet Gynecol 1970;108:1141.

Hohenfellner R, Petri E. Sling procedures. In: Stanton SL, Tanagho E, eds. Surgery of Female Incontinence. New York: Springer-Verlag, 1980.

Jarvis GJ. Detrusor muscle instability: A complication of surgery? Am J Obstet Gynecol 1981;139:219.

Jarvis GJ, Hall S, Stamp S, Millar DR, Johnson A. An assessment of urodynamic examination in incontinent women. Br J Obstet Gynaecol 1980;87:893.

Krantz K. Marshall-Marchetti-Krantz procedure. In: Stanton SL, Tanagho E, eds. Surgery of Female Incontinence. Heidelberg: Springer, 1980:47.

Langer R, Ron-El R, Newman M, Herman A, Caspi E. Detrusor instability following colposuspension for urinary stress incontinence. Br J Obstet Gynaecol 1988;95:607.

McGuire EJ, Savastano JA. Stress incontinence and detrusor instability/urge incontinence. Neurourology and Urodynamics 1985;4:313.

Pereyra AJ. A simplified surgical procedure for the correction of stress incontinence in women. West J Surg 1959;67:223.

Quinn MJ, Beynon J, Mortenson NM, Smith PJB. Transvaginal endosonography in the assessment of urinary stress incontinence. Br J Urol 1988;62:414.

Quinn MJ, Beynon J, Mortenson NM, Smith PJB. Vaginal endosonography in the postoperative assessment of colposuspension. Br J Urol 1989;63:295.

Quinn MJ, Farnsworth BA, Pollard WJ, Smith PJB, Stott MA. Vaginal ultrasound in the diagnosis of stress incontinence: A prospective comparison to urodynamic investigations. Neuro Urodynam 1989;8: 291.

Raz S. Modified bladder neck suspension for female stress incontinence. Urology 1981;18:82.

Richardson DA. Value of the cough pressure profile in the evaluation of patients with stress incontinence. Am J Obstet Gynecol 1986;155:808.

Richmond DH, Sutherst JR, Brown MC. Screening of the bladder base and urethra using linear array transrectal ultrasound scanning. J Clin Ultrasound 1986; 14:647.

Shah PJR. The assessment of patients with a view to urodynamics. In: Mundy A, Wein A, Stephenson T, eds. Urodynamics: Principles, Practice and Application. Edinburgh: Churchill-Livingstone, 1984:53.

Stamey T. Endoscopic suspension of the vesical neck. In: Stanton SL, Tanagho E, eds. Surgery of Female Incontinence. Heidelberg: Springer, 1980:77.

Stanton SL. What is the place of urodynamic investigations in a district general hospital? Br J Obstet Gynaecol 1983;90:97.

Stanton SL, Cardozo L. Results of the colposuspension operation for incontinence and prolapse. Br J Obstet Gynaecol 1979;86:693.

Stanton SL, Krieger MS, Ziv E. Videocystourethrography: Its role in the assessment of incontinence in the female. Neurourol Urodynam 1988;7:155.

Versi E, Cardozo L. Perineal pad weighing versus videographic analysis in genuine stress incontinence. Br J Obstet Gynaecol 1986;93:364.

Transvaginal Sonography: A Clinical Atlas, Second Edition,
edited by Arthur C. Fleischer and Donna M. Kepple.
J.B. Lippincott Company, Philadelphia, © 1995.

CHAPTER **10**

Cervix and Lower Uterine Segment

Donna M. Kepple, RT, RDMS
Arthur C. Fleischer, MD

INTRODUCTION

Transabdominal sonography (TAS) has been the traditional sonographic method for evaluation of the cervix and lower uterine segment. This technique uses the distended urinary bladder as an acoustic window and, for many years, was considered the method of choice for evaluation of the cervix. However, inaccuracies in evaluation of cervical length were often experienced due to compression of the lower uterine segment and cervix from the distended urinary bladder. The cervix and lower uterine segment may also be obscured transabdominally by maternal obesity, overlying fetal parts, or oligohydramnios.

The development and acceptance of transvaginal (TVS) and transperineal sonography (TPS) offer alternatives to the transabdominal approach and provide increased resolution of the cervix, accurate cervical length measurements, and increased resolution of fetal parts in the lower uterine segment (Fig. 10-1) (Hertzberg and coworkers, 1991; Jeanty and coworkers, 1986; Mahony and coworkers, 1990). The transperineal approach to cervical evaluation is performed using the same transducer

as for transabdominal imaging. Transabdominally, the cervix is oriented in a vertical plane, with the vagina in a horizontal orientation. Transperineal orientation of the cervix is such that the cervix is horizontal and perpendicular to the ultrasound beam, with the vagina oriented in a more vertical plane. When TVS is contraindicated, transperineal sonography (TPS), which has no known complications, is particularly beneficial in evaluating virginal patients or those with vaginal atrophy, vaginal anomalies, or premature rupture of membranes (PROM).

The uterus is a thick-walled muscular organ that lies within the true pelvis. The uterus is comprised of three regions: the fundus, the corpus, and the cervix. The fundus is the convex, superior portion of the organ, which extends beyond the tubal ostia and is predominately composed of myometrium. The corpus, or uterine body, is inferior to the fundus and superior to the internal os of the cervix. The term cervix means "neck" and refers to the narrow inferior portion of the uterus that is contiguous with the vagina. In adult premenopausal women, the corpus is longer than the cervix, whereas the converse is true in prepubescent girls. In newborns,

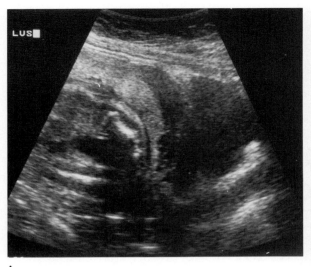

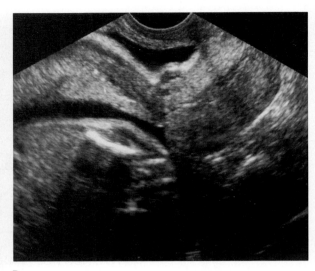

A   B

FIGURE 10-1
Normal cervix. (**A**) TAS showing low-lying placenta, but its relationship to the internal cervical os is
not clear. (**B**) TVS showing the placenta to extend to the internal cervical os. The cervix is long, and
the endocervical canal closed.

the relation of the cervix to the corpus and fundus is 1:1. After puberty, the ratio becomes 1:2 and remains constant throughout menopause.

The main uterine arteries that arise from the hypogastric arteries supply blood flow to the uterus and cervix. At the level of the cervicocorporal junction of the uterus, the uterine artery bifurcates into an ascending and descending branch. The ascending branch courses upward to supply blood to the corpus and fundus of the uterus. The descending branch courses inferiorly to supply blood to the cervix and upper vagina.

CERVICAL EVALUATION OF THE GYNECOLOGIC PATIENT

The normal cervical length in nongravid patients is 2.5 to 4 cm. Frequently, the endocervical canal may be identified by an echogenic linear interface on the sagittal plane of the cervix (Fig. 10-2). Increased fluid content of the mucous within the endocervical canal during the periovulatory period may be normally seen as a hypoechoic interface.

Nabothian cysts (small cervical inclusion cysts), caused by obstructed and dilated endocervical glands are the most common finding in reproductive age women (Fig. 10-3). Rarely symptomatic, nabothian cysts are typically thin-walled and measure

less than 1 cm. They are frequently multiple and are sometimes confused with other cystic cervical structures such as a cervical ectopic pregnancy, extruding products of a spontaneous uterine abortion, or a cystic adnexal mass (Janus and Wagner, 1989).

Solid masses of the cervix include cervical fibroids, prolapsed uterine fibroids, cervical polyps, endometrial polyps prolapsing into the cervix, and cervical carcinoma. Eight percent of all fibroids are cervical in origin. Typically, leiomyomas are small and asymptomatic. Larger fibroids may cause pain or bleeding or produce bowel and bladder symptoms. TVS may demonstrate an irregular cervical canal, which may lead to suspicion of a cervical mass in asymptomatic patients.

Cervical stenosis may be appreciated with TVS or TPS. Cervical stenosis is an obstruction at the level of either the external or internal cervical os, caused by iatrogenic manipulations such as obstetric trauma, conization, cryotherapy, or radiation. Premenopausal patients typically experience dysmenorrhea, with oligomenorrhea or amenorrhea as their primary symptom for referral for pelvic sonography.

Hematometrocolpos occurs as a result of the obstruction and appears as low-level echoes within the distended uterine cavity on TVS. The postmenopausal patient may experience cervical stenosis and usually exhibits fewer symptoms than menstruating

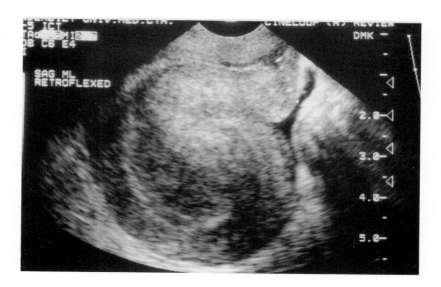

FIGURE 10-2
TVS showing a normal cervix in a severely retroflexed uterus.

women because the accumulation of blood and secretions within the endometrial cavity is significantly less.

Cervical carcinoma accounts for 18% of all female gynecologic malignancies and 30% of all deaths due to female malignancies. Although approximately 13,000 new cases of cervical carcinoma are diagnosed each year in the United States, the mortality rate has decreased significantly as the result of widespread screening using the Papanicolaou smear (PAP smear). Ultrasound has not played a major role in the staging of cervical carcinoma, although TVS is helpful in identifying hypoechoic and hyperechoic masses within the cer-

vix. Transrectal sonography may assist in determining the depth of cervical invasion because the transducer is farther away from the cevix than the vaginal transducer is, and it is frequently less affected by near-field artifacts (Meanwell, 1987).

CERVICAL EVALUATION OF THE GRAVID PATIENT

Patients who present with a positive pregnancy test and nondiagnostic endometrial findings require additional evaluation of the adnexa and cervix for the detection of an ectopic gestation. Cervical pregnan-

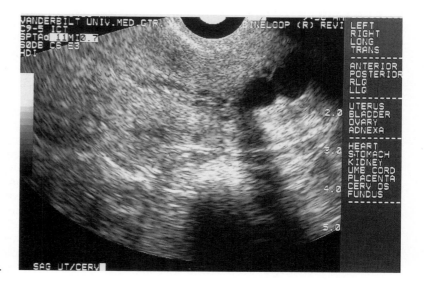

FIGURE 10-3
TVS showing cervical inclusion cysts.

cies are rare, with an occurrence rate between 1:10,000 and 1:16,000 pregnancies. Previous cervical or uterine instrumentation predisposes the cervix as a site for implantation. Congenital uterine malformations and diethylstilbestrol (DES) exposure may also increase the risk. Cervical ectopic pregnancies demonstrate the sonographic appearance of a gestational sac within the endocervical canal that is embedded within the cervical muscle (Sherer and coworkers, 1991; Rosenberg and Williamson, 1992). A spontaneous intrauterine abortion in progress may mimic the appearance of the cervical ectopic pregnancy; however, contractions with expulsion of the pregnancy usually assist in the differential diagnosis. Nabothian cysts or cervical carcinoma may also be confused with a cervical ectopic gestation.

Evaluation of the maternal cervix is an essential component of the obstetric sonographic examination, particularly in the detection of placenta previa, placenta accreta, or cervical incompetence and in those patients who present with preterm labor. Transabdominal evaluations are extremely limited in the third trimester because overlying fetal parts obstruct visualization of the cervix. Visualization is improved with overdistension of the maternal bladder; however, the cervix may become compressed and true cervical length may be distorted. Placing the patient in the Trendelenburg position or manual manipulation of the fetal head may aid in increased visualization of the cervix. TVS can provide accurate cervical evaluations but may be contraindicated in patients with PROM because there is a potential risk of ascending infection. Experience is required when evaluating a patient with bleeding and a suspected placenta previa. In such patients, the transducer must not touch the cervix. TPS is often the preferred method for cervical evaluations in these cases because there are no known contraindications for the examination. Wiping of the perineum after voiding may introduce air into the vagina, which obscures the cervical anatomy. Consequently, we routinely encourage our patients not to use toilet tissue after voiding.

Sonographically, the gravid cervix appears as a distinct soft tissue structure (see Fig. 10-1). The mucous plug appears as an echogenic line within the endocervical canal. After loss of the mucous plug, the echogenic line may be absent or thin. Cervical measurements are obtained between the external and internal cervical os. The internal os is the point at which the cervix comes into contact with the amniotic membranes, and the external os is the point at which the cervical canal can no longer be visualized. Normal cervical lengths should be greater than 3 cm for a positive outcome of the pregnancy (Smith and coworkers, 1983; Harris and Barth, 1993).

During pregnancy, the cervix infrequently demonstrates dynamic changes, with the internal os appearing to open and close during the sonographic evaluation. Diagnostic pitfalls may occur when narrowing of the lower uterine segment is visualized due to a focal contraction which may mimic a "dilated" or "funneled" cervix associated with cervical incompetency (Fig. 10-4) (Karis and coworkers, 1991). Because contractions are transient, delayed sonograms following resolution of the contraction will demonstrate a normal cervix and lower uterine segment.

One maneuver used to assess the integrity of the cervix is to put pressure on the fundus while the transvaginal probe is adjacent to the cervix. If cervical incompetency is suspected, it will demonstrate shortening and effacement.

Preterm labor is the most frequent cause of poor neonatal outcome. Those patients at risk for preterm cervical effacement and dilatation include:

Preterm labor or previous history of preterm labor
Incompetent cervix or following cerclage placement
DES exposure
PROM
Multiple gestations

Cervical incompetence accounts for more than 15% of preterm deliveries and occurs in .05% to 1% of all pregnancies. Cervical incompetence is a functional condition, usually is not associated with labor, and classically results in a history of recurrent and usually painless second trimester spontaneous abortions. Sonographic findings include a cervix measuring less than 3 cm in length, open internal os, and "funneling" or an "hourglass" appearance of the patient's membranes into the endocervical canal.

A cervical cerclage is commonly placed in women with recurrent histories of cervical incompetence. Other patients who may require a cerclage for improved pregnancy outcomes include those with cervical hypoplasia or congenital abnormalities resulting from DES exposure. The cerclage is ideally placed before 16 weeks of gestational age, under elective circumstances; however, cerclages have been performed as late as 24 weeks in emergent situations.

Sonographic visualization of the sutures of the cerclage are identified as echogenic foci within the cervical stroma (Fig. 10-5). The cerclage is typically

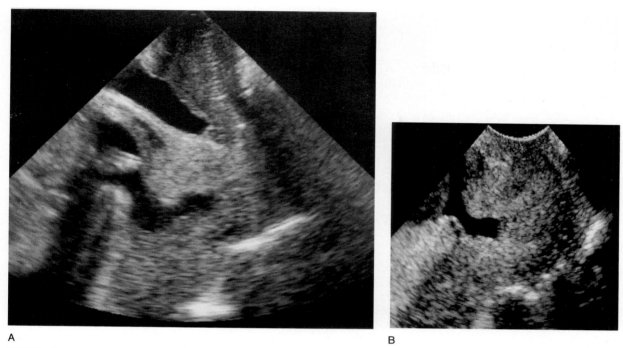

A   B

FIGURE 10-4
''Funneling'' of the cervix. (**A**) TPS suggests early funneling and opening of the internal cervical os.
(**B**) TVS better depicts the funneling.

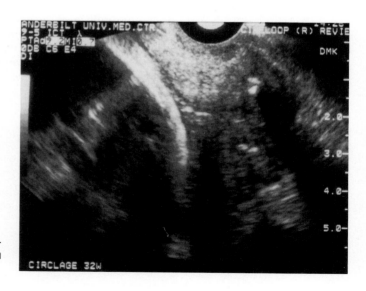

FIGURE 10-5
Midsagittal TVS of the cervix showing echogenic sutures within the anteroposterior portion of the cervix in a 32-week pregnancy.

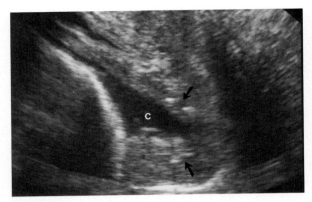

FIGURE 10-6
TPS showing dilatation of the endocervical canal in a patient with a cerclage in place (*arrows* show sutures).

positioned midway between the internal and external os. Transrectal sonography may be performed during the operative procedure to assist in the placement of the cerclage (Fleischer and coworkers, 1989). Dilatation of the internal os or shortening of the cervix on subsequent sonograms may indicate an early sign of impending cerclage failure (Fig. 10-6). Most importantly, the sonographic information may demonstrate dilatation of the internal os before clinical palpation and detection.

The site of placental implantation is related to the location of blastocyst implantation in early pregnancy. Patients with placenta previa typically present with painless vaginal bleeding in the third trimester, due to thinning of the lower uterine segment which leads to tears in the marginal and basilar veins. Massive vaginal bleeding with mortal-

ity to the mother and fetus can occur as a result of an attempted vaginal delivery when a previa is undiagnosed. Advanced maternal age, multiparity, and prior uterine surgery (most commonly from a previous cesarean section) contribute to the incidence of placenta previa. Approximately 20% of previas are complete previas, with the placenta implanted on both sides of the internal cervical os. A partial previa is identified when one side of the placenta is implanted over the internal cervical os. A marginal previa implants adjacent to the internal os but does not cover it and is difficult to diagnose transabdominally (Fig. 10-7). Additional life-threatening circumstances include a vasa previa, which is the result of an extra-amniotic vessel positioned on the placental surface over the internal os and between the presenting part of the fetus. Color Doppler sonographic evaluation of the internal os greatly assists in the diagnosis of a vasa previa.

A false-positive diagnosis may occur with TAS when an overdistended urinary bladder compresses an anterior placenta or when focal myometrial contractions are present, mimicking a previa. TPS and TVS play an important role in the diagnosis of these conditions; both examinations are performed with a nondistended maternal urinary bladder. When TVS is performed, the transducer can be placed in the mid-vagina, away from the cervix (Hertzberg, 1992).

Additional placental abnormalities may also be evaluated with TVS and color Doppler evaluations. Placenta accreta is the abnormal growth of the placenta into the myometrium without intervening decidua. When the chorionic villi are attached to the myometrium without invasion, the condition is termed "placenta accreta." Further invasion of the

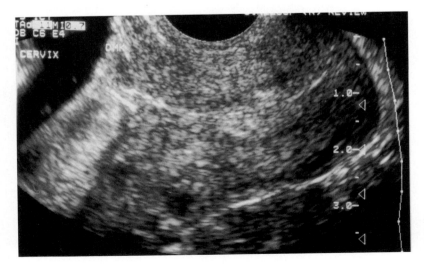

FIGURE 10-7
TVS showing a closed cervix with the placenta covering the cervical os.

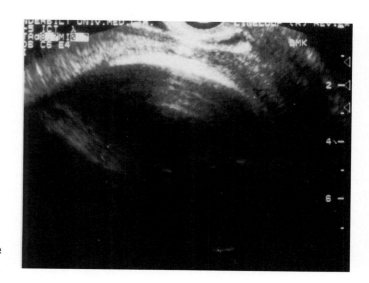

FIGURE 10-8
TVS showing total dilatation and effacement of the cervix.

villi into the myometrium is termed "placenta increta." Penetration of the villi through the myometrium to the serosal surface of the uterus or invasion into the urinary bladder wall is termed "placenta percreta." The incidence of placenta accreta is increased with multiparity and previous uterine surgery, most commonly prior cesarean section. Placental attachment over a scar predisposes the patient to this condition. There is also an increased association with a placenta previa. The predelivery diagnosis is necessary due to the increased morbidity of patients with a placenta accreta that is not diagnosed before delivery. Severe bleeding occurs because the placenta is difficult, if not impossible, to extract after delivery. Patients may require emergency hysterectomy after delivery to correct severe hemorrhage.

Suspicion for a placenta accreta, increta, or percreta arises when the sonographic findings demonstrate absence of the normal hypoechoic myometrium beneath the placenta. Multiple sonolucent areas within the placenta demonstrate vascular spaces both on color and pulsed Doppler evaluations.

SUMMARY

Evaluation of the cervix is an important component that is often underutilized or inadequately assessed in pelvic and obstetric sonograms. Recognition of possible abnormalities of the cervix is critical in the complete assessment of pelvic sonography (Fig. 10-8). Because there are a variety of techniques, the cervix can nearly always be optimally visualized.

REFERENCES

Fleischer A, Lombardi S, Kepple D. Transrectal sonography for guidance during cerclage. J Ultrasound Med 1989;8:589.

Harris RD, Barth RA. Sonography of the gravid uterus and placenta: Current concepts. AJR 1993;160:455.

Hertzberg BS, Bowie JD, Weber TM, et al. Sonography of the third trimester cervix: Value of transperineal scanning. AJR 1991;157:73.

Hertzberg BS, Bowie JD, Carroll BA, et al. Diagnosis of placenta previa during the third trimester. Role of transperineal sonography. AJR 1992;159:83.

Janus C, Wagner L. Nabothian cysts stimulating an adnexal mass. Clin Imaging 1989;13:157.

Jeanty P, D'Alton M, Romero R, et al. Perineal scanning. Am J Perinatol 1986;3:289.

Karis JP, Hertzberg BS, Bowie JD. Sonographic diagnosis of premature cervical dilatation—potential pitfall due to lower uterine segment contractions. J Ultrasound Med 1991;10:83.

Mahony BS, Nyberg DA, Luthy DA, et al. Translabial ultrasound of the third trimester uterine cervix: Correlation with digital examination. J Ultrasound Med 1990;9:717.

Meanwell CA, Rolfe EB, Blackledge G, et al. Recurrent female pelvic cancer: Assessment with transrectal ultrasonography. Radiology 1987;162:278.

Rosenberg RD, Williamson MR. Cervical ectopic pregnancy: Avoiding pitfalls in the ultrasonographic diagnosis. J Ultrasound Med 1992;11:365.

Sherer DM, Abramowicz JS, Thompson HO, et al. Comparison of transabdominal and endovaginal sonographic approaches in the diagnosis of a case of cervical pregnancy successfully treated with methotrexate. J Ultrasound Med 1991;10:409.

Smith CV, Anderson JC, Matamoros A, et al. Transvaginal sonography of cervical width and length during pregnancy: The vertical cervix. AJR 1983;140:737.

Transvaginal Sonography: A Clinical Atlas, Second Edition,
edited by Arthur C. Fleischer and Donna M. Kepple.
J.B. Lippincott Company, Philadelphia, © 1995.

CHAPTER **11**

Second and Third Trimester: Applications of Transvaginal Sonography

Jodi P. Lerner, MD
Ana Monteagudo, MD
Ilan E. Timor-Tritsch, MD

INTRODUCTION

Evaluation of the pregnant patient who is in the second or third trimester of pregnancy has always been within the realm of transabdominal sonography (TAS). The evaluation of fetal anatomy and search for anomalies by transabdominal scanning is the standard of care for obstetric patients. The advent of transvaginal sonography (TVS) and use of its high-frequency, high-resolution probes began a new phase of sonographic evaluation. The most complete fetal assessments using TVS are performed in the first trimester of pregnancy, but new applications of the vaginal technique are increasingly used later in gestation. In addition to better visualization of the fetal head, TVS may be used for other obstetric indications, including cervical as-

sessment, placenta previa localization, and fetal evaluation when oligohydramnios is present or when the patient is morbidly obese and the transabdominal view is sharply limited.

GENERAL FETAL ANATOMY

Early to Mid Second Trimester

An early fetal anatomic evaluation may be easily performed using TVS in the 13- to 16-week gestational age period (Fig. 11-1). Anomalies that are present at this gestational age are better delineated transvaginally than transabdominally. Many later-appearing anomalies may not be excluded, however, and the resolution of transabdominal probes is insufficient for the anomaly survey when it is per-

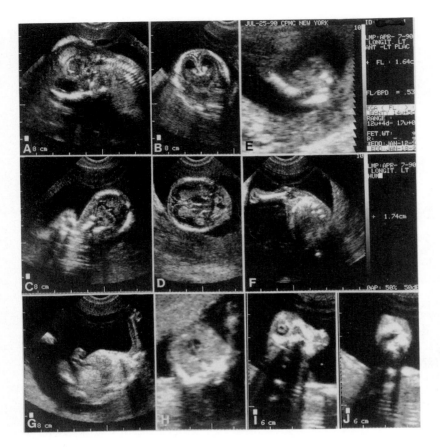

FIGURE 11-1
A sample of anatomic structures in a TVS examination at 15 weeks gestational age. (**A**) Sagittal view of brain and cervical spine. (**B–D**) Multiple views of brain. (**E**) Femur. (**F**) Humerus and partial transverse view of thorax. (**G**) Cord insertion. (**H**) Four chamber heart view. (**I**) Face and eye lens. (**J**) Lips and open mouth.

formed at a gestational age of less than 18 weeks. Achiron and Tadmor (1991) evaluated 800 patients between 9 and 13 weeks of gestation by both transabdominal and transvaginal sonography. The transvaginal approach was found to be superior to the transabdominal approach in both identification and characterization of anomalies. The limitation of the technique was that several anomalies not seen at this initial scan were present when the patients returned for the follow-up transabdominal scan at 18 to 20 weeks of gestation.

A large study recently completed by Bronshtein (1994) screened 19,150 low-risk pregnancies at 14 to 16 weeks of gestation using TVS over the time period 1987 to 1994. The detection rate for congenital anomalies was 1 in 45 pregnancies; some of the anomalies were transient and might have resolved by the time of the 18- to 22-week transabdominal study. Although 29 false-negative and four false-positive cases were encountered, more than 94% of the anomalies could be identified at this early gestational age. Bronshtein's conclusion is that TVS of the patient with a 14- to 16-week-old fetus will replace the traditional first transabdominal obstetric screen, which is conventionally performed in the late second trimester.

Timor-Tritsch and coworkers (1992) performed a study that evaluated the ability of the high-frequency transvaginal scanning method to consistently image first and early second trimester fetal structures. Ninety-seven low-risk pregnancies were scanned from the 9th through 14th week of gestation. Fingers, face and palate, feet and toes, and the four-chamber heart view were structures detected consistently in the 12- to 14-week group. The group concluded that transvaginal scanning can detect anomalies in the early second trimester, although not all malformations manifest themselves or can be detected at 14 to 15 weeks of gestation.

Selective transvaginal sonographic examination of fetal parts in both low- and high-risk pregnancies is feasible, and if an anomaly is detected, early counseling or intervention may be implemented. Transvaginal echocardiographic examination in the early second trimester is feasible, with a four-chamber heart view obtainable in 70% to 100% of cases and the extended fetal cardiac examination identifiable in 63% to 100% of cases (Paladini and

Palmieri, 1992; Achiron and coworkers, 1994; Johnson and coworkers, 1992; Gembruch and coworkers, 1993). Gembruch and coworkers (1993) report that the four-chamber heart view, including both atria, atrioventricular valves, and ventricles as well as the origin and double crossing, or aorta and pulmonary trunk, can be demonstrated beginning at the 13th week of gestation. Achiron and coworkers (1994) diagnosed six fetuses with cardiac defects in a study performed transvaginally in 660 patients with fetuses between 13 and 15 weeks of gestation. Three cardiac anomalies were undetected in this group: two of the fetuses had a minor ventricular septal defect diagnosed postnatally, and the third had multiple cardiac rhabdomyoma diagnosed in the third trimester. Early second trimester transvaginal echocardiographic assessment is feasible and accurate, especially when both the four-chamber heart view and the outflow tracts are evaluated. The high cost and high training demands of accurate early transvaginal echocardiography may preclude this modality from screening low-risk populations. One author suggests restricting use of transvaginal echocardiography to cases in which other anomalies are detected, to high-risk patients in whom congenital heart disease was present in a previous pregnancy, or to pregestational diabetic patients (Gembruch and coworkers, 1993).

Other anomalies, including ocular defects, skeletal dysplasias, and cleft lip and palate, have been identified in the early second trimester using TVS (Bronshtein and coworkers, 1991a, 1991b, 1993c).

In conclusion, TVS is an important tool for the early detection of structural fetal anomalies, and the number and variety of conditions that are being diagnosed is increasing.

Mid Second Trimester to Term

Although the performance of TVS in the general evaluation of the fetus late in gestation would overcome the limitation of late-occurring anomalies, the large size of the fetus and the distance of fetal parts from the range of the vaginal probe usually prohibit a complete fetal survey performed in this manner. Obstetric scans rely on the clarity of the images obtained. This clarity depends on the presence of amniotic fluid around the fetus. The clearly identifiable boundaries at the tissue–fluid interface make this examination clinically significant. There is a clear demarcation of fluid around body parts and organs. In gynecologic scans using TAS, no such clear interphases exist; high-frequency TVS probes provide better organ definition. Similarly, in those pregnancies in which there is a severe lack of fluid, it is almost impossible to obtain diagnostic-

quality images using TAS. In these extreme cases of oligohydramnios, it is worthwhile to use a 5- or 6.5-MHz transvaginal probe.

Transvaginal sonography is used in special circumstances late in gestation such as in cases of oligohydramnios or in obese patients when the view using TAS is inadequate. In addition, TVS is an ideal approach for the detailed evaluation of the vertex fetal head, as discussed in the next section.

Fetal position determines the particular anatomy that TVS shows. In terms of scanning capability, the tradeoff of the high-frequency, high-resolution probe is diminished penetration. It may become evident that only the fetal structures or organs closest to the cervix will be well visualized using the transvaginal approach. In a vertex presentation, the detailed cranial anatomy, face, neck, and upper spine are imaged. Bronshtein and coworkers (1993a) differentiated septated and nonseptated nuchal cystic hygroma using TVS in the second trimester of pregnancy. This discrimination is important for counseling and follow-up because the prognosis is different between the septated and nonseptated types of hygroma. In a fetus who is in the breech presentation, the sacral spine, genitalia, bladder, bowel, and kidneys may be evaluated for abnormalities. The differential diagnosis of the nonvisualized fetal urinary bladder in the second trimester of pregnancy was evaluated using TVS in a combined low-risk and high-risk group of patients who underwent 13,458 ultrasound examinations (Bronshtein and coworkers, 1993b). The group concluded that persistent nonvisualization of the bladder is an indication for a careful examination of the fetal kidneys, and the characterization of kidney morphology leads the clinician to the correct diagnosis. Fetal intraabdominal cysts have been detected in the second trimester of pregnancy by TVS and serially followed over the course of the gestation for progress or resolution (Zimmer and Bronshtein, 1991).

In conclusion, transvaginal sonographic evaluation of the fetus in the second trimester of pregnancy may replace the low-risk transabdominal survey due to the better resolution afforded by the vaginal probe and clearer identification and characterization of anomalies. In special cases, such as oligohydramnios or low fetal position, TVS is the only option for these diagnoses and greatly enhances diagnostic accuracy.

FETAL HEAD AND BRAIN

The fetal brain can be imaged using both transabdominal and transvaginal sonography during the second and third trimesters of pregnancy. In 1989,

Benacerraf and Estroff first reported the use of TVS to measure the deeply engaged fetal head. In 1991, Monteagudo and coworkers used TVS in the systematic study of the fetal brain.

The customary approach to scanning the fetal brain was and, in many places, is the transabdominal route (Pasto and Kurtz, 1986; Filly and coworkers, 1989, 1991; Nyberg, 1989; Romero and coworkers, 1988). Over the last several years, however, it has become evident that the vaginal scanning technique yields better quality images (Fig. 11-2) and, therefore, more clear diagnoses (Monteagudo and coworkers, 1991; Timor-Tritsch and coworkers, 1991; Timor-Tritsch and Monteagudo, 1991). The improved resolution of the TVS images is the direct result of the fetal brain being scanned through one of the fetal fontanelles, usually the anterior one. The fontanelles act as an acoustic window into the fetal brain, thus avoiding the need to scan through the fetal cranial bones. However, because there are limitations in obtaining all desired sections and planes transvaginally, a combination of transabdominal and transvaginal sonography should be used to optimally image the fetal brain. It is important to use both techniques when a fetal brain anomaly is encountered. In addition to describing the lesion, it is important to attempt to establish the most likely diagnosis or differential diagnoses. Determining

that a structure or an organ is normal is more difficult than confirming the presence of an anomaly. Therefore, the added information provided by the higher resolution of TVS allows greater accuracy in assessing normalcy.

The following discussion describes the sonographic anatomy of the normal fetal brain during the second and third trimesters of pregnancy. The anatomy is described using coronal and sagittal sections similar to those used in neonatal brain scans.

Fetal brain scanning can be performed anytime during the gestation if the fetus is in a cephalic presentation. If the fetus is in a breech presentation, the sagittal and coronal views may be obtained transabdominally. The ideal transvaginal probe for performing transvaginal–transfontanelle imaging of the fetal brain is an end-firing 5.0- to 7.5-MHz probe that is placed in one of the vaginal fornices, usually the posterior fornix (Fig. 11-3). Once the transvaginal probe is in place, clear images can usually be obtained by moving the probe until its tip is in line with the fetal anterior fontanelle. Even though the anterior fontanelle is most commonly used (Fig. 11-4), the posterior fontanelle may also be used. On occasion, after placing the transducer probe in the posterior fornix of the vagina, the image obtained is of poor quality. This is most likely the result of neither fontanelle being in line with the probe and

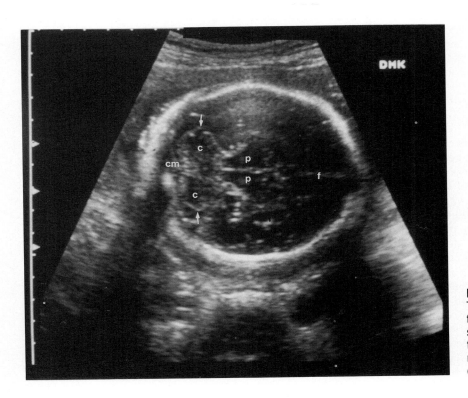

FIGURE 11-2
Transvaginal image of the brain obtained in the slightly posteriorly slanted axial plane, highlighting the posterior fossa. (*cm*, cisterna magna; *c*, cerebellum; *p*, pedunculi; *f*, falx)

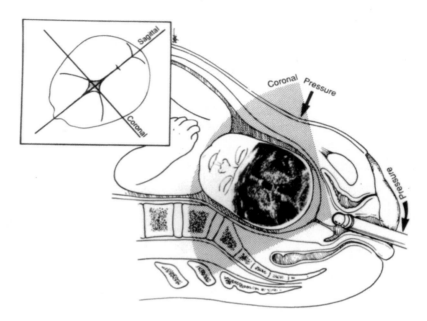

FIGURE 11-3
The technique of TVS during the second and third trimesters. (*Inset*) The planes obtained by rotation of the transducer. (From Monteagudo A, Reuss ML, Timor-Tritsch IE: Imaging the fetal brain in the second and third trimester using transvaginal sonography. Obstet Gynecol 1991; 77:27.)

the scanning taking place through the cranial bones. To correct this situation, the fetal head may be manipulated through the maternal abdomen with the free hand of the sonologist or sonographer. Once a clear image is obtained, the scanning begins.

The coronal and the sagittal planes are obtained by rotating the probe 90° around its axis over the anterior fontanelle. For example, if a coronal section is apparent on the video monitor, then, by rotating the probe 90°, the sagittal section is imaged. Serial coronal sections are obtained by slowly sweeping the probe from anterior to posterior and back again (away from the face and toward the occiput or vice versa). Serial sagittal sections are obtained by tilting

or angling the probe laterally toward the right and left ears of the fetus. The anatomy described in the following paragraphs represents the major anatomic landmarks as shown by TVS.

Normal Intracranial Anatomy

Normal intracranial anatomy is presented in detail in a series of coronal and sagittal sections. In the coronal plane, the anatomy is described from the most anterior to the most posterior section (Fig. 11-5). Although the anatomy is described in three planes (anterior, midline, and posterior), many more planes can be imaged depending on how thin or thick the sections of the brain are made. By using these three coronal sections, normal development can be assessed and most congenital abnormalities that affect the developing fetal brain can be identified. The sagittal anatomy is described in two planes: a median sagittal section and a parasagittal section. The combination of imaging in these five planes results in a thorough study of the fetal brain. A transabdominal axial section may complement this neuroanatomic examination of the fetus.

Coronal Sections
Anterior Coronal Section. The first (anterior) coronal section passes through the parenchyma of the frontal lobes (Fig. 11-6). The frontal lobes of the brain are separated into the right and left lobes by the interhemispheric fissure. The interhemispheric fissure appears as a bright echogenic midline structure. Several structures can be imaged below the

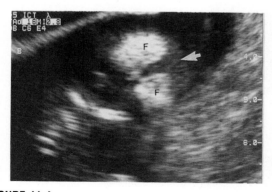

FIGURE 11-4
Tangential picture of the anterior fontanelle (*arrow*). The two frontal bones (*F*).

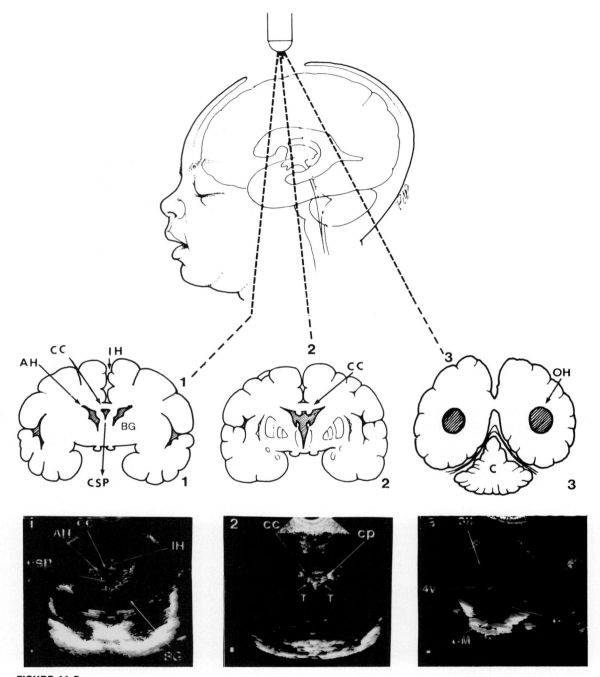

FIGURE 11-5
Serial coronal sections of the fetal head at 30 weeks gestation. (*Panel 1*) A mid-coronal section.
Visible on this plane are the cavum septi pellucidi (*csp*), the basal ganglia (*BG*), the inter-hemispheric
fissure (*IH*), the corpus callosum (*CC*), and the anterior horn (*AH*). (*Panel 2*) A more posterior
coronal section, on which the corpus callosum (*CC*) and the anterior horns containing the choroid
plexus (*cp*) are shown above the thalami (*T*). The foramina Monroe are marked by small arrows.
(*Panel 3*) The posterior or occipital coronal section is depicted. *OH,* occipital horn; *4V,* 4th ventricle;
c, cerebellum; *CM,* cisterna magna.

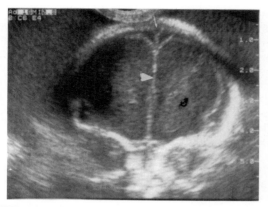

FIGURE 11-6
This extremely anterior coronal section, not depicted in Fig. 11-4, shows the typical steer's head configuration. The orbits are seen. The interhemispheric fissure and the falx are marked by an arrowhead, and the small arrow points to the superior sagittal sinus.

bright echogenic rim of the cranium. Immediately below the cranium, the superior sagittal sinus can be seen as a slightly triangular structure, through which, using a high frame rate or color Doppler sonography, blood flow can be observed. Below the superior sagittal sinus, the subarachnoid space appears as a hypoechoic area above the cerebral cortex. This space becomes less prominent with the progressive brain growth over the term of pregnancy.

Midcoronal Section. The midcoronal section contains parts of the lateral ventricular system as well as the corpus callosum and cavum septi pellucidi, which are important midline structures (Fig. 11-7A and B). At the base of the interhemispheric fissure and at right angles to it, the hypoechoic corpus callosum is located. Although the corpus callosum starts developing early in the second trimester of pregnancy, it is not consistently imaged until the 20th week of gestation. To the right and left side of

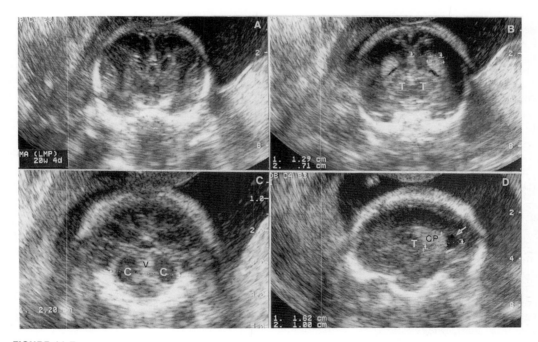

FIGURE 11-7
A coronal and sagittal section of the brain at 20 weeks (*Panel A and B*). Two mid-coronal sections. *Panel A* is slightly more anterior than *Panel B*. On *Panel A* the anterior horns and the cavum septi pellucidi is seen. On *Panel B* the hyper-echoic choroid plexi are seen on top of the thalami (*T*). (*Panel C*) A posterior coronal section depicting the hyper-echoic cerebellar vermis (*V*) and the cerebellar hemispheres (*C*). The bi-cerebellar diameter in this case is 2.2 cm. (*Panel D*) A paramedian sagittal section showing the occipital horn (*arrow*), the choroid plexus (*CP*), and the thalamus (*T*). Some of the measurements of the ventricles and the thickness of the choroid plexus are shown on this figure.

the interhemispheric fissure, the anterior horns of the lateral ventricles appear as linear, bilateral fluid-filled structures. As the fetus matures, the lateral ventricles become narrower and sometimes are difficult to image. The ventricles approximate each other in the midline and contain within them the echogenic choroid plexus. The choroid plexus fills the cavities of the lateral ventricles. In the midline, located between the anterior horns and below the corpus callosum, the cavum septi pellucidi are seen. The entrance of the choroid plexus into the third ventricle through the foramina of Monro can be seen on a coronal plane. The cavum is separated from the ventricles by a thin septum. The thalami are located below the cavum septi pellucidi. In the midline between the thalami, the third ventricle can occasionally be imaged as a narrow longitudinal slit. The third ventricle usually is not imaged unless an abnormality such as ventriculomegaly or hydrocephalus is suspected. If imaged in an unusually high position, below the interhemispheric fissure, absence of the corpus callosum and of the cavum septi pellucidi must be ruled out (Pilu and coworkers, 1993).

Posterior Coronal Section. In the most posterior coronal section, the occipital horns of the lateral ventricle, the cerebellum, and the tentorium above the cerebellum are imaged (see Fig. 11-7C). The occipital horns appear as perfectly rounded sonolucent structures, giving the impression of an owl's eye or face. In the posterior fossa, the cerebellum is imaged. Above the cerebellum, the sonolucent fourth ventricle can be imaged. Below the cerebellum, an equally sonolucent cisterna magna is present. In most cases of open spinal defects, the cisterna magna is obliterated in this section.

Sagittal and Parasagittal Sections
Median Sagittal Section. The median sagittal section reveals two simple-to-locate structures: the corpus callosum and the sonolucent cavum septi pellucidi. The corpus callosum develops in an anterior to posterior fashion and is fully developed by 18 to 20 weeks of gestation (Fig. 11-8). Toward the 25th to 28th week of gestation, the vaginal scanning approach yields clear images of clinical diagnostic value (Figs. 11-9 through 11-11). The corpus callosum is a prominent hypoechoic, semilunar midline structure located above the cavum septum pellucidum. It has three parts: the anterior, or knee (genu); middle, or body (corpus); and posterior, or tail (splenium). Therefore, by determining the shape of the corpus callosum, the sonographer can determine which direction the fetus is facing. Above and parallel to the corpus callosum, the cingulate gyrus is progressively easier to identify as the gesta-

tion advances. Below the corpus callosum, the cavum septum pellucidum appears as a large prominent hypoechoic structure. Located above and covering the thalamus, the bright echogenic tela choroidea (choroid plexus) of the third ventricle can be imaged. In the direction of posterior fossa, the cerebellum and the hyperechoic vermis appear below the tentorium. The cisterna magnae are hypoechoic structures surrounding these structures. The triangularly shaped hypoechoic fourth ventricle can be seen at times indenting the cerebellum anteriorly. Abnormalities of the posterior fossa (e.g., arachnoid cysts or megacisterna magnae) can be easily diagnosed in this section.

Paramedian Sagittal Section. By tilting the transvaginal probe slightly to the right or left, a paramedian sagittal section is obtained. This section reveals the anterior horn, the body of the lateral ventricles, which includes the choroid plexus within it, and the occipital horn, which is a prominent sonolucent structure.

Because of their lateral position, the temporal horns can be seen only when the transducer is angled to obtain an extremely lateral section, usually impossible by TVS. If all parts of the lateral ventricles (anterior, posterior, and temporal horns) are imaged on the same paramedian section, ventriculomegaly or hydrocephalus must be suspected. In both the midline and parasagittal sections, the gyri and sulci can be imaged. During the first and second trimesters of pregnancy, the surface of the brain is smooth, but with the growth spurt that occurs at approximately 28 to 30 weeks of gestation, the number of gyri and sulci increases rapidly (Chi and coworkers, 1977; Dorovini-Zis and Dolman, 1977). The sonographic appearance of the brain surface then changes from a smooth one to one with an interlacing network of hyperechoic lines.

If the probe is tilted somewhat more toward the fetal ear, an extreme paramedian sagittal section reveals the insula (see Fig. 11-11). The midcerebral artery can be found in this anatomic area.

Fetal Spine

The fetal spine and the spinal cord can be imaged on both the sagittal and coronal planes. Figure 11-12 depicts a normal cervical spine. Sagittal and transverse sections may reveal spina bifida with or without extruding spinal cord (Fig. 11-13).

Detection of Ventriculomegaly and Hydrocephalus

Transvaginal sonography can be used to detect a wide variety of brain malformations or diseases that

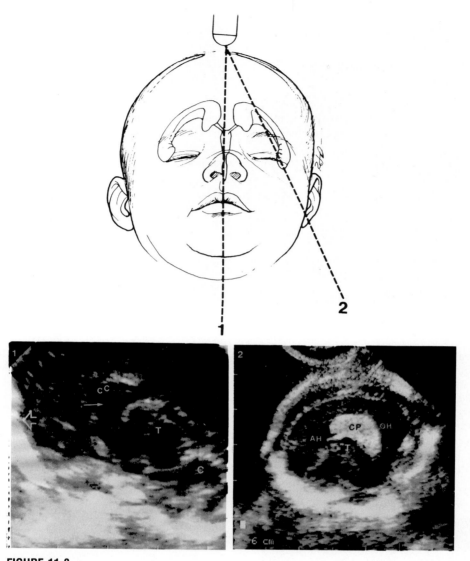

FIGURE 11-8
A median sagittal and paramedian sagittal section of the brain at 18 weeks . (*Panel 1*) The median sagittal image showing the corpus callosum (*CC*), the cavum septi pellucidi marked by an arrow, the thalamus (*T*), and the cerebellum (*C*). The frontal direction is marked by an open arrow. (*Panel 2*) The paramedian sagittal section depicting the anterior horn (*AH*), the occipital horn (*OH*), the thalamus (*T*) and the hyper-echoic choroid plexus (*CP*).

exhibit anatomic brain manifestations. This chapter presents a sample of the more common pathologic conditions to illustrate the potential of TVS as an important diagnostic tool.

Transvaginal sonography is an excellent tool to image the brain in the presence of any congenital brain malformation, but in the presence of ventriculomegaly and hydrocephalus it can provide infor-

mation not readily available with conventional TAS. Therefore, the result of adding TVS to the conventional transabdominal scan is that the fetal brain is imaged in the three scanning planes (axial, coronal, and sagittal), enabling the sonologist or sonographer to reconstruct a more accurate three-dimensional image of the abnormality. Hydrocephalus and ventriculomegaly refer to dilatation of the

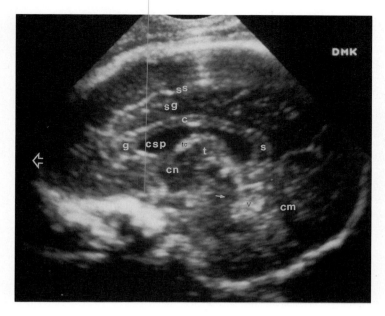

FIGURE 11-9

This represents a median sagittal section of the brain at 28 weeks. The frontal direction is marked by an open arrow. The structures seen on this image are the three parts of the corpus callosum, the knee (*g*, genu), the body (*c*, corpus) and the tail (*s*, splenium). The cavum septi pellucidi (*csp*) and the thalamus (*t*), above which the tela choroidea (*tc*) is seen. The head of the caudal nucleus is seen anterior to the thalamus (*cn*), the vermis of the cerebellum is hyper-echoic (*v*), the arrow points to the fourth ventricle, and the cisterna magna (*cm*) also is seen posteriorly. Above the corpus callosum, the cingulate gyrus (*cg*) and the cingulate sulcus (*cs*) are seen.

fetal lateral ventricles with or without enlargement of the cranium (Fig. 11-14). In hydrocephalus, the dilatation of the cerebral ventricles is the result of an increased amount of cerebrospinal fluid with an accompanying increase in intraventricular pressure. Fetuses with hydrocephalus usually have a head circumference or biparietal diameter that is larger than expected for their gestational age. In general, the greater the discrepancy, the worse the degree of hydrocephalus that is present. In contrast, ventriculomegaly refers to dilatation of the fetal lateral ventricles in the presence of normal fetal intraventricular pressures. In these cases, the fetal head circumference may be within the normal range for gestational age (Filly and coworkers, 1991; Rumack and Johnson, 1984). Although most cases of ventriculomegaly or hydrocephalus are bilateral, unilateral hydrocephalus is a rare condition that can affect

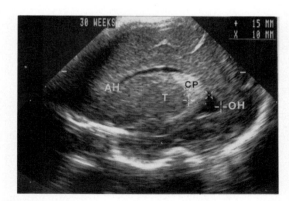

FIGURE 11-10

A paramedian sagittal section depicting the anterior horn (*AH*), the occipital horn (*OH*), and the thalamus (*T*) on which the choroid plexus is seen (*CP*) filling the antrum of the lateral ventricle. The measurements depict the thalamus to the tip of the occipital horn distance which is 15mm and the height of the occipital horn, which is 10mm. This image was taken in a fetus of 30 weeks.

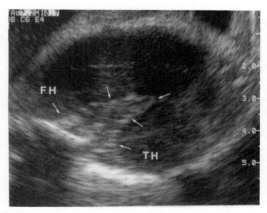

FIGURE 11-11

This is an extreme paramedian sagittal section revealing the insula outlined by small arrows. This image was seen in a 26 week fetus. However, towards term, the gaping insula is slowly obliterated and presents as a discreet line marking the meeting line between the frontal and temporal horns (*FH* and *TH*).

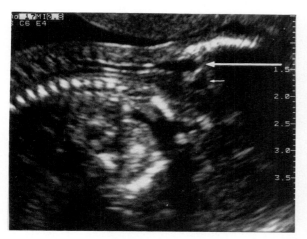

FIGURE 11-12
This is a sagittal section of the cervical and upper thoracic spine showing the spinal cord. The long arrow points toward the cisterna magna and the small arrow points to the fourth ventricle.

the fetus and usually results from unilateral obstruction of the foramina of Monro (Patten and coworkers, 1991; Chari and coworkers, 1993).

If a concomitant meningomyelocele is present (Chiari type II), the fetal skull may exhibit a distorted shape called the "lemon sign." This is due to the low intracranial pressure, which renders a caved-in shape of the temporal horn (Fig. 11-15).

The estimated incidence of hydrocephalus is 0.5 to 3 per 1000 live births. The incidence of isolated hydrocephalus is between 0.4 and 0.9 per 1000 live births (Habib, 1981). The most common cause of hydrocephalus is the obstruction of the cerebrospinal fluid along its route of circulation. Using TVS, ventriculomegaly or hydrocephalus may be diagnosed by several different methods. Qualitative methods include the search for changes in the shape of the lateral ventricles. In the presence of hydrocephalus, the anterior horns are imaged in the first coronal section, when only brain parenchyma is normally present in this view. In the midcoronal section, progressive rounding or bulging of the superior and lateral aspects of the frontal horns may be seen. In the parasagittal plane, all three components of the lateral ventricle are imaged in the same section in the presence of ventriculomegaly or hydrocephalus; in their absence, only the anterior and posterior (occipital) horns are imaged. In cases of hydrocephalus or ventriculomegaly, the choroid plexus thins and may be sonographically seen "dangling" or floating freely within the dilated ventricle.

Quantitative methods to assess ventriculomegaly or hydrocephalus have been based on widely accepted nomograms of the fetal lateral ventricles (Jeanty and coworkers, 1981; Pretorius and coworkers, 1986; Cardoza and coworkers, 1988; Pilu and coworkers, 1989; Siedler and Filly, 1987; Denkhaus and Winsberg, 1979; Johnson and coworkers, 1980). All of the commonly used nomograms of the fetal

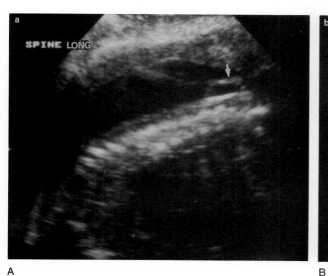
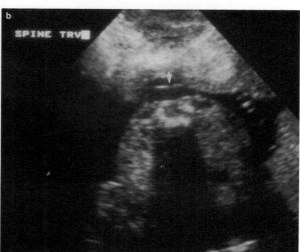

A   B

FIGURE 11-13
A case of spina bifida with meningocele. (**A**) A longitudinal section of the upper spine. The arrow points to the bulging meninges. (**B**) A cross-section at the same level.

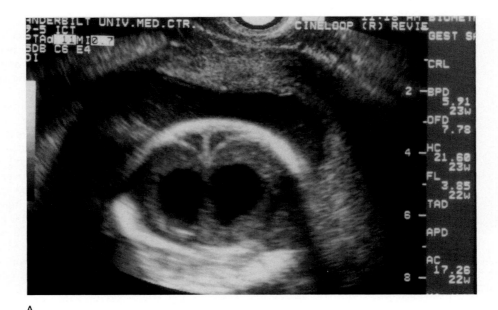

A

B

FIGURE 11-14
Hydrocephalus at 22 weeks gestation. (**A**) A coronal section showing the distended lateral ventricles. (**B**) A sagittal section showing tne dilated lateral ventricles with anterior, posterior and temporal horns (*AH, OH, TH,* respectively).

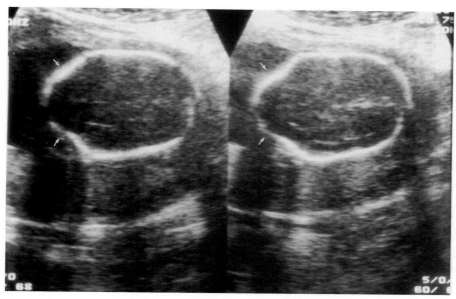

FIGURE 11-15
The lemon-shaped skull is shown. The temporal bones are concave (*arrows*).

lateral ventricle were generated using measurements obtained transabdominally in the axial plane. Therefore, when scanning the fetal brain transvaginally in coronal and sagittal sections, these nomograms cannot be applied. Using TVS, we recently developed nomograms of the fetal lateral ventricles (Monteagudo and coworkers, 1993, 1994). The main difference between our nomograms and those previously published is that we performed all our measurements transvaginally using coronal and sagittal sections. Nine nomograms were developed using 347 fetuses between 14 and 40 weeks of gestation. A total of seven measurements of the fetal lateral ventricles were used to generate the nomograms. In addition, two ratios were calculated using three of the seven measurements. Serial follow-up of 36 cases of patients carrying fetuses with hydrocephalus was carried out. As expected, all parts of the lateral ventricles increased with progressing ventriculomegaly or hydrocephalus. The only exception was the thickness of the choroid plexus, which decreased as ventriculomegaly progressed (Monteagudo and coworkers, 1993, 1994).

The outcome of prenatally detected hydrocephalus is closely related to the presence of associated anomalies. The reported incidence of anomalies in this group ranges from 70% to 83% (Drugan and coworkers, 1989; Pretorius and coworkers, 1985; Chevernak and coworkers, 1985; Nyberg and co-

workers, 1987; Hudgins and coworkers, 1988). In presence of other anomalies, the prognosis for the fetus/neonate is poor, and developmental delay varying from mild to severe can be expected (Drugan and coworkers, 1989). Isolated hydrocephalus has a better prognosis for the neonate, and the reported incidence of "normal" outcome ranges from 54.5% to 80% (Drugan and coworkers, 1989; Glick and coworkers, 1984).

ASSESSMENT OF THE CERVIX

The high-frequency transvaginal ultrasound probes excel in producing high-resolution images at the expense of shallow penetration; the cervix is a logical target of TVS. The probe can be placed close to the cervix, with the region of interest lying within 3 to 5 cm, a span that matches the focal zone of the transvaginal probes.

Before 1986, imaging of the cervix was performed exclusively by the transabdominal route. This mode of scanning traditionally requires a full bladder, which then enables a reactively clear image of the lower uterine segment. However, such imaging leads to unnatural distortion of compression of the cervical lips, leading to a falsely perceived normal appearance of the compressed lower segment or to a false-positive diagnosis of placenta previa. In contrast, TVS is performed with the patient's bladder being empty or almost empty, which enables cervical imaging without such distortion.

In pregnant patients, the shape of the cervical internal os area changes, as does the cervical length, as a function of periodic uterine contractions. The "behavior" of the cervix modulated by uterine activity should be observed.

Literature Review

A chronologic reading of the literature reflects not only the constant expansion of theoretic and practical knowledge concerning the clinical importance of the uterine cervix, but also the rapidly improving imaging techniques of the cervix. Palpatory (digital) evaluation of the cervix to assess its status before induction of labor leads to the most widely used "scoring system," that is, the Bishop score (Bishop, 1964).

Sonographic evaluation of the cervix was begun in the late 1970s (Sarti and coworkers, 1979). Many articles about using TAS to assess the cervix, primarily in the first half of the pregnancy term, have been published (Bernstine and coworkers, 1981; Redford and coworkers, 1981; Brook and coworkers, 1981; Fried, 1981; Parulekar and Kiwi, 1982, 1988; Bowie and coworkers, 1983; Vaalamo and Kivikoski, 1983; Bartolucci and coworkers, 1984; Feingold and coworkers, 1984; Confino and coworkers, 1986; Varma and coworkers, 1986a, 1986b; Zemlyn, 1978; Mason, 1989; O'Leary and Ferrell, 1986; Ayers and coworkers, 1988; Michaels and coworkers, 1986; Podobnik and coworkers, 1988; Ludmir, 1988; Lorenz and coworkers, 1990; Brown and coworkers, 1986).

Observations by Brook and coworkers as well as by Feingold and coworkers suggested that the cervical length and its dilation should be measured to diagnose cervical incompetence. Diameters of 19 mm and 15.8 mm, respectively, were considered to be consistent with cervical incompetence. The positive and negative effects of the patient's full bladder on the transabdominal sonographic determination of cervical anatomy have been observed (Brook and coworkers, 1981; Bowie and coworkers, 1983; Confino and coworkers, 1986; Varma and coworkers, 1986b; Zemlyn, 1978; Mason, 1989). The introduction of TVS resulted in a new wave of reports which, at first, practically duplicated some of the previous works performed using TAS. Brown and coworkers were the first to report on the shape of the internal os (Y, U, and V shapes) seen with a transvaginal probe. Kushnir and coworkers (1990), Soneck and coworkers (1990), and Andersen and coworkers (1990, 1991a, 1991b) have reported on

precisely measuring cervical length and attempting to predict premature labor. It was concluded that TVS not only better defined cervical anatomy but also represented a better clinical evaluation of the cervix than the palpatory digital cervical examination (Paterson-Brown and coworkers, 1991). Other articles comparing TVS and digital palpation of the cervix confirmed these observations (Lim and coworkers, 1992; Jackson and coworkers, 1992; Okitsu and coworkers, 1992; Raner and Davis Harrigan, 1990; Quinn, 1992; Jaffe and coworkers, 1992; Smith and coworkers, 1992).

Sonographic Anatomy and Scanning Technique

Scanning is performed in the sagittal plane and must show the entire length of the cervical canal. Using the proper equipment, the sonographic anatomy of the cervix is self-explanatory. The most important issue is to understand the orientation of the image. If the scanning orientation uses the apex of the "pie" pointing upward, then the transducer tip approaches the top of the image and shows the cervix from that point of view. By convention, the anatomy of the area of interest in the sagittal plane consists of:

1. Anterior to the vagina (to the left of it on the image or video screen) and parallel to it is the urethra. Somewhat deeper is the bladder. Posterior to the vagina (to the right of it) is the hyperechoic rectum.
2. If the uterus is anteverted (i.e., the fundus of the uterus is immediately adjacent and below the bladder), then the cervical canal is almost at a right angle to the vagina. At the right end of the cervical canal is the external os. At this point, the transducer is close to the anterior lip of the cervix.

Transducer positioning is extremely important, and its depth within the vagina should be adjusted to reveal the entire cervix within the focal range of the transducer. The best possible image should be "negotiated" by tilting the probe or by slightly pushing and pulling or rotating it to align the cervical canal with the scanning plane. Steerable scanning angles present some advantage in cervical imaging. At or after a cervical dilatation of 2 to 3 cm with total effacement, it is virtually impossible to image the cervix.

The following anatomic landmarks can be detected on the sagittal section obtained by TVS: the internal and external ossa, the posterior vaginal wall, the cervical canal, and the anterior and posterior cervical lips (Fig. 11-16).

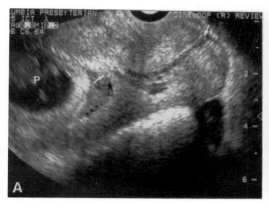 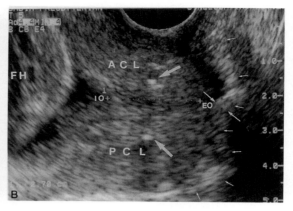

FIGURE 11-16
(A) Sagittal TVS image of a normal cervix. The cervical canal can be seen between the two arrows. (*P*, early intrauterine pregnancy at 8 weeks.) **(B)** On the sagittal image from the left to the right, the following structures are seen: the fetal head (*FH*); anterior and posterior cervical lips (*ACL, PCL*); the internal and the external os (*IO* and *EO*); and the posterior vaginal wall, followed by small arrows, the thickness of the vagina shown between the two middle-sized arrows. The cross-section of correctly-placed cervical sutures are also shown (*large arrows*). The cervical length is 2.7cm.

The following measurements of the cervix in the sagittal plane are possible:

1. Cervical length is measured from the external to the internal os. The thickness of the vagina (which is anatomically close to the external os) should not be included in the cervical length measurement. At times, the cervical canal curves upward, or anteriorly, on the image. In this case, two measurements should be taken and combined to follow the cervical anatomy. Tables 11-1 and 11-2 summarize the cervical measurements reported by different authors using TAS and TVS, respectively.

2. Cervical width or thickness is measured from the anterior lip to the posterior lip, including the entire tissue width.

3. Cervical dilatation is measured anywhere along the distal half of the cervical canal (Fig. 11-17).

The most important dimension of cervical anatomy is the cervical length. By averaging the figures published in most articles, it seems that the normal cervical length during early pregnancy is 32.5 to 52 mm. The cervix apparently shortens somewhat in the second trimester to approximately 38 to 47 mm and arrives at a final length of approximately 33 to

TABLE 11-1
Reported Normal Cervical Length by Transabdominal Sonography During Pregnancy

Author	Year	No. of Patients	Cervical length (mm)*			Mean for Entire Pregnancy (mm)*
			I Trim	*II Trim*	*III Trim*	
Zemlyn	1981	100	29	38	38	37
Bowie	1983					
Bladder empty		30				32.5
Bladder full		32				46
Varma	1986	30	32	37	33	
Podobnik	1988	80	49	47	44	
Ayers	1988					52 ± 6
Andersen	1990	135	53	43	39	

* The measurements are rounded to the closest mm.

Adapted from Andersen HF. Transabdominal and transvaginal sonography of the uterine cervix during pregnancy. J Clin Ultrasound 1991a;19:77–82.

TABLE 11-2
Reported Normal Cervical Length by Transvaginal Sonography During Pregnancy

Author	Year	No. of Patients	Cervical length (mm)*			Mean for Entire Pregnancy (mm)*
			I Trim	*II Trim*	*III Trim*	
Kushnir	1990	166	43	45	42	
Andersen	1990	177	40	42	32	
Smith	1992	132	35	37	40	36
Murakawa	1993	177	37	35	30	33

* The measurements are rounded to the closest mm.

Adapted from Andersen and Ansbacher. Ultrasound: A new approach to the evaluation of cervical ripening. Semin Perinatol 1991b;15(2):140–148.

44 mm during the third trimester. These sonographic measurements are known to be accurate secondary to work done on the nongravid uterine cervix prior to surgery. The nongravid uterine cervix was found to be 38 ± 10 mm by TVS, which matched the actual ruler measurements of the same cervices after hysterectomy (38.4 ± 7 mm).

Clinically, one of the most important anatomic features of the cervix in the pregnant patient is the shape of the internal os. As proposed by Brown and coworkers (1986), the shape of the os is easily recognized. These internal os areas include the Y shape; the U, or ballooning, shape; and the V, or funneling, shape (Figs. 11-18 and 11-19). The clinical significance of cervical funneling is discussed later in this section in relation to prediction of premature labor and inducibility of the cervix at term.

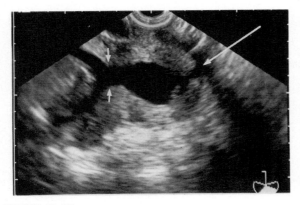

FIGURE 11-17
A ballooning cervix is shown. The long arrow points to the slightly dilated external os. The short arrows point to an area in the cervix which may be demonstrating a contraction sweeping through the lower segment of the cervix (Courtesy of Dr. R. Nir, Haifa, Israel).

Cervical glands flank the cervical canal and appear as slightly sonolucent structures. With less than adequate imaging, such as with faulty focusing or the use of low-frequency probes, the glands may create the faulty appearance of cervical dilatation. Echogenic material seen within the internal os area represents the mucous plug and may obliterate the view of a funneling cervical os.

Digital Versus Transvaginal Sonographic Evaluation

Because TAS is now considered an inadequate tool to evaluate cervical anatomy, studies comparing the digital palpatory cervical examination are compared with the more precise, objective TVS studies. Andersen (1990, 1991a) concluded that digital evaluation of cervical length underestimated the length by an average of 2.1 cm. Jackson and coworkers (1992) found an underestimation of 1.36 cm of the cervix by digital evaluation compared with TVS and a ruler measurement on the subsequent hysterectomy specimens. Soneck and coworkers (1990) found an underestimation in 87% of cases by digital examination when compared with TVS; the average difference was 14.1 mm. Okitsu and coworkers (1992) encountered similar results in their reported series. In a recent study by Boozarjomehri and coworkers (1994), no relationship betweeen TVS and digitial assessment of the cervical length was found.

The main reason for the discrepancy between the palpatory digital examination of the cervix and measurements made by TVS is that the digital examination can only evaluate the lower half (i.e., the vaginal portion) of the anterior cervical lip. This digital examination cannot evaluate the upper cervical segment, which is situated below the bladder. Additionally, the digital examination cannot evaluate the internal os in a closed cervix.

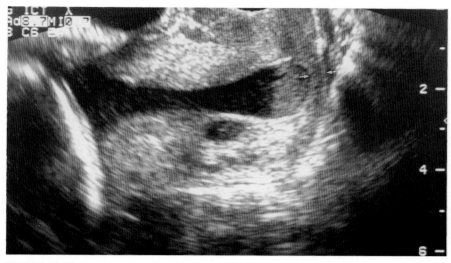

FIGURE 11-18
Sagittal image of a ballooning cervix. Note the thinning of the cervix to less than 0.5cm between the two arrows.

Clinical Applications of Cervical Ultrasonography

Prediction and Evaluation of Cervical Competence

An early and accurate diagnosis of cervical incompetence would enable active management of this problem and possibly prevent premature labor.

Researchers differ in their sonographic criteria to establish cervical incompetence; some use the criteria of a shortened cervix of less than 3.4 cm at 15 weeks of gestation, others use the criteria of cervical dilatation greater than 1.9 cm (Brook and coworkers, 1981; Podobnik and coworkers, 1988). Several authors use strict criteria in which any shortening of the cervical length below 4 cm is considered a pathologic finding (Ayers and coworkers, 1988). Andersen (1991a) suggests that it is not enough to measure the cervical length or dilatation on the sagittal TVS view, but the internal os should be evaluated for the presence of funneling or ballooning (Fig. 11-20, and see Figs. 11-17 through 11-19). It is sonographically easy to detect the placement of cervical sutures on the vaginal image or to follow

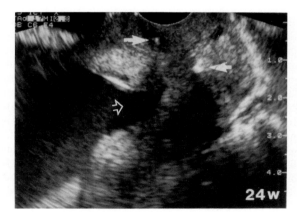

FIGURE 11-19
Wedging of the internal os area at 24 weeks is shown (*open arrow*). The white arrows show the cross-section of previously-placed cervical sutures.

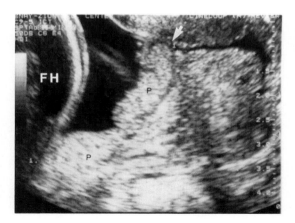

FIGURE 11-20
A normally-shaped internal os of a patient at 27 weeks of gestation, in the somewhat shortened (1.8cm) cervix. The placenta (*P*) reaches the level of the internal os marked by an arrow. The fetal head is seen (*FH*).

up the subsequent cervical changes that may occur (Fig. 11-21, and see Figs. 11-16 and 11-19). The location of the suture seen on the image can be used as a landmark for changes in the dimensions and the configuration of the cervix. Fleischer and coworkers (1989) suggest the use of a linear transrectal probe to intraoperatively guide the placement of the suture.

In addition to scrutinizing the cervix for signs of incompetence, it is practical to scan the cervix in each case in which TVS is used for any obstetric or gynecologic indication. In addition to detecting cervical fibroids and endocervical polyps, subchorionic hematomas or frank blood clots may be sonographically imaged close to the internal os. The possibility of a cervical pregnancy should be considered and, despite its low prevalence, systematically ruled out.

Prediction of Cervical Inducibility

Several authors have reported on the poor performance of the Bishop score alone in the prediction of cervical response to labor induction (Friedman and coworkers, 1966; Hughes and coworkers, 1976; Dhall and coworkers, 1987). The most important variable in predicting inducibility appears to be dilatation of the cervix (Paterson-Brown and coworkers, 1991). Since Brown and coworkers (1986) described the possibility of evaluating the area of the internal os, attention has been focused on the use of the shape of this area in predicting the patient's response to induced labor.

Boozarjomehri and coworkers (1994) showed that the total duration of labor and the duration of the latent phase were both significantly associated with the presence of cervical wedging (funneling)

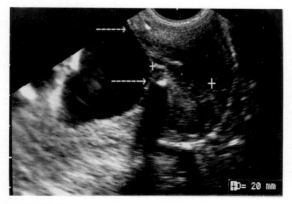

FIGURE 11-21
A shortened cervix (20mm). Cervical sutures placed earlier (*arrows*) are now close to the inner wall of the cervix/uterus. No contractions were felt by the patient. The sutures were left in place and presumably are holding the cervix closed.

seen on TVS, but not associated with the result of digital examination (effacement or dilatation). A similar study was conducted by Gomez and coworkers (1994) in which several measurements of the funneled cervix were obtained, including presence of funneling, funnel width, and funnel length. A specially constructed cervical index proved to be the best predictor of preterm labor and delivery.

More research to support these observations on inducibility is needed.

Prediction of Premature Labor

Premature labor and delivery is probably the greatest challenge of modern perinatology. Overtreatment and wasting of resources are the results of the inability to accurately diagnose and predict those patients who are truly at high risk for this complication.

The definition of preterm labor is the detection of change in the effacement (length) and in the dilatation of the cervix over a short period of time in the presence of uterine contractions at a preterm gestational age. Both aspects of this evaluation are subjective and depend on the observer's experience and the prevalence of this condition in the patient population. The false-positive rate of diagnosing true preterm labor is high; unnecessary hospitalization, wasted provider time, and the administration of potent and potentially dangerous drugs are the rule when the patients are evaluated as such.

The first attempts to correctly diagnose true preterm labor were made using TAS. The criteria used to establish the diagnosis included the presence of cervical shortening, where cervical length was measured as less than 3 cm, cervical dilatation was measured in excess of 1 cm, and there were bulging membranes through a thin lower uterine segment (Fried, 1981; Bartolucci and coworkers, 1984). The sonographic presence of the above mentioned signs predicted premature delivery in a large percentage of the patients studied. These digital and sonographic signs are still considered to be the gold standard in establishing the risk for preterm labor (Stubbs and coworkers, 1986; Papiernik and coworkers, 1986; Murakawa and coworkers, 1993). In articles by Andersen and coworkers (1990), Soneck and coworkers (1990), and Okitsu and coworkers (1992), it was concluded that the risk for premature labor was higher with a shorter cervical length as measured by sonography. They also concluded that TVS was superior to TAS and to digital examination in establishing the characteristics of the cervix.

Guzman and coworkers (1994) suggested a technique whereby application of transfundal pressure under real-time observation is used in mid-trimester pregnancies at risk for preterm labor. The sagittal cervical image is obtained by TVS, and cervical changes observed as a response to transfundal pressure were then treated by cervical cerclage.

It appears that the transvaginal sonographic evaluation of the cervix has the potential to serve as a screening tool for the identification of preterm labor leading to preterm delivery. Correct identification of preterm labor may enable more judicious use of hospitalization and hospital personnel, and, in many cases, avoid unnecessary medication of patients.

We believe that TVS should be widely used in the diagnosis of the cervix and its abnormal conditions. Technically, it is easily applicable to all patients in the office, emergency room, and delivery suites. This relatively short examination is easy to learn and to administer. It is particularly well suited to patients who are hard to evaluate or examine, including obese patients and those patients with long vaginal vaults. In a busy labor and delivery suite where expedient patient triage is important, TVS can help shorten diagnostic evaluations. Digital palpatory examination of the cervix should be followed by TVS of the cervix in the previously described situations.

PLACENTA PREVIA AND ACCRETA

Placenta previa is a common complication of pregnancy, occurring in approximately 1 in 200 to 250 births. Placenta previa is largely a problem of parous women. The highest risk group includes those women with a prior placenta previa and multiple prior cesarean sections. In this group, the recurrence risk may be as high as 4% to 8% (Green, 1989). Placenta accreta, strongly associated with placenta previa, is a considerable contributor to maternal morbidity and mortaltiy. The presence of placenta accreta, including the associated variants of placenta increta and percreta, has been essentially undiagnosed in the antepartum period; it is most often realized with the attempt at placenta removal at the time of cesarean section. Severe hemorrhage ensues, often necessitating multiple blood transfusions and hysterectomy.

The first use of TVS in this setting was in the diagnosis of placenta previa (Fig. 11-22) when the gold standard of TAS was found to be inadequate, especially when visualizing a posterior placenta (Farine and coworkers, 1990; Cunningham and coworkers, 1989). TVS was found to be superior to TAS in diagnosing placenta previa and invariably correct in ruling it out (Farine and coworkers, 1990). The advantages of the transvaginal route over the transabdominal route are many: the higher frequency probe is used, the probe is proximal to the internal os, and there are technical limitations of TAS in such settings as posterior placenta, obese patients, and low fetal head. TVS is associated with increased clarity of diagnosis, decreased time of scanning, and no increased incidence of hemorrhage (Cunningham and coworkers, 1989). TVS correctly identified placenta previa in 29 of 34 patients compared with only 16 of 34 identified transabdominally (Farine and coworkers, 1990). This group clearly identified the cervical canal and internal os in all 77 cases by TVS, whereas only 70% (54 cases) were identified by TAS. Although classic obstetric teaching has prohibited any vaginal manipulation in the presence of placenta previa, the safe use of TVS in patients with placenta previa has been confirmed (Farine and coworkers, 1990; Sherman and coworkers, 1992; Guy and coworkers, 1990; Timor-Tritsch and Yunis, 1993). Timor-Tritsch and Yunis

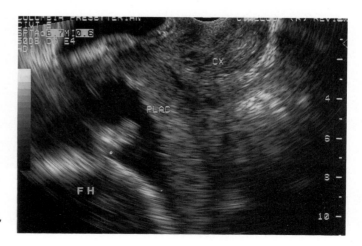

FIGURE 11-22
Sagittal TVS image of placenta previa. *Cx*, cervix; *Plac*, placenta; *FH*, fetal head.

(1993) measured the angle between the axis of the cervix and that of the vaginal probe and concluded that the angle between the cervix and probe was at least 44°, an angle which is sufficient to prevent the probe from inadvertently slipping into the cervix.

Observance of turbulent blood flow within the placenta or at the uteroplacental junction has been described using gray scale TVS in an attempt to differentiate placenta previa from placenta accreta (Sherman and coworkers, 1992; Guy and coworkers, 1990). Guy and coworkers (1990) first used TVS to antenatally diagnose placenta accreta in a group of 16 patients with suspected placenta previa at term. The presence of lacunar flow in seven of the 16 patients predicted a higher incidence of blood loss, transfusion requirement, abnormally implanted placenta, and cesarean hysterectomy when compared with the patients in whom no lacunar flow patterns were seen. These authors have speculated that this leads to "carved out" areas that serve as blood conduits and which may bleed extensively at delivery. With the recent development of color-coded blood flow and Doppler studies, the evaluation of uteroplacental blood flow patterns of abnormally located and suspected adherent placentas is a logical next step. A recent study performed by our group evaluated the efficacy of TVS and color-coded blood flow and found it valuable in the prediction of placenta accreta (Lerner and coworkers, 1994). A pattern of intense and turbulent blood flow extending from the placenta into the surrounding uterine and cervical tissues should alert the physician to the possibility of placenta accreta (Fig. 11-23).

Vasa previa, in which a placental blood vessel crosses the cervix in the area of the internal os, is another complication of pregnancy that may be able to be diagnosed using TVS and color Doppler studies (Fig. 11-24). Although no placenta previa may be present in this situation, timely antenatal diagnosis is important to ensure a successful clinical outcome.

The implication of diagnosing placenta previa, vasa previa, and placenta previa with accreta antenatally is that the patient may be extensively counseled and an appropriate surgical plan made; the incidence of these placental abnormalities does not decrease with this knowledge. TVS improves the diagnostic accuracy in the prediction of both placenta previa and accreta and should replace TAS as the gold standard diagnostic modality for these indications.

SUMMARY

Transvaginal sonography has become the gold standard imaging modality in gynecology and early pregnancy. It appears from the preliminary work of Bronshtein and other researchers that TVS is feasible for the structural evaluation of the fetus at an earlier gestational age than is possible by the traditional transabdominal approach. Due to its inherent limitations, TVS applied during the second and third trimesters of pregnancy has been limited and specific in its goals, for example, in a patient with oligohydramnios. Even though TVS cannot replace the transabdominal approach in all settings during the second and third trimesters of pregnancy, the expanding experience points to diverse uses.

One of the important uses of TVS during the second and third trimester of pregnancy is high-

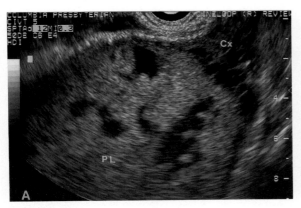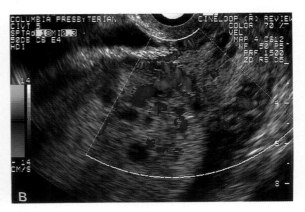

FIGURE 11-23
Grey scale (**A**) and color-enhanced (**B**) TVS images of placenta previa accreta. (**A**) Multiple placental lakes are seen and there is no clear placental-myometrial interface. *Cx*, cervix; *Pl*, placenta. (**B**) These placental lakes are highlighted by color Doppler TVS.

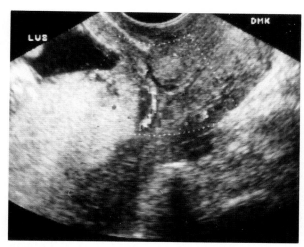

FIGURE 11-24
Transvaginal color Doppler study showing placenta previa with a blood vessel overlying the internal cervical os (placenta vasa previa).

resolution imaging of the fetal intracranial structures in the sagittal and coronal planes. Although these planes can often be obtained with TAS as well, there may be technical difficulties in TAS imaging due to maternal or fetal factors precluding adequate visualization. We believe that this new approach will become part of the routine fetal neurologic examination, especially when a previous history of a fetal nervous system anomaly or predisposing factors for such conditions are present.

There is renewed interest in the study of different aspects of cervical anatomy using TVS. More research regarding prediction of inducibility at term or prediction of preterm labor is needed to corroborate the limited but well-documented literature on the subject.

Clearly superior to TAS for the evaluation of abnormally located placentae, TVS is now being employed consistently for this indication.

The future role of TVS in the second and third trimesters of pregnancy is developing, and may become universally used and fully integrated into our diagnostic program.

REFERENCES

Achiron R, Tadmor O. Screening for fetal anomalies during the first trimester of pregnancy: Transvaginal versus transabdominal sonography. Ultrasound Obstet Gynecol 1991;1:186.

Achiron R, Weissman A, Rotstein Z, Lipitz S, Mashiach S, Hegesh J. Transvaginal echocardiographic examination of the fetal heart between 13 and 15 weeks' gestation in a low-risk population. J Ultrasound Med 1994;13:783.

Andersen HF. Transabdominal and transvaginal sonography of the uterine cervix during pregnancy. JCU 1991a;19:77.

Andersen HF, Ansbacher R. Ultrasound: A new approach to the evaluation of cervical ripening. Semin Perinatol 1991b;15(2):140.

Andersen HF, Nugent CE, Wanty SD, et al. Prediction of risk for preterm delivery by ultrasonographic measurement of cervical length. Am J Obstet Gynecol 1990;163:589.

Ayers J, DeGrood R, Compton A, Barclay M, Ansbacher R. Sonographic evaluation of the cervical length in pregnancy: Diagnosis and management of preterm cervical effacement in patients at risk for premature delivery. Obstet Gynecol 1988;71:939.

Bartolucci L, Hill W, Katz M, Gill P, Kitzmiller J. Ultrasonography in preterm labor. Am J Obstet Gynecol 1984;149:52.

Benacerraf BR, Estroff JA. Transvaginal sonographic imaging of the low fetal head in the second trimester. J Ultrasound Med 1989;8:325.

Bernstine RL, Lee SH, Crawford WL, et al. Sonographic evaluation of the incompetent cervix. JCU 1981;9:417.

Bishop EH. Pelvic scoring for elective induction. Obstet Gynecol 1964;24:266.

Boozarjomehri F, Timor-Tritsch IE, Chao CR, Fox HE. Transvaginal sonographic evaluation of the cervix in labor: Presence of cervical wedging is associated with shorter duration of induced labor. Am J Obstet Gynecol 1994;171(4):1081.

Bowie JD, Andreotti RF, Rosenberg EL. Sonographic appearance of the uterine cervix in pregnancy: The vertical cervix. Am J Roentgenology 1983;737.

Bronshtein M. Transvaginal assessment of fetal anomalies. Presented at the Fourth Congress of the International Society of Ultrasound in Obstetrics and Gynecology, Budapest, October 20, 1994.

Bronshtein M, Bar-Hava I, Blumenfeld I, Bejar J, Toder V, Blumenfeld Z. The difference between septated and nonseptated nuchal cystic hygroma in the early second trimester. Obstet Gynecol 1993a;81(5):683.

Bronshtein M, Bar-Hava I, Blumenfeld Z. Differential diagnosis of the nonvisualized fetal urinary bladder by transvaginal sonography in the early second trimester. Obstet Gynecol 1993b;82(40):490.

Bronshtein M, Keret D, Deutsch M, Liberson A, Bar-Hava I. Transvaginal sonographic detection of skeletal anomalies in the first and early second trimesters. Prenat Diagn 1993c;13:597.

Bronshtein M, Mashiah N, Blumenfeld I, Blumenfeld Z. Pseudoprognathism: An auxiliary ultrasonographic sign for transvaginal ultrasonographic diagnosis of cleft lip and palate in the early second trimester. Am J Obstet Gynecol 1991a;165:1314.

Bronshtein M, Zimmer E, Gershoni-Baruch R, Yoffe N, Meyer H, Blumenfeld Z. First and second trimester diagnosis of fetal ocular defects and associated anomalies: Report of eight cases. Obstet Gynecol 1991b; 77(3):443.

Brook I, Feingold M, Schwartz A. Ultrasonography in the diagnosis of cervical incompetence in pregnancy: A new diagnostic approach. Br J Obstet Gynecol 1981; 88:640.

Brown JE, Thiema GA, Shah DM, Fleischer AC, Boehm FH: Transabdominal and transvaginal endosonography: Evaluation of the cervix and lower uterine segment in pregnancy. Am J Obstet Gynecol 1986;155: 721.

Cardoza JD, Goldstein RB, Filly RA. Exclusion of fetal ventriculomegaly with a single measurement of the width of the lateral ventricular atrium. Radiology 1988;169:711.

Chari R, Bhargava R, Hammond I, et al. Antenatal unilateral hydrocephalus. Can Assoc Radiol J 1993;44:57.

Chevernak FA, Berkowitz RL, Tortora M, et al. The management of fetal hydrocephalus. Am J Obstet Gynecol 1985;151:933.

Chi JG, Dooling EC, Gilles FH. Gyral development of the human brain. Ann Neurol 1977;1:86.

Confino E, Mayden KL, Giglia RV, et al. Pitfalls in sonographic imaging of the incompetent uterine cervix. Acta Obstet Gynecol Scand 1986;65:593.

Cunningham FG, MacDonald PC, Gant NF, eds. Obstetrical hemorrhage: Placenta previa. In: Williams Obstetrics. Norwalk, CT: Appleton & Lange, 1989:714.

Dhall K, Mittal SC, Kumar A. Evaluation of pre-induction scoring systems. Aust N Z J Obstet Gynaecol 1987; 27:309.

Denkhaus H, Winsberg F. Ultrasonic measurement of the fetal ventricular system. Radiology 1979;131:781.

Dorovini-Zis K, Dolman CL. Gestational development of brain. Arch Pathol Lab Med 1977;101:192.

Drugan A, Krause B, Canady A, et al. The natural history of prenatally diagnosed cerebral ventriculomegaly. JAMA 1989;261:1785.

Farine D, Peisner DB, Timor-Tritsch IE. Placenta previa: Is the traditional diagnostic approach satisfactory? JCU 1990;18:328.

Feingold M, Brook I, Zakut H. Detection of cervial incompetence by ultrasound. Acta Obstet Gynecol Scand 1984;63:407.

Filly RA, Cardoza JD, Goldstein RB, Barkovich AJ. Detection of fetal central nervous system anomalies: A practical level of effort for a routine sonogram. Radiology 1989;172:403.

Filly RA, Goldstein RB, Callen PW. Fetal ventricle: Importance in routine obstetric sonography. Radiology 1991;181:1.

Fleischer AC, Lombardi S, Keppze DM. Guidance for cerclage using transrectal sonography. J Ultrasound Med 1989;8:589.

Fried A. Bulging amnion in premature labor: Spectrum of sonographic findings. Am J Roentgenology 1981; 136:181.

Friedman EA, Niswander KR, Bayonet-Rievera NP, et al. Relation of prelabor evaluation to inducibility and the course of labor. Obstet Gynecol 1966;28:495.

Gembruch U, Knopfle G, Bald R, Hansmann M. Early diagnosis of fetal congenital heart disease by transvaginal echocardiography. Ultrasound Obstet Gynecol 1993;3:310.

Glick PL, Harrison MR, Nakayama KD, et al. Management of ventriculomegaly in the fetus. J Pediatr 1984; 105:97.

Gomez R, Galasso M, Romero R, et al. Sonographic examination of the uterine cervix is a better predictor of the likelihood of preterm delivery than digital examination of the cervix in preterm labor with intact membranes. Am J Obstet Gynecol 1994;171(4):956.

Green JR. Placenta previa and abruptio placentae. In: Creasy R, Resnick R, eds. Maternal Fetal Medicine: Principles and Practice. Philadelphia: WB Saunders, 1989:592.

Guy GP, Peisner DB, Timor-Tritsch IE. Ultrasonographic evaluation of uteroplacental blood flow patterns of abnormally located and adherent placentas. Am J Obstet Gynecol 1990;163:723.

Guzman ER, Rosenberg JC, Houlihan C, Ivan J, Waldron R, Knuppel R. A new method using vaginal ultrasound and transfundal pressure to evaluate the asymptomatic incompetent cervix. Obstet Gynecol 1994;83:248.

Habib Z. Genetics and genetic counselling in neonatal hydrocephalus. Obstet Gynecol Surv 1981;36:529.

Hudgins RJ, Edwards MSB, Goldstein R, et al. Natural history of fetal ventriculomegaly. Pediatrics 1988;82: 692.

Hughes MJ, McElin TW, Bird CC. An evaluation of pre-induction scoring systems. Obstet Gynecol 1976;48: 635.

Jackson GM, Ludmir J, Bader TJ. The accuracy of digital examination and ultrasound in the evaluation of cervical length. Obstet Gynecol 1992;79:214.

Jaffe GM, Dee Valle GO, Izquierdo LA, et al. Diagnosis of cervical change in pregnancy by means of transvaginal sonography. Am J Obstet Gynecol 1992; 166:986.

Jeanty P, Dramaix-Wilmet M, Delbeke D, et al. Ultrasonic evaluation of fetal ventricular growth. Neuroradiology 1981;21:127.

Johnson ML, Dunne MG, Mack LA, et al. Evaluation of fetal intracranial anatomy by static and real-time ultrasound. JCU 1980;8:311.

Johnson P, Sharland G, Maxwell D, Allan L. The role of transvaginal sonography in the early detection of congenital heart disease. Ultrasound Obstet Gynecol 1992;2:248.

Kushnir O, Vigil DA, Izquierdo L, Schiff M, Curet LB. Vaginal sonographic assessment of cervical length changes during normal pregnancy. Am J Obstet Gynecol 1990;162:991.

Lerner JP, Deane S, Timor-Tritsch IE. Characterization of placental pathology by using transvaginal sonography and color-coded blood flow. Ultrasound Obstet Gynecol 1994;4:1.

Lim BH, Mahmood TA, Smith NC, Beat I. A prospective comparative study of transvaginal ultrasonography and digital examination of cervical assessment in the third trimester of pregnancy. JCU 1992;20:599.

Lorenz RP, Comstock CH, Bottoms SF. Randomized prospective trial comparing ultrasonography and pelvic examination for preterm labor surveillance. Am J Obstet Gynecol 1990;162:1603.

Ludmir J. Sonographic detection of cervical incompetence. Clin Obstet Gynecol 1988;31:101.

Mason G. Ultrasound assessment of the cervix: The bladder effect (Abstract). Proceedings of the British Medical Ultrasound Society Meeting. December 1989; 119.

Michaels WH, Montgomery C, Karo J, Temple J, Ager J, Olson J. Ultrasound differentiation of the competent from the incompetent cervix: Prevention of preterm delivery. Am J Obstet Gynecol 1986;154:537.

Monteagudo A, Reuss ML, Timor-Tritsch IE. Imaging the fetal brain in the second and third trimester using transvaginal sonography. Obstet Gynecol 1991; 77:27.

Monteagudo A, Timor-Tritsch IE, Moomjy M. In utero detection of ventriculomegaly during the second and third trimesters by transvaginal sonography. Ultrasound Obstet Gynecol 1994;4:193.

Monteagudo A, Timor-Tritsch IE, Moomjy M. Nomograms of the fetal lateral ventricles using transvaginal sonography. J Ultrasound Med 1993;5:265.

Murakawa H, Utami T, Hasegawa I, Tanaka K, Fuzimori R. Evaluation of threatened preterm delivery by transvaginal ultrasonographic measurement of cervical length. Obstet Gynecol 1993;82:829.

Nyberg DA. Recommendations for obstetric sonography in the evaluation of the fetal cranium. Radiology 1989; 172:309.

Nyberg DA, Mack LA, Hirch J, et al. Fetal hydrocephalus: Sonographic detection and clinical significance of associated anomalies. Radiology 1987;82:692.

Okitsu O, Mimura T, Nakayama T, Aono T. Early prediction of preterm delivery by transvaginal ultrasonography. Ultrasound Obstet Gynecol 1992;2:402.

O'Leary JA, Ferrell RE. Comparison of ultrasonographic and digital cervical examination. Obstet Gynecol 1986; 68:718.

Paladini D, Palmieri S. Fetal echocardiography: Transabdominal versus transvaginal approach. Ultrasound Obstet Gynecol 1992;2:145.

Papiernik E, Bonyer J, Collin D, et al. Precocious cervical ripening and preterm labor. Obstet Gynecol 1986;238.

Parulekar SG, Kiwi R. Ultrasound evaluation of sutures following cervical cerclage for incompetent cervix uteri. J Ultrasound Med 1982;1:223.

Parulekar S, Kiwi R. Dynamic incompetent cervix uteri: Sonographic observations. J Ultrasound Med 1988; 7:481.

Pasto ME, Kurtz AB. I. Fetal neurosonography. Ultrasonography of the normal fetal brain. Neuroradiology 1986;28:380.

Paterson-Brown S, Fisk NM, Rodeck CH, Rodeck E. Preinduction cervical assessment by Bishop's score and transvaginal ultrasound. Eur J Obstet Gynecol Reprod Biol 1991;40:17.

Patten RM, Mack LA, Finberg HJ. Unilateral hydrocephalus: Prenatal sonographic diagnosis. AJR 1991;156: 359.

Pilu G, Reece EA, Goldstein I, et al. Sonographic evaluation of the normal developmental anatomy of the fetal cerebral ventricles: II. The atria. Obstet Gynecol 1989;73:250.

Pilu G, Sandri F, Perolo A, et al. Sonography of fetal agenesis of the corpus callosum: A survey of 35 cases. Ultrasound Obstet Gynecol 1993;3:318.

Podobnik M, Bulic M, Smiljanic N, et al. Ultrasonography in the detection of cervical incompetency. JCU 1988; 13:383.

Pretorius DH, Davis K, Manco-Johnson ML, et al. Clinical course of fetal hydrocephalus: 40 cases. AJR 1985; 144:827.

Pretorius DH, Drose JA, Manco-Johnson ML. Fetal lateral ventricular ratio determination during the second trimester. J Ultrasound Med 1986;5:121.

Quinn MJ. Vaginal ultrasound and cervical cerclage: A prospective study. Ultrasound Obstet Gynecol 1992; 2(6):410.

Raner J, Davis Harrigan JT. Improving the outcome of cerclage by sonographic follow-up. J Ultrasound Med 1990;9:275.

Redford DHA, Nicol BD, Willman BK. Diagnosis by real time ultrasound of hourglass herniation of the fetal membranes. Br J Obstet Gynecol 1981;88:73.

Romero R, Pilu G, Jeanty P, et al. The central nervous system. In: Prenatal Diagnosis of Congenital Anomalies. Norwalk, CT: Appleton & Lange, 1988:1.

Rumack CM, Johnson ML. Hydrocephalus. In: Rumack CM, Johnson ML, eds. Perinatal and Infant Brain Imaging. Role of ultrasound and Computed Tomography. Chicago: Year Book, 1984:155.

Sarti DA, Sample WF, Hobel CJ, Staisch KJ. Ultrasonic visualization of dilated cervix during pregnancy. Radiology 1979;130:417.

Sherman SJ, Carlson DE, Platt LD, Medearis AL. Transvaginal ultrasound: Does it help in the diagnosis of placenta previa? Ultrasound Obstet Gynecol 1992;2:256.

Siedler DE, Filly RA. Relative growth of higher fetal brain structures. J Ultrasound Med 1987;6:573.

Smith CV, Anderson JC, Matamoros A, Rayburn WF. Transvaginal sonography of cervical width and length during pregnancy. J Ultrasound Med 1992; 11:465.

Soneck JD, Iams JD, Blumenfeld M, Johnson F, Landon M, Gabbe S. Measurement of cervical length in pregnancy: Comparison between vaginal ultrasonography and digital examination. Obstet Gynecol 1990; 76:172.

Stubbs TM, Van Dorsten P, Miller MC. The preterm cervix and preterm labor: Relative risk, predictive values and change over time. Am J Obstet Gynecol 1986; 155:829.

Timor-Tritsch IE, Monteagudo A. Transvaginal sonographic evaluation of the fetal central system. Obstet Gynecol Clin North Am 1991;18(4):713.

Timor-Tritsch IE, Monteagudo A, Peisner DB. High-frequency transvaginal sonographic examination for the potential malformation assessment of the 9-week to 14-week fetus. JCU 1992;20:231.

Timor-Tritsch IE, Monteagudo A, Warren WB. Transvaginal ultrasonographic definition of the central nervous system in the first and early second trimesters. Am J Obstet Gynecol 1991;164:497.

Timor-Tritsch IE, Yunis R. Confirming the safety of transvaginal sonography in patients suspected of placenta previa. Obstet Gynecol 1993;81:742.

Vaalamo P, Kivikoski A. The incompetent cervix during pregnancy diagnosed by ultrasound. Acta Obstet Gynecol Scand 1983;62:19.

Varma TR, Patel RH, Pillai U. Ultrasonic assessment of cervix in "at risk" patients. Acta Obstet Gynecol Scand 1986a;65:147.

Varma TR, Patel RH, Pillai U. Ultrasonic assessment of cervix in normal pregnancy. Acta Obstet Gynecol Scand 1986b;65:229.

Zemlyn S. The effect of the urinary bladder in obstetrical sonography. Radiology 1978;169:169.

Zimmer E, Bronshtein M. Fetal intra-abdominal cysts detected in the first and early second trimester by transvaginal sonography. JCU 1991;19:564.

Transvaginal Sonography: A Clinical Atlas, Second Edition,
edited by Arthur C. Fleischer and Donna M. Kepple.
J.B. Lippincott Company, Philadelphia, © 1995.

CHAPTER **12**

Transvaginal Color Doppler Sonography in Gynecologic Disorders

Arthur C. Fleischer, MD
Donna M. Kepple, RDMS
Jeanne A. Cullinan, MD

INTRODUCTION

The ability to assess the flow to and within pelvic masses expands the capability of diagnostic sonography to include pathophysiologic parameters (Fig. 12-1). Although differential diagnosis of pelvic masses by their morphology can achieve accuracies in the 80% to 90% range, a secondary test such as transvaginal color Doppler sonography (TV-CDS) is occasionally needed to further characterize masses that have nonspecific morphologic sonographic features (Fig. 12-2) (Granberg and coworkers, 1989). Ovarian masses can be distinguished from uterine masses by depiction of their vascular supplies. In addition, areas of abnormal vascularity (tumor neovascularity) can be used as a means to distinguish benign from malignant masses.

As greater experience with color Doppler sonography (CDS) is obtained, its role in the evaluation of pelvic masses is becoming more clear. Its practical role as an adjunct to morphologic assessment by traditional transvaginal sonography (TVS) in the evaluation of pelvic masses has been verified in several studies (Bourne and coworkers, 1989; Kurjak and coworkers, 1991; Fleischer and coworkers, 1991; Weiner and coworkers, 1992; Kawai and coworkers, 1992; Natori and coworkers, 1992). One study indicated that CDS added important clinical information in approximately 40% of patients being scanned for a pelvic mass (Fleischer and coworkers, 1993).

The information obtained from CDS can potentially add to the clinical management of patients by:

1. Adding confidence for the observation that a mass may be hemorrhagic and may spontaneously regress
2. Confirming the sonographic diagnosis of ovarian torsion that requires immediate surgical intervention
3. Differentiating those patients whose masses

359

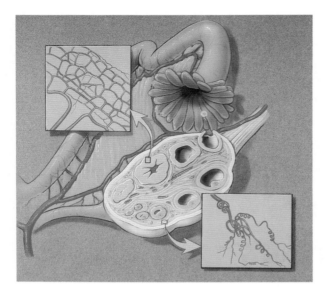

FIGURE 12-1
Diagram showing ovarian arterial vascularity. The ovary has a dual blood supply from the adnexal branch of the uterine artery, which courses along the ovarian ligament, and the main ovarian artery, which courses along the infundibulopelvic ligament. These feeding vessels give off branches that penetrate the capsule of the ovary. The configuration of intraovarian vascularity depends on the presence of follicular development. In areas that do not contain developing follicles, the intraovarian vessels are tortuous and coiled, whereas, if they are within the wall of the corpus luteum, a low impedance vascular arcade develops.

may be treated with a minimally invasive approach (such as pelvoscopic surgery) from those who need standard laparotomy and extensive cancer surgery.

This chapter emphasizes those areas in which Doppler sonography can significantly assist in the differential diagnosis of pelvic masses beyond that information obtained with conventional transabdominal or transvaginal sonography. Other applications, such as evaluation of the endometrium and vascularity of fibroids before and after medical treatment, are discussed. The use of TV-CDS in infertility and early pregnancy is discussed in Chapters 6, 7 and 8.

INSTRUMENTATION AND TECHNIQUE

Doppler sonography can be performed with either transabdominal or transvaginal transducer-probes. Once a line of sight is established, the sample volume should be tailored to the size of the vessel examined. Large feeding vessels should have their entire volume sampled, whereas small intraparenchymal vessels need only the smallest sample volume that encompasses the entire vessel. The waveform shape gives a rough indication of the type of flow within the vessel. With major feeding vessels, the flow has a more uniform velocity, giving a thin-

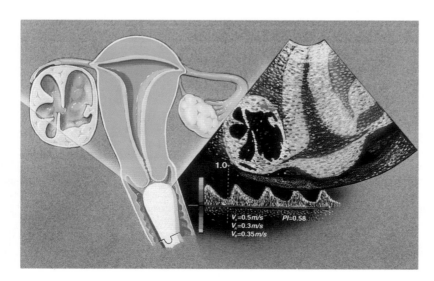

FIGURE 12-2
Diagram of TV-CDS showing three components: transvaginal sonographic image, pulsed-gated Doppler, and waveform analysis.

ner frequency envelope; with smaller intraparenchymal vessels, the flow is more turbulent, giving a larger range of velocities, which is shown by the wider waveform. Resistance is typically higher as the blood flows further into the parenchymal bed.

Maximum systolic velocity can be estimated if the Doppler angle is kept between 20° and 60° of the actual course of the vessel. When the vessel is visualized, angle correction is recommended. Wall filters should be set at a minimum so that the lowest velocities can be determined.

Analysis of waveforms can be accomplished using standard indices such as the resistive index (RI) (maximum systolic velocity minus diastolic peak velocity divided by maximum systolic velocity) or pulsatility index (PI) (maximum systolic velocity minus diastolic velocity divided by the mean velocity). There is some debate concerning which index is more accurate; however, both are sufficient if diastolic flow is present. If diastolic flow is absent or reversed, RI cannot be used and PI is needed. We prefer using PI because it takes into account more of the shape of the waveform. Other indices that can be used include the perfusion index, which is the area under the waveform in systole divided by the area under the waveform in diastole.

Future systems may allow assessment of the relative perfusion similar to that on a scintigraphic camera, with quantification of the number of excited pixel elements per unit time. Infusion of contrast media may also be useful in assessment of perfusion by CDS. Color Doppler power mode is now available on some scanners and provides an overall depiction of vascularity (both arterial and venous).

Transvaginal approach is recommended if the lesion is within 5 to 10 cm of the cul-de-sac. Transabdominal scanning is needed if the lesion is more than 10 cm in size or is superior to the uterine fundus. Gentle pressure can be applied to the mass to determine whether it is intrauterine or extrauterine, adherent or freely mobile.

BASIC DIAGNOSTIC PRINCIPLES

The waveform obtained from Doppler assessment of flow indicates the relative resistance to flow within an organ or area within a particular structure (Fig. 12-3). Waveforms can be analyzed by their RI or PI location and distribution of vessels, maximum systolic velocity, and presence of a diastolic notch.

Figure 12-2 demonstrates TV-CDS of abnormal vessels within an ovarian tumor. Normal arterioles have a layer of muscular lining that is not present in tumors. This muscular lining has a role in regulating

parenchymal perfusion; it is typically associated with a flow pattern that has relatively high pulsatility. With a paucity of this muscular lining seen in tumor vessels, there is continuous diastolic flow and less of a difference in systolic and diastolic peaks and low pulsatility. There usually is a lack of a diastolic notch as well. The presence of a notch usually indicates that the vessel has a muscular layer and, therefore, is a major feeding vessel. When a vessel is vasodilated, the pulsatility is reduced as a reflection of decreased resistance to forward flow. This pattern simulates that of a tumor vessel, although a diastolic notch is typically present.

Tumor vessels typically have high diastolic flow related to the multiple areas of stenosis and vasodilatation within the network of tumor vessels. The velocities may also be increased related to the requirements of tumor perfusion and arteriovenous communications within the network of tumor vessels.

A clear understanding of these principles is needed in analysis of pelvic masses with Doppler sonography. Some nonneoplastic tumors may demonstrate blood flow characteristics of truly malignant masses (Tables 12-1 and 12-2).

Future developments may include more precise determination of the blood flow characteristics of these vessels as depicted by their Doppler waveforms. Also, smaller vessels will be depicted as the resolution and power mode imaging improves. With these improvements, the smaller intraparenchymal borders of the uterus and ovaries, as well as masses within those organs, will become more apparent.

ACCURACY AND SPECIFICITY

Diagnostic accuracies of 90% and higher have been reported in several series in differentiating benign from malignant ovarian lesions using these diagnostic principles (Table 12-3) (Kurjak and coworkers, 1991; Fleischer and coworkers, 1991). In general, true positive (percentage of malignant masses with low impedance) is 90% to 95%, whereas false positives (percentage of benign lesions with low PI) ranges from 0.2% to 20% (Fig. 12-4). Even though TV-CDS may not improve actual detection of mass, it seems to improve specificity in differentiating benign from malignant masses. The figures from these studies substantiate the use of TV-CDS in selected cases as a means to differentiate benign versus malignant masses.

(text continues on page 364)

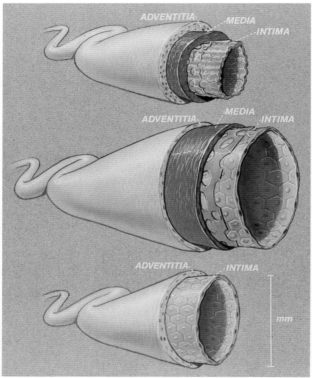
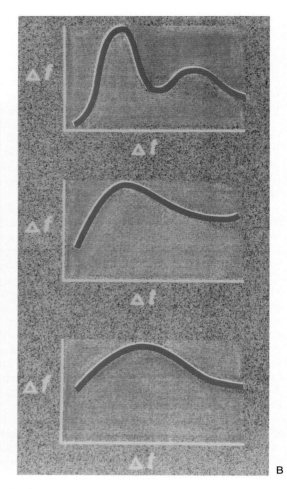

FIGURE 12-3
Correlation of vessels and waveforms. (**A**) Normal small arterioles containing a muscular media that regulates intraparenchymal flow. This thins out as the arteriole progresses distally but is absent in vessels associated with tumors. (**B**) Waveforms. In normal arterioles, there is a significant difference between systolic and diastolic velocity peaks and a "notch" indicating initial resistance to forward flow. On the contrary, tumor vessels have relatively high diastolic flow relative to systolic flow and do not have a notch. Vasodilated vessels have waveforms somewhere between the two extremes.

TABLE 12-1
Typical TV-CDS Parameters

Benign	PI greater than 1.0 (high-impedance flow)
	Flow seen in periphery, not in center
	Diastolic "notch"
Malignant	PI less than 1.0 (low-impedance flow)
	Flow in periphery and center
	Absent diastolic "notch"

PI, pulsatility index.

TABLE 12-2
Typical Impedance of Ovarian Masses

High (PI greater than 1.5)
  Cystadenomas
  Hemorrhagic cysts

Intermediate or variable (PI between 1.0 and 1.5)
  Dermoid cyst
  Endometrioma*

Low (PI less than 1.0)
  Ovarian malignancies
  Inflammatory masses
  Metabolically "active" masses
  Corpus luteum

*May vary with menstrual cycle.

PI, pulsatility index.

362

TABLE 12-3
TV-CDS of Ovarian Masses: Reported Series

PI (Yr)	Number of Patients	Malignant (M)/ Benign (B)	Index	Cut-off Value	Mean RI (PI) (Range) Malignant	# of Stage I CaO	Mean RI (PI) (Range) Benign	Sensitivity (%)	Specificity (%)	Positive Predictive Value (%)	Negative Predictive Value (%)	Accuracy (%)
Kurjak (1989)	20	5/15	RI	0.4	0.33 ± 0.08	5	—	100	97	87	100	98
Bourne (1989)	18	8/10	PI	—	0.3 – 0.9	3	3.2 – 7.0	—	—	—	—	—
Kurjak (1991)	680	56/624	RI	0.4	0.28 – 0.40	16	>0.40	96	99	98	99	99
Fleischer (1991)	43	11/32	PI	1.0	0.8 ± 0.6 (0.7 – 1.0)	7	1.8 ± 0.8 (0.7 – 1.0)	B: 90 M: 100	83	95 73	71 100	92 100
Fleischer (1991)	26	3/23	PI	1.0	0.7 ± 0.2 (0.7 – 1.0)	7	1.9 ± 0.7 (0.6 – 2.8)	B: 90 M: 100	83	95 73	71 100	92 100
Campbell (1992)	7	7/0	PI RI	— —	0.61 (0.40 – 0.96) 0.46 (0.33 – 0.78)	5	— —	—	—	—	—	—
Weiner (1992)	53	17/36	PI	1.0	0.75 – 0.81	4	—	94	97	97	94	—
Kawai (1992)	24	9/15	PI	1.25	0.93 ± 0.65		1.45 ± 0.05	—	—	—	—	—
Hata (1991)	20	8/12	RI	—	0.50 ± 0.12		0.88 ± 0.22	—	—	—	—	—
Timor-Tritsch (1992)	80	13/67	PI RI	— —	0.45 0.48	2	1.15 0.64	—	—	—	—	—
Tekay (1992)	72	11/61	RI RI	0.6 0.5	0.4 – 0.6	1	0.4 – 1.0	82 46	72 89	35 42	96 90	74 82
Kurjak (1992)	83	29/54	PI RI	— 0.4	0.5 – 0.9 0.37 ± 0.08	18	0.5 – 3.5 0.62 ± 0.11	90	95	96	95	—
Hamper (1992)	31	6/24	PI		0.77 ± 0.33 (0.31 – 1.09)		1.93 ± 1.02 (0.23 – 3.99)	97	100	100	99	99
Schneider (1993)	55	16/39	RI	0.8				94	56	47	76	—
Lin (1994)	370	90/280	RI	0.4		21		69	97	89	91	—
Bromley (1993)	33	12/21	RI	0.6		24		91	52	—	—	—
Valentin (1994)	149	28/121	Velocity; PI; morphology			4		—	—	—	—	—
Brown (1994)	44	24/36	PI RI RI	1.0 0.4 0.4				100 50	46 96	—	—	—
Levine (1994)	36	19/17	RI	0.4	0.47 ± 0.1 (0.32 – 0.66)		0.57 ± 0.17 (0.33 – 0.87)	—	—	—	—	—
Wu (1994)	410	103/307	RI	0.4	0.41		0.23 – 0.82	68	97	—	—	—
Wu (1994)	222	70/152	RI	0.4 × epithelial germ cell met Stage I, II, III, IV	0.40 0.36 0.49 0.40		0.68 (follicular) 0.41 (luteal)	—	—	—	—	—
Carter (1994)	167	88/79	Morph. + RI + PI	0.4 1.0	0.6 ± 0.2 2.3 ± 1.5		0.8 ± 0.2 1.1 ± 0.6	83	95	91	90	—

PI, pulsatility index; *RI*, resistive index.

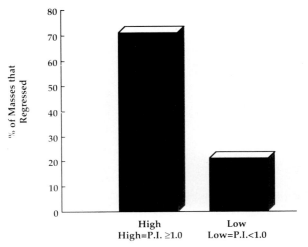

FIGURE 12-4
Initial PI versus regression.

Using cutoff values of PI less than 1.0 as indicative of malignancies, our series documented a high negative predictive value of 98% and nearly as high a positive predictive value of 85% (Fig. 12-5) (Fleischer and coworkers, 1991). Thus, TV-CDS seems to accurately exclude the possibility of malignancy, thereby allowing for less minimally invasive surgery such as pelvoscopic surgery to be considered. Analysis of multiple parameters such as vessel location, maximum systolic velocity, and presence of a notch may also enhance specificity (Fig. 12-6) (Fleischer and coworkers, 1991).

Retrospective analysis of 93 patients who underwent surgery and pathologic evaluation of the excised tissue after TVS and CDS indicates that, in approximately 40% of cases studied, CDS provided enhanced specificity concerning organ of origin and histologic type of mass over those obtained with TVS (Fleischer and coworkers, 1993). In particular, the enhanced specificity of CDS was most evident in detection of the presence of ovarian malignancy, adnexal torsion, and ectopic pregnancy. In 40% of the cases, the specificity of CDS and TVS were considered equal, whereas in 6% of cases, TVS was more specific than CDS. In 14% of cases however, neither CDS nor TVS was histologically specific. These cases included a patient in whom a 2-mm metastatic ovarian cancer was not diagnosed and a necrotic leiomyosarcoma was misdiagnosed as an ovarian neoplasm. Detection of abnormal flow is related to this presence and the extent to which tumor neovascularity is elicited. In lesions less than 3 to 5 mm or in slowly growing areas, neovascularity is not as extensive as in larger and more rapidly growing ones.

The true sensitivity of CDS awaits studies that compare preoperative to postoperative findings in women undergoing surgery for conditions not related to the ovary. This will require studies similar to those done with conventional TVS in women undergoing urologic surgery or hysterectomy and oophorectomy secondary to endometrial carcinoma (Rodriques and coworkers, 1988; Fleischer and coworkers, 1990). In general, the added specificity afforded by CDS substantiates its use in selected cases in which TVS is equivocal or nondiagnostic (Fleischer and coworkers, 1993; Tekay and Jouppila, 1992; Timor-Tritsch and coworkers, 1993; Kurjak and Predanik, 1992; Schneider and coworkers, 1993; Valentin and coworkers, 1994; Bromley and coworkers, 1994).

OVARIAN MASSES

The ovary is the source of a variety of pelvic masses ranging from benign cysts to solid neoplasms (Figs. 12-7 through 12-10). It can also be the site of metastases, usually from gastrointestinal tract primaries. Some pelvic masses may also simulate the appearance of an ovarian mass. These include endometriomas and paraovarian cysts that are adjacent to but not within the substance of the ovary.

The waveforms seen in the ovary vary in women of reproductive age according to the phase of the menstrual cycle. During the menstrual and follicular phase, there is high-resistance flow. With formation of the corpus luteum, low-resistance waveforms are seen as the result of newly formed vessels within the walls of the corpus luteum.

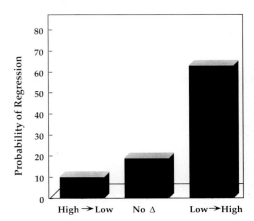

FIGURE 12-5
Change in PI versus probability of regression.

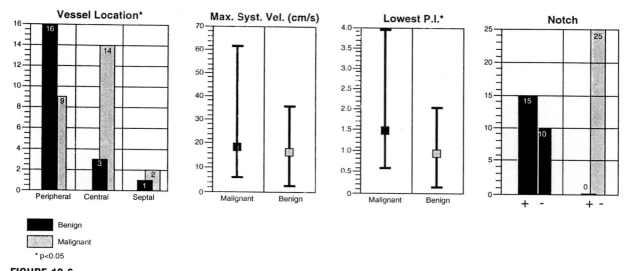

FIGURE 12-6
Malignant masses tended to have central flow, higher maximum systolic velocities, lower PI, and lacked a diastolic notch. (Fleischer A. J Ultra Med, 1993;12:41.)

Although the morphology as depicted by conventional TVS can be used in most cases to determine their probable histologic composition, there are overlaps that an adjunctive test such as CDS can be helpful in further clarifying the cause of some pelvic masses. For example, complex masses containing cystic and solid areas may represent either benign hemorrhagic corpus lutea or ovarian tumors (see Figs. 12-7 through 12-9). Some irregularities in the wall of a mass may be due to benign causes such as dermoid cysts or may be a reflection of malignant change. Thus, CDS is most useful in cases that have nonspecific morphologic features as well as in cases in which torsion is suspected.

The waveforms obtained from vessels using Doppler sonography give a general impression on the distribution and characterization of blood flow to and within ovarian masses. The feeding arteries, mainly the adnexal branch of the uterine artery, and the main ovarian artery have a muscular coating that is present in both benign and malignant lesions. However, vessels located within the mass typically are low-flow, high-impedance, except the corpus luteum. In the corpus luteum, vessels along the wall have a paucity of muscular lining and high diastolic flow, which is suggestive of tumor neovascularity.

In patients in whom a corpus luteum is suspected clinically, it is highly recommended that these patients be rescanned in the late menstrual phase of the next cycle to exclude the possibility of a corpus luteum. If low-impedance flow persists after rescanning or cessation of hormone replacement medications, an abnormal mass is probably present and surgery indicated. Alternatively, patients with persistent masses may be given a trial of norethenrone, a luteolytic agent that can accelerate involution of corpora lutea.

A variety of lesions may demonstrate low-impedance, high-diastolic flow (see Table 12-2). These include inflammatory masses (e.g., tubo-ovarian abscesses), actively hemorrhaging luteal cysts, and some dermoid cysts. These masses have in common enlarged and vasodilated normal vessels that can simulate the flow pattern seen in some ovarian tumors (see Fig. 12-9). It is important to determine whether the waveform has a diastolic notch because this is an indication that there is initial resistance to forward flow offered by the muscular lining of the arteriole. Because resistance typically decreases as the vessel courses toward the center of an organ, the absence of a notch in a feeder vessel may have higher predictive value than if the waveform was obtained from an intraparenchymal branch.

Malignancies tend to demonstrate color Doppler flow in the solid areas in the center portion of the mass or in papillary excrescences or irregular areas of the wall (see Fig. 12-9). This flow typically has low pulsatility (PI <1.0) that lacks a diastolic notch (Fleischer and coworkers, 1993). Some metabolically active tumors and germ cell tumors demonstrate this pattern as well.

A group of lesions demonstrates a range of Doppler flow from high resistance to low resistance.

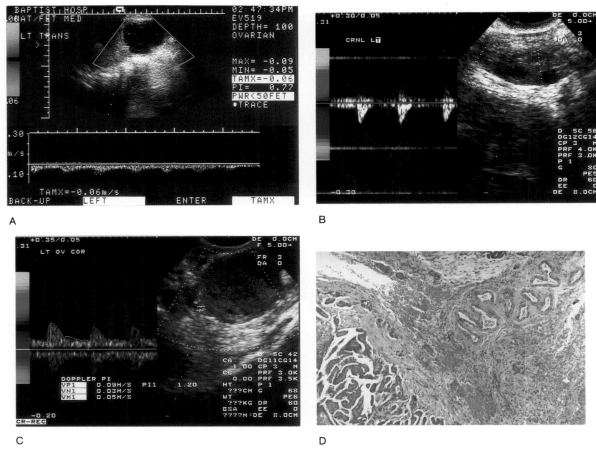

FIGURE 12-7
Hemorrhagic cysts. (**A**) A 3-cm hypoechoic mass with relatively low impedance. (**B**) Same patient as in *A* followed up after 6 weeks. There is high-impedance flow within the ovary and total regression of the hemorrhagic mass. (**C**) Hypoechoic area within an enlarged ovary containing areas of intermediate-impedance flow. (**D**) Low-power photomicrograph of *C* showing hemosiderin deposits indicative of chronic hemorrhage.

These lesions include dermoid cysts and endometriomas. Dermoid cysts may have low-impedance flow when they are actively dividing cells within the dermoid cysts as opposed to their relatively stagnant growth in established masses. Endometriomas may demonstrate low-impedance flow when there is hemorrhage in the menstrual phase of the cycle.

Although there are only approximately 50 stage I cancers detectable by CDS, most of these are recognizable by their characteristic low pulsatility flow patterns (Kurjak and coworkers, 1991, 1993). In one study, 16 of 17 malignancies had a PI less than 1, whereas benign lesions had a PI greater than 1 in 35 of 36 examples (Weiner and coworkers, 1992). The overall accuracy of color Doppler sonography appears to be better than that of CA-125 testing and probably is greatest in rapidly growing tumors that require significant blood flow, such as in some aggressive stage I and II lesions.

EXTRA-OVARIAN MASSES

A variety of lesions may mimic the morphologic and Doppler features of ovarian masses (Figs. 12-11 and 12-12). These include pedunculated uterine fibroids, some tubal masses, paraovarian cysts, and, rarely, bowel lesions (see Fig. 12-12). Gentle pressure with the probe may be used between the uterus and the mass to differentiate pedunculated uterine lesions

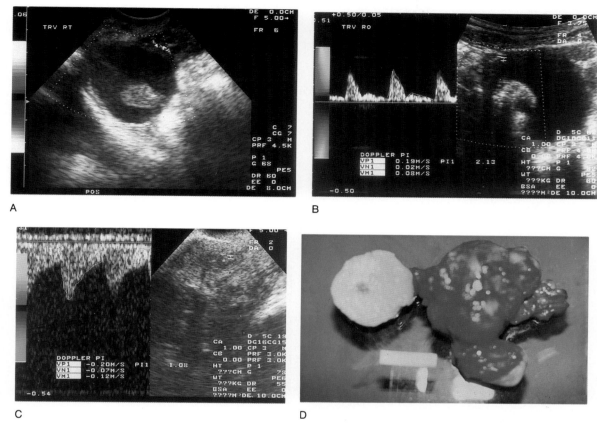

FIGURE 12-8
Dermoid cysts. (**A**) Hypovascular dermoid cyst with solid plug showing minimal flow within the wall. (**B**) Mildly vascular dermoid cyst containing echogenic solid plug and high-impedance flow in the periphery. (**C**) Solid dermoid cyst with low-impedance flow. (**D**) Gross specimen of C showing solid areas.

from those arising in the adnexa. Vascular fibroids tend to have low pulsatility characteristics similar to ovarian neoplasms. Tubal cancers, although rare, may also demonstrate low pulsatility. Paraovarian lesions tend to be cystic and, when infected, may have low pulsatility. Some bowel lesions may simulate the appearance of adnexal pathology due to their multiloculated appearance if matted. Diverticular abscesses and inflammatory bowel lesions may also have low-impedance flow.

ADNEXAL OVARIAN TORSION

One of the major applications of CDS is in the diagnosis of ovarian torsion. Although the ovary has a dual blood supply, torsion typically affects flow from both the ovarian artery and the adnexal branch of the uterine artery. Typically, there is absent arterial flow within an enlarged ovary. This may demonstrate irregular solid areas related to hemorrhage, which may precipitate the torsion initially (Fig. 12-13). There may be high-resistance flow in the hilar vessels and, in some cases, venous flow in the capsular vessels as well.

The optimal time for diagnosing ovarian torsion is before development of gangrenous changes. This may result in some hypoperfused lesions to be overdiagnosed as torsion, but these lesions may be amenable to early surgical intervention anyway.

(text continues on page 377)

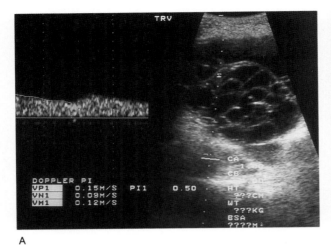

A

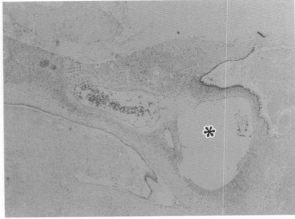

B

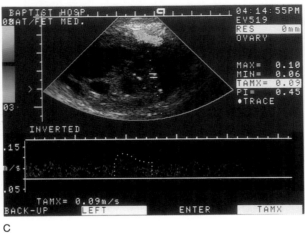

C

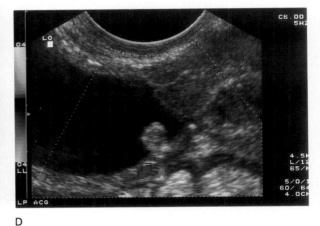

D

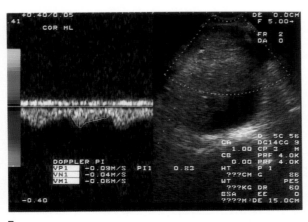

E

FIGURE 12-9
Ovarian tumors. (**A**) Cystadenocarcinoma shown by low-impedance flow within an irregular septum. (**B**) Low-power photomicrograph of *A* showing abnormal vessel (*asterisk*) within septation, which lacks a muscular media. (**C**) Solid tumor with low-impedance flow in a granulosa cell tumor. (**D**) Cystadenofibroma with solid papillary excrescence demonstrating focal area of flow at the base of the excrescence. (**E**) Cystadenocarcinoma with solid area showing low-impedance flow. (*continued*)

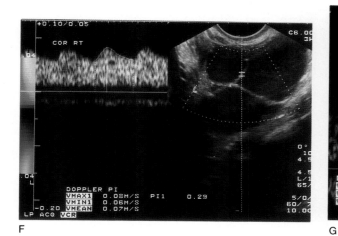

F

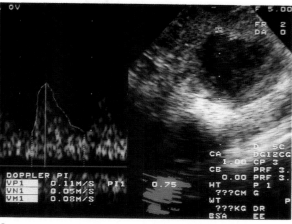

G

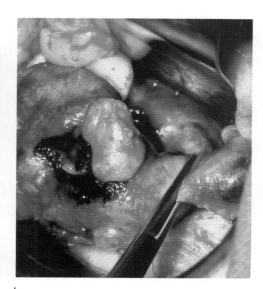

I

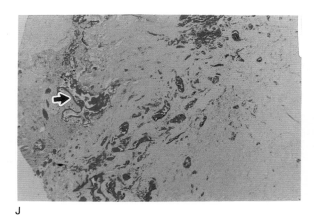

H

J

FIGURE 12-9 *(Continued)*
(F) Mucinous cystadenoma with focal area of low impedance within septation in a pregnant patient. **(G)** Mildly enlarged ovary containing irregular solid areas with low-impedance flow. **(H)** Same patient as in *G* showing extension of tumor into dilated left fallopian tube. **(I)** Intraoperative photograph of same patient as in *G* and *H* showing enlarged dilated tube and tumor. **(J)** Low-power photomicrograph showing abnormal vessels *(arrow)*. *(continued)*

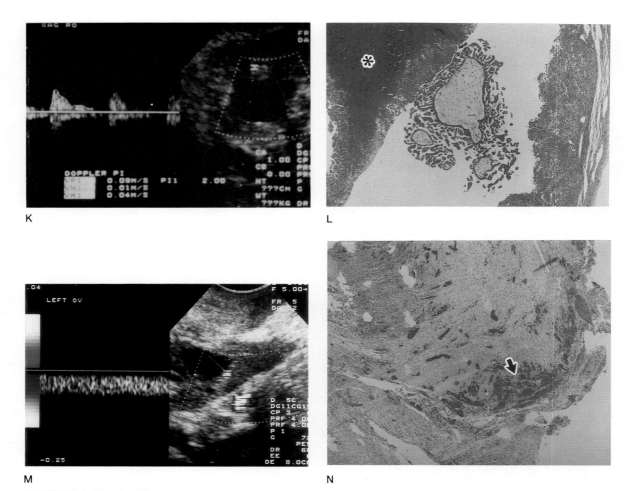

FIGURE 12-9 *(Continued)*
(**K**) Area of high-impedance flow surrounding a follicle in a patient with bowel mass and elevated CA-125 level. (**L**) Low-power photomicrograph showing tumor (*asterisk*) within the wall of the follicle. (**M**) Cystic mass with irregular solid wall demonstrating venous-like flow. (**N**) Low-power photomicrograph of mass in *M* showing tumor sinusoids (*arrow*).

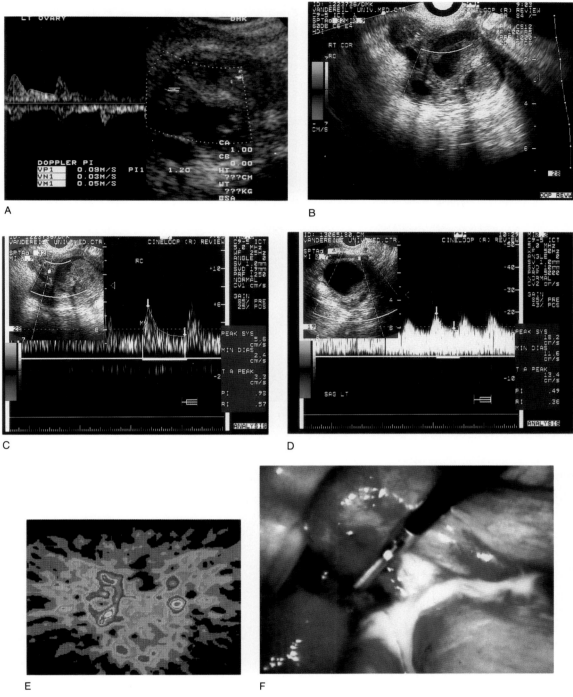

FIGURE 12-10

Inflammatory masses. (**A**) Tubo-ovarian abscess showing intermediate-impedance flow within a solid area. Note the notch in the diastole. (**B**) CDS showing flow within the wall of a multiloculated right adnexal mass. (**C**) Triplex image of *B* showing low-impedance flow. (**D**) Triplex image of *B* and *C* showing low-impedance flow. (**E**) Position emission tomography (PET) scan showing hypermetabolic (blue colored) areas in bilateral tubo-ovarian abscesses. (**F**) Intraoperative photograph showing pus exuding from a tubo-ovarian abscess.

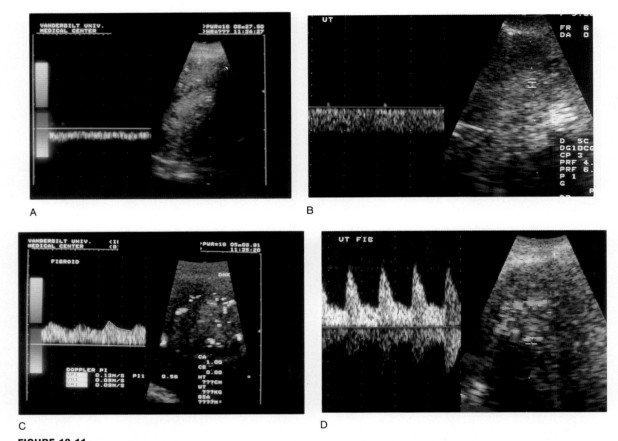

FIGURE 12-11
Uterine disorders. (**A**) Thickened endometrium and venous flow in hyperplastic endometrium. (**B**) Similar findings in a patient with dilatation and curettage proven endometrial carcinoma. (**C**) Relatively vascular intramural fibroid. (**D**) Submucosal fibroid with intermediate-impedance flow. (*continued*)

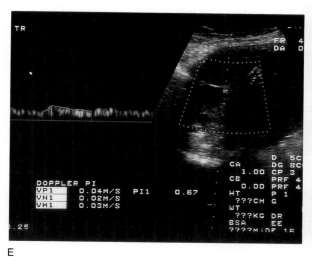

E

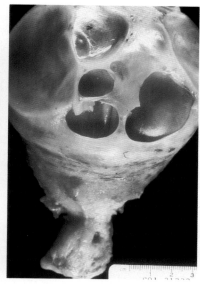

F

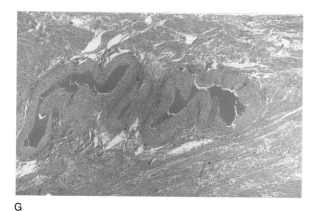

G

FIGURE 12-11 *(Continued)*
(E) Cystic uterine mass with low-impedance, low-velocity flow.
(F) Gross specimen of *D*. **(G)** Low-power photomicrograph of
D and *E* showing dilated vessels with muscular media. **(H)**
Intraligamentous leiomyoma with low-impedance flow. **(I)**
Same patient as in *H* showing dilated vessels (*curved arrow*).

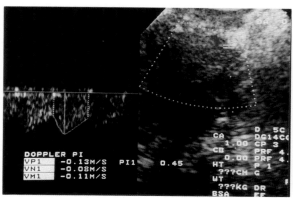

H

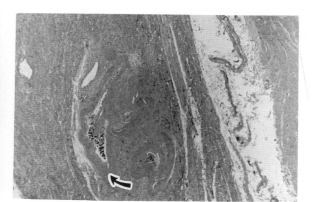

I

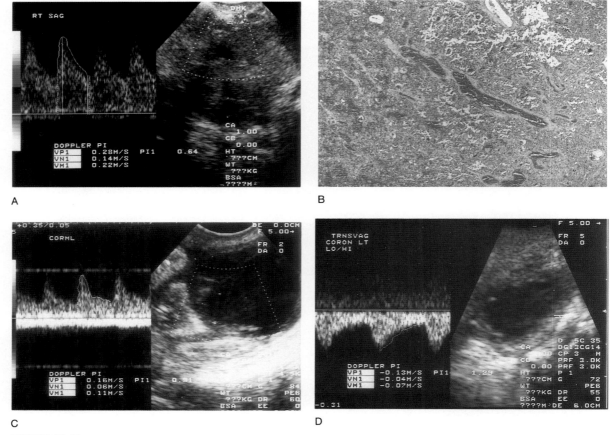

FIGURE 12-12
Miscellaneous disorders. (**A**) Hypervascular solid mass arising from the omentum, representing omental metastases. (**B**) Low-power photomicrograph showing numerous vessels. (**C**) Cystic mass related to bowel showing low-impedance flow, representing an appendiceal abscess. (**D**) Diverticular abscess showing low-impedance flow within its wall.

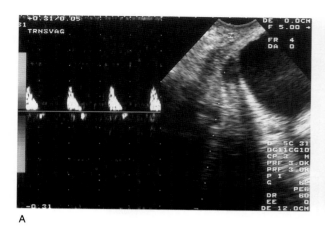

A

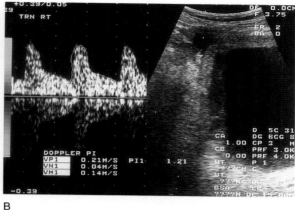

B

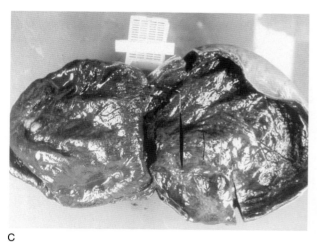

C

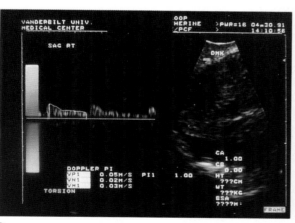

D

FIGURE 12-13
Ovarian torsion. (**A**) Complex mass showing high-impedance flow along the periphery. (**B**) Same patient as in *A* showing intermediate-impedance flow. (**C**) Twisted hemorrhagic ovary. (**D**) Enlarged ovary showing low-impedance, low-velocity flow in adnexal branch. (**E**) Gangrenous ovary of the patient shown in *D*. (*continued*)

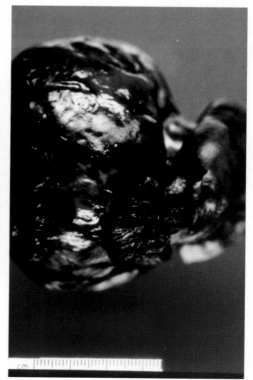

E

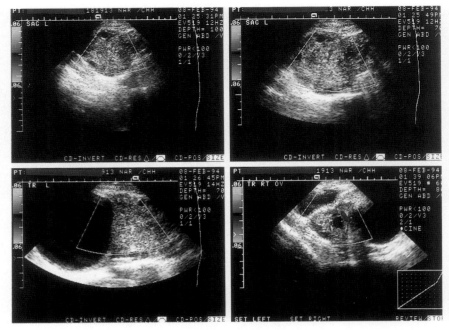

F

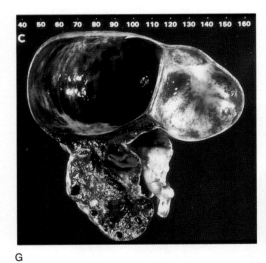

G

FIGURE 12-13 *(Continued)*
(F) Composite TV-CDS showing a cysic mass arising from an enlarged left ovary. The right ovary was normal and depicted in bottom right frame. Both ovaries demonstrate flow. **(G)** Sectioned specimen through the left ovary of the patient in *F* showing a multiloculated ovarian tumor that was twisted. (Courtesy of Mary Warner, M.D.)

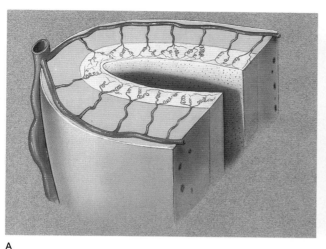

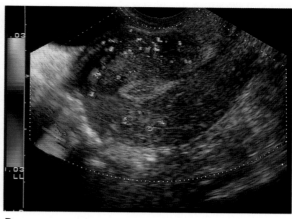

A   B

FIGURE 12-14
Uterine arterial perfusion. (**A**) The main uterine artery gives off arcuate branches that course in a spoke wheel configuration. The radial branches course through the myometrium, ending in spiral branches within the endometrium. (**B**) TVS in a normal uterus showing flow within arcuate and radial branches.

UTERINE DISORDERS

Transvaginal color Doppler sonography can depict hypovascular areas within the endometrium and myometrium associated with endometrial cancer. It can also display the relative vascularity of submucosal fibroids or polyps (Fig. 12-14; see Fig. 12-11). In general, relatively vascularized fibroids tend to be more responsive to GnRH analog treatment than hypovascular ones (Matta and coworkers, 1988).

SUMMARY

Color Doppler sonography is most useful in differentiating morphologically similar masses such as hemorrhagic corpora lutea from ovarian neoplasms. It has a primary role in evaluating ovarian torsion. The areas of overlap in benign versus malignant lesions tend to involve masses that contain vasodilated vessels or those that are actively hemorrhaging. Future developments include more sensitive

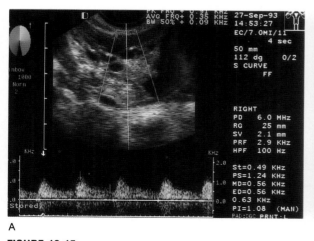

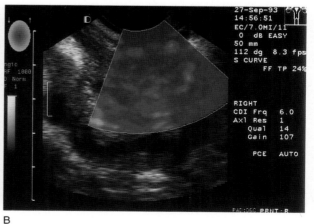

A   B

FIGURE 12-15
Color Doppler energy mode imaging. (**A**) Conventional TV-CDS of an enlarged right ovary containing areas of low-impedance flow. (**B**) Color Doppler flow imaging of the same ovary. The lighter areas of color represent intraovarian flow.

detection of vessels so that overall areas of perfusion can be studied (Fig. 12-15).

REFERENCES

Bourne T, Campbell S, Steer C, Whitehead MI, Collins WP. Transvaginal color flow imaging: A possible new screening technique for ovarian cancer. BMJ 1989; 299:1367.

Bromley B, Goodman H, Benacerraf BR. Comparison between sonographic morphology and Doppler waveform for the diagnosis of ovarian malignancy. Obstet Gynecol 1994;83:434.

Fleischer A, Cullinan J, Kepple D, Williams L. Conventional or color Doppler sonography of pelvic masses: Relative specificity. J Ultrasound Med 1993;12:705.

Fleischer AC, Kepple DM, Rodgers W. Color Doppler sonography of ovarian masses: A multiparameter analysis. J Ultrasound Med 1993;12:41.

Fleischer AC, McKee MS, Gordon AN, et al. Transvaginal sonography of postmenopausal ovaries with pathologic correlation. J Ultrasound Med 1990;9:637.

Fleischer AC, Rodgers WH, Rao BK, et al. Assessment of ovarian tumor vascularity with transvaginal color Doppler sonography. J Ultrasound Med 1991;10:563.

Granberg S, Wikland M, Jansson I. Macroscopic characterization of ovarian tumors and the relation to the histological diagnosis: Criteria to be used for ultrasound evaluation. Gynecol Oncol 1989;35:139.

Kawai M, Kano T, Kikkawa F, Maeda O, Oguchi H, Tomoda Y. Transvaginal Doppler ultrasound with color flow imaging in the diagnosis of ovarian cancer. Obstet Gynecol 1992;79:163.

Kurjak A, Predanic M. New scoring system for prediction of ovarian malignancy based on transvaginal color Doppler sonography. J Ultrasound Med 1992;11:631.

Kurjak A, Shalan H, Matijevic R, Predanic M, Kupesic-

Urek A. Stage I ovarian cancer by transvaginal color Doppler sonography: A report of 18 cases. Ultrasound Obstet Gynecol 1993;3:1.

Kurjak A, Zalud I, Alfirevic Z. Evaluation of adnexal masses with transvaginal color ultrasound. J Ultrasound Med 1991;10:295.

Matta WH, Stabile I, Shaw RW, Campbell S. Doppler assessment of uterine blood flow changes in patients with fibroids receiving the gonadotrophin releasing hormone agonist buserelin. Fertil Steril 1988;49:1083.

Natori M, Kouno H, Nozawa S. Flow velocity waveform analysis for the detection of ovarian cancer. Medical Review 1992;40:45.

Rodriques MH, Platt LD, Medearis AL, Lacarra M, Lobo RA. The use of transvaginal sonography for evaluation of postmenopausal ovarian size and morphology. Am J Obstet Gynecol 1988;159:810.

Schneider VL, Schneider A, Reed KL, Hatch KD. Comparison of Doppler with two-dimensional sonography and CA 125 for prediction of malignancy of pelvic masses. Obstet Gynecol 1993;81:983.

Tekay A, Jouppila P. Validity of pulsatility and resistance indices in classification of adnexal tumors with transvaginal color Doppler ultrasound. Ultrasound Obstet Gynecol 1992;2:338.

Timor-Tritsch IE, Lerner JP, Monteagudo A, Santos R. Transvaginal ultrasonographic characterization of ovarian masses by means of color flow-directed Doppler measurements and a morphologic scoring system. Am J Obstet Gynecol 1993;168:909.

Valentin L, Sladkevicius P, Marsal K. Limited contribution of Doppler velocimetry to the differential diagnosis of extrauterine pelvic tumors. Obstet Gynecol 1994; 83:425.

Weiner Z, Thaler I, Beck D, Rottem S, Deutsch M, Brandes JM. Differentiating malignant from benign ovarian tumors with transvaginal color flow imaging. Obstet Gynecol 1992;79:159.

Transvaginal Sonography: A Clinical Atlas, Second Edition,
edited by Arthur C. Fleischer and Donna M. Kepple.
J.B. Lippincott Company, Philadelphia, © 1995.

CHAPTER **13**

Transvaginal Color Doppler Sonography in Early Pregnancy

Arthur C. Fleischer, MD
Donna M. Kepple, RDMS
Jeanne A. Cullinan, MD

INTRODUCTION

Transvaginal color Doppler sonography (TV-CDS) affords delineation of choriodecidual and corpus luteum flow in normal intrauterine pregnancy. It can also demonstrate vascularity within the adnexa associated with ectopic pregnancies (Tekay and coworkers, 1993; Emerson and coworkers, 1992; Atri and coworkers, 1992; Kurjak and coworkers, 1994). The relative activity of trophoblasts can be implied by the vascularity as depicted by TV-CDS. In addition, TV-CDS can depict abnormal placental invasion of the myometrium. This chapter discusses applications of TV-CDS in early pregnancy, namely the detection of abnormal pregnancies, including ectopic and nonviable intrauterine pregnancies.

The power intensities used in TV-CDS are less than the limits established by the Food and Drug Administration (i.e., 94 mW/cm²). The use of CDS may actually decrease the overall exposure levels because the colorized areas are targeted for pulsed Doppler interrogation rather than being searched blindly with a sample volume over the same area.

INTRAUTERINE PREGNANCY

Before an embryo is detected, CDS shows a relative increase in flow to the myometrium and endometrium (Kurjak and coworkers, 1994). Specifically, endometrial veins are most readily identified near the developing choriodecidual sac. Between 6 and 12 weeks of gestation, there is a gradual increase in maximum systolic velocities in the arterioles within the choriodecidua. However, this increase in systolic velocity cannot be used in differentiating types of failed intrauterine pregnancies, such as incomplete abortions or molar pregnancies (Arduini and coworkers, 1990).

Once an embryo is identified, flow within the fetal heart and umbilical cord can be identified. In the fetus of more than 10 weeks, flow within the

cranium, specifically, arteries comprising the circle
of Willis, can be seen. The major visceral vessels
such as the abdominal aorta or inferior vena cava
can also be seen. The flow within umbilical arteries of the cord demonstrates absent or reversed
diastolic flow, typically until the 12th to 14th
week. Figures 13-1 and 13-2 show intrauterine pregnancies.

ECTOPIC PREGNANCY

Transvaginal color Doppler sonography provides an
adjunct to the conventional evaluation for ectopic
pregnancy with transvaginal sonography (TVS)
(Emerson and coworkers, 1992). CDS provides flow
information concerning the endometrium, myometrium, and adnexa.

In the adnexa, a vascular ring of flow, which is
separate from the ovary, is seen in ectopic pregnancies. The actual waveform can demonstrate a variety
of patterns, including high-resistance to low-
resistance type flow. CDS findings of the corpus
luteum should not be mistaken for an ectopic pregnancy. Corpora lutea can be identified within the
ovary as areas of low-impedance flow that are
within the ovary.

The transformed decidua within the uterus in
ectopic pregnancies demonstrates high-resistance
flow; arterioles within the decidua in an intrauterine
pregnancy demonstrate increased diastolic flow.

The diagnostic sensitivity of sonography for the
detection of ectopic pregnancies can be improved
by using TV-CDS (Emerson and coworkers, 1992).
In addition, abnormal early pregnancies can be distinguished from failing intrauterine pregnancies.
Figure 13-3 shows ectopic pregnancies.

TROPHOBLASTIC DISEASE

Complete hydatidiform moles may demonstrate
vesicular changes within the myometrium. This
is usually accompanied by increased flow as evidenced on TV-CDS (Tekay and coworkers, 1993).
This finding is also seen in cases of recurrent trophoblastic disease with invasion within the myometrium. Figure 13-4 depicts trophoblastic disease.

ABNORMAL PLACENTATION

Transvaginal color Doppler sonography is useful in
the detection of placenta accreta, and percreta (see
Fig. 13-4E). These conditions vary as to the extent of
myometrial invasion by placental vessels. On CDS,
areas of increased flow are seen within the lower
uterine segment. Hypoechoic areas representing
vascular lakes may also be present.

SUMMARY

Transvaginal color Doppler sonography has its major impact in the detection of ectopic pregnancies
that may not be apparent on conventional TVS. Additional applications include evaluation of nonviable intrauterine pregnancies, trophoblastic disease,
and abnormal placental invasion.

REFERENCES

Arduini D, Rizzo G, Boccolini MR, et al. Functional assessment of utero-placental and fetal circulations by
means of color Doppler ultrasonography. J Ultrasound Med 1990;9:249.
Atri M, Bret P, Tulandi T, Senterman MK. Ectopic pregnancy: Evolution after treatment with transvaginal
methotrexate. Radiology 1992;185:749.
Emerson DS, Cartier MS, Altieri LA, et al. Diagnostic efficacy of endovaginal color Doppler flow imaging in
an ectopic pregnancy screening program. Radiology
1992;183:413.
Kurjak A, Zalud I, Predanic M, Kupesic S. Transvaginal
color and pulsed Doppler study of uterine blood flow
in the first and early second trimesters of pregnancy:
Normal versus abnormal. J Ultrasound Med 1994;
13:43.
Tekay A, Martikainen H, Heikkinen H, Kivela A, Jouppila
P. Disappearance of the trophoblastic blood flow in
tubal pregnancy after methotrexate injection. J Ultrasound Med 1993;12:615.

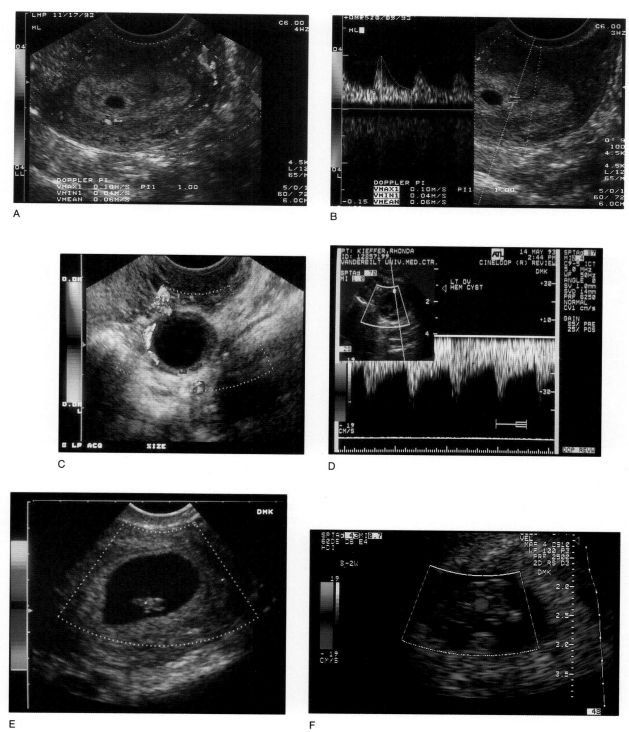

FIGURE 13-1
Normal intrauterine pregnancy. (**A**) TV-CDS showing flow within the myometrium and choriodecidua in a 5-week intrauterine pregnancy. (**B**) Waveform from arteriole within choriodecidua for patient in A. (**C**) Flow within the wall of a corpus luteum in early pregnancy. (**D**) TV-CDS showing low impedance high diastolic flow within this hemorrhagic corpus luteum. (**E**) Flow within the heart of a 6-week embryo. (**F**) Same embryo as in E at 8 weeks, 2 days. (*continued*)

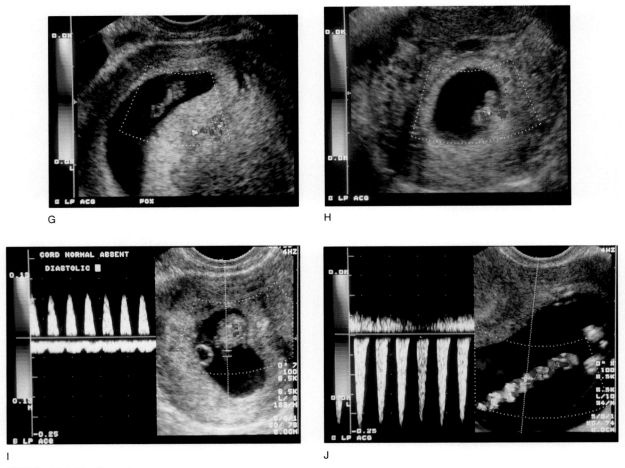

FIGURE 13-1 *(Continued)*
(**G**) CDS demonstrating flow within the cord and yolk sac of a 7-week embryo/fetus. (**H**) Same embryo/fetus as in *G* showing flow within the embryo itself. (**I**) Absent diastolic flow within the cord in a 9-week fetus. (**J**) Absent diastolic flow within the cord of a 10-week fetus. *(continued)*

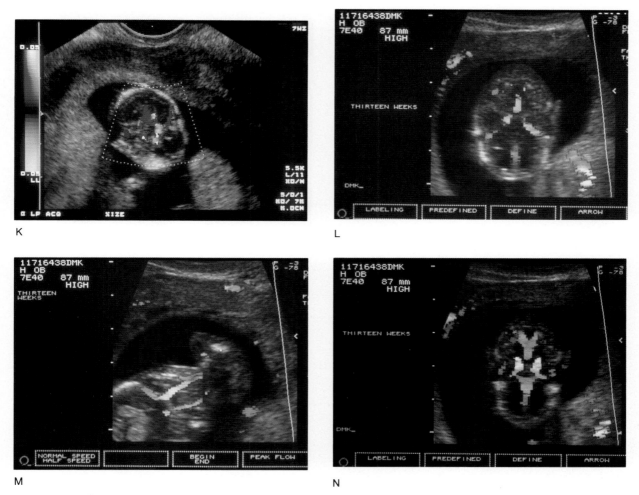

K   L

M   N

FIGURE 13-1 *(Continued)*
(**K**) Flow within the fetal brain of a 12-week fetus. (**L**) Flow within the major intracranial vessels in a 13-week fetus. (**M**) Flow within both right and left common carotids of the fetus in *L*. (**N**) Basilar, middle cerebral, and anterior communicating arteries within the brain of a 13-week fetus.

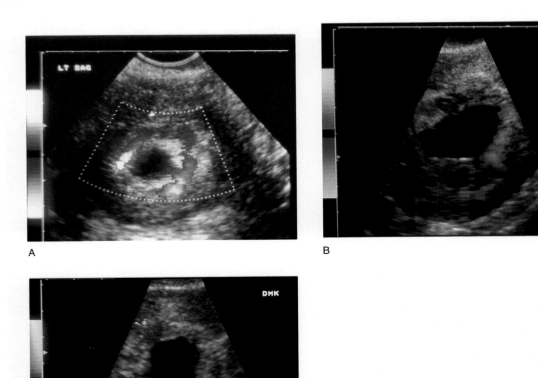

FIGURE 13-2
Nonviable intrauterine pregnancies. (**A**) Increased venous flow surrounding choriodecidua in a failing intrauterine pregnancy. (**B**) Increased venous flow within the choriodecidua surrounding a deflated gestational sac. (**C**) No detectable flow within the irregular choriodecidua of a missed abortion.

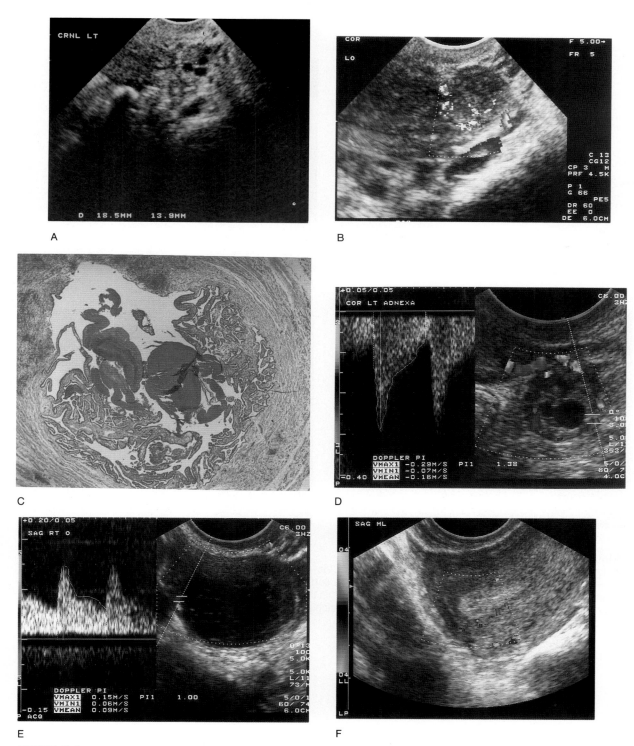

FIGURE 13-3

Ectopic pregnancies. (**A**) TVS of left adnexa demonstrating the left ovary, which contained several 3- to 5-mm follicles. (**B**) CDS of the same patient as in *A* demonstrating a ring around the ectopic pregnancy separate from the ovary. (**C**) Low-power photomicrograph of the patient shown in *A* and *B* demonstrating a 3-mm ectopic pregnancy. (**D**) Ectopic pregnancy in the left adnexa demonstrating high systolic peak flow within the wall of the ectopic pregnancy. (**E**) Same patient as in *D* with the right ovary containing a hemorrhagic corpus luteum with low-impedance flow. (**F**) Same patient as in *D* and *E* demonstrating decreased myometrial flow. (*continued*)

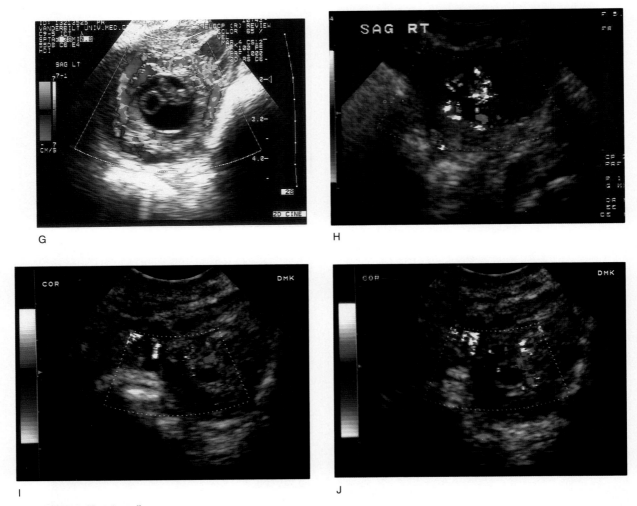

FIGURE 13-3 (Continued)
(G) Hypervascularity surrounding an ectopic pregnancy within the left fallopian tube at 7 weeks since last menstrual period. (H) Ectopic pregnancy adjacent to the corpus luteum in the right ovary. (I) Ectopic pregnancy demonstrating an area of increased flow within the fallopian tube. (J) Same patient as in I showing another area of flow around an unruptured ectopic pregnancy. (continued)

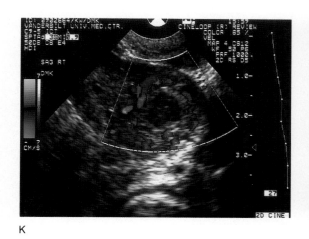

K

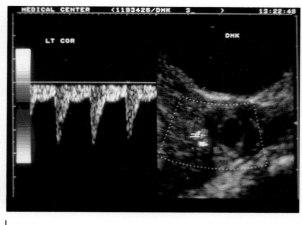

L

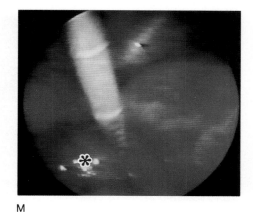

M

FIGURE 13-3 *(Continued)*
(**K**) Ring-like vascularity within the hemorrhagic corpus luteum. (**L**) CDS suggesting possibility of interstitial ectopic pregnancy. (**M**) Image taken at laparoscopy of patient shown in *L* showing fibroma of round ligament (*asterisk*).

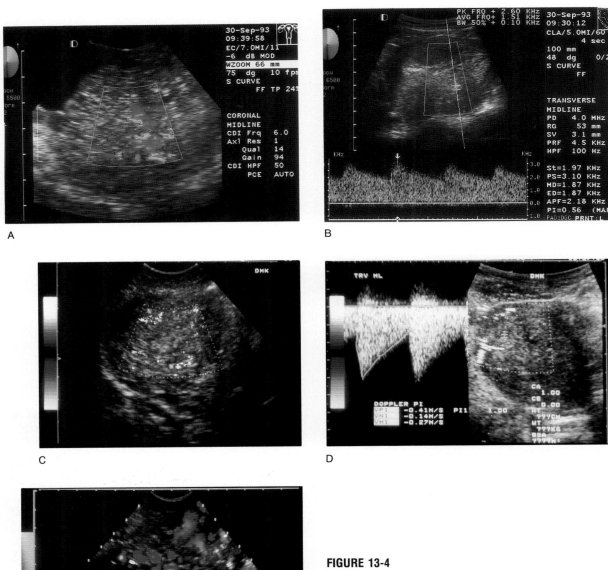

FIGURE 13-4
Trophoblastic disease. (**A**) Focal areas of increased flow within the placenta. (**B**) Same patient as in *A* demonstrating increased diastolic flow in a partial mole. (**C**) Increased flow within an echogenic area within the myometrium in a patient with a history of evacuation of a hydatidiform mole. (**D**) Waveform from vessels within the echogenic mass shown in *C* showing low-impedance, high-velocity flow representing an area of invasive trophoblastic disease. (**E**) Placenta previa percreta shown by increased flow within the myometrium in a patient who had a placenta previa and had a history of previous cesarean section.

Transvaginal Sonography: A Clinical Atlas, Second Edition,
edited by Arthur C. Fleischer and Donna M. Kepple.
J.B. Lippincott Company, Philadelphia, © 1995.

CHAPTER **14**

Transperineal Scanning

Patricia C. Freeman, RDMS, RDCS
Joyce Kelly, RT, RDMS

INTRODUCTION

Delineation of the cervix is part of every obstetric or gynecologic sonographic study. Obstetric patients who have third trimester bleeding should have the region of the internal os evaluated for placenta previa, yet many physicians are wary of introducing a transvaginal transducer into the vagina in these patients. Transabdominal sonography (TAS) often fails to give the details necessary to rule out a placenta previa. Transperineal sonography (TPS) can also help in the evaluation of cervical abnormalities, such as in the incompetent cervix. First described in 1986, TPS has added a new diagnostic dimension to sonographic imaging of the cervical region (Jeanty and coworkers, 1986).

TECHNIQUE

Only minimal preparation of the transducer is necessary to perform a transperineal scan. A small amount of coupling gel is placed in a commercially available condom. The transducer is placed in the condom, and air bubbles are squeezed away from the face of the transducer. If necessary, a rubber band may be used to secure the condom around the neck of the transducer (Fig. 14-1).

To perform a transperineal scan, the patient is positioned in the lithotomy position with legs bent and adducted (frog position). If the examination table has stirrups, they should be used to support the patient's legs. If condoms are not available or do not fit over the transducer, alternative covers are examination gloves or plastic bags.

It is necessary during perineal scans for the patient to have an empty bladder. This allows better visualization of the anatomy and prevents side lobe artifacts as well as anatomic displacement caused by the distended urinary bladder. Because wiping with toilet tissue after voiding may introduce air into the vagina, the patient should be instructed not to wipe after urinating.

The transducer is placed directly on the vestibule with the beam directed in a sagittal scan plane orientation. Better contact is obtained by placing the coupling gel directly on the patient rather than on the probe because the gel is lost going through the pubic hair.

The orientation for this procedure is different from that for TAS and is the same as that for transvaginal sonography (TVS). In the sagittal scan plane, the urinary bladder appears in the upper left position of the screen. The patients's feet are at the top of the screen (i.e., inferior) and the patient's head is at the bottom of the screen (i.e., superior). Anterior is to the left of the screen, and posterior to the right.

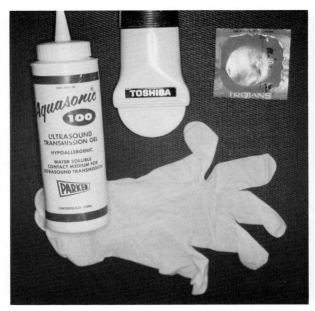
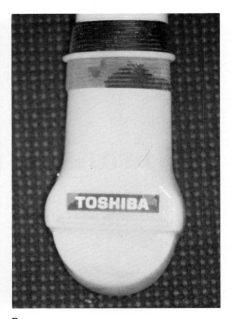

A   B

FIGURE 14-1
(**A**) Materials needed to perform TPS. (**B**) Transducer prepared for TPS.

NORMAL ANATOMY

The orientation for a transperineal scan is shown in Figure 14-2. The pubic bone is in the upper left corner of the image. If a true sagittal scan is taken, the transducer beam readily passes through the symphysis pubis, which is composed of fibrocartilage and hyaline cartilage. If the transducer is on the bone instead of cartilage, acoustic shadowing results, greatly degrading the image.

Directly below the pubic bone, an echo-free area is seen. This is the urinary bladder. Its size depends on the amount of urine present in the bladder at the time of the examination. Preferably, the bladder is almost empty, because a distended bladder displaces the area of interest out of the image. The urethra appears as a hypoechoic tract that exits the bladder toward the perineum at the top of the image.

The vagina is located to the right of the symphysis pubis and urethra. Like the urethra, it is a vertical hypoechoic structure. The hypoechoic portion corresponds to the muscular layer of the vaginal wall. The lumen is echogenic. If possible, a pelvic examination should not be performed before the transperineal scan because a pelvic examination in-

troduces air that is trapped in the rugae of the vaginal canal. The trapped air causes shadowing, resulting in a suboptimal scan.

To the right (posterior) of the vagina is the rectum. The rectum may be filled with a variety of echo patterns depending on its contents.

The cervix is below the vagina, facing the urinary bladder or the transducer. It is recognizable by the typical biconcave shape. The endocervical canal is seen as a thin, echogenic line. A rounded, hypoechoic area can be seen to each side of the canal, joining the isthmus of the uterus.

Only the isthmus of the uterus and cervix can be identified. When information regarding the body or fundus of the uterus is needed, TAS or TVS should be performed.

INDICATIONS FOR A TRANSPERINEAL SCAN

The transperineal scan is a useful adjunct to TAS. It is most beneficial when imaging the cervix, lower uterine segment, or a retroflexed uterus. TAS is better when the fundus of the uterus needs to be evalu-

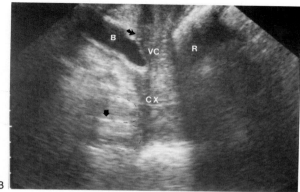

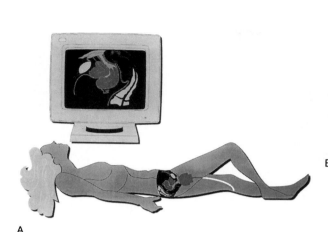

A

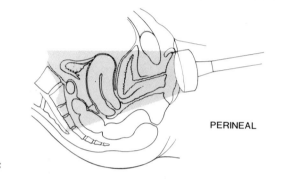

FIGURE 14-2
Transperineal sonography. (**A**) Orientation for TPS. Caudal is at the top of the image and cranial is at the bottom. Anterior is to the left of the image and posterior to the right. (**B**) TPS image. *B*, bladder; *VC*, vaginal canal; *R*, rectum; *CX*, cervix; *arrow*, endocervical canal; *curved arrow*, urethra. The image is displayed as if it is rotated 90°. (**C**) Anatomy shown in TPS. Remember, the image is displayed as if rotated 90°.

C

ated. TVS is excellent for examining the lower uterine segment, adnexa, or early pregnancy, but is contraindicated in a patient with premature rupture of membranes because there is a risk of inducing an ascending infection. TVS may be used in cases of third trimester bleeding and suspicion of placenta previa, but the operator must be careful not to touch the cervix with the transducer.

Several clinical problems may be solved by using TPS. Incompetent cervix during pregnancy is a difficult diagnosis to make. Figure 14-3A demonstrates TAS on a patient with an incompetent cervix. The cervix cannot be clearly visualized. Figure 14-3B is the transperineal scan on the same patient. The dilated proximal endocervical canal can be clearly seen with a cerclage suture in place. Figure 14-3C is the same patient 7 weeks later. Again, the dilated cervix with the cerclage suture in place is noted in Figure 14-3D. Figure 14-4 demonstrates an incompetent cervix on TPS that was not apparent on TAS (see Chap 10).

Placenta previa can be difficult to rule out if the fetal head shadows the lower uterine segment. Figures 14-5 and 14-6 are transperineal scans per-

formed to rule out placenta previa. In Figure 14-6, the fetal head is shown to be snug against the internal os with no placenta previa. At times, TAS cannot delineate the margin of the placenta (Fig. 14-7A). TPS demonstrates a space of 2.4 cm between the inferior edge of the placenta and the internal os, excluding the diagnosis of placenta previa (Fig. 14-7B). Figure 14-8 is an example of a transperineal scan performed on a patient with a complete placenta previa. The internal os is completely covered by the placenta. In the presence of placenta previa, the sonographer should consider placenta accreta. Clinical indications that place the patient at an increased risk include previous cesarean section, myomectomy, dilation and curettage, or any other uterine surgery. There are three degrees of placental invasion of the myometrium. In placenta accreta, the placenta attaches to the myometrium. In placenta increta, the placenta invades the myometrium, and in placenta percreta, the placenta invades through the wall of the myometrium and may even attach to the bladder or other pelvic structures. Figure 14-5E is a perineal scan demonstrating an

(text continues on page 396)

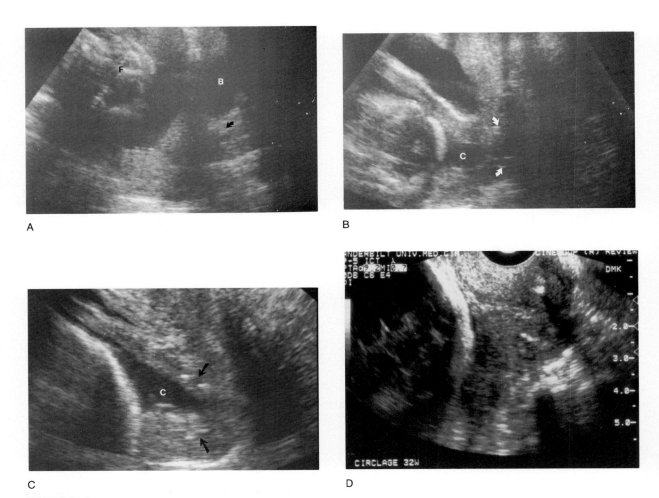

FIGURE 14-3

(A) TAS of a patient with incompetent cervix. The cervix (*curved arrow*) is not well evaluated. *B*, maternal bladder; *F*, fetus. (B) TPS on the same patient as in *A* demonstrating a dilated endocervical canal (*C*) with a cerclage suture in place (*arrows*). (C) Same patient 7 weeks later. Note the dilated endocervical canal with the cerclage sutures. (D) TVS showing sutures of cerclage to be approximately 1 cm deep to the cervix.

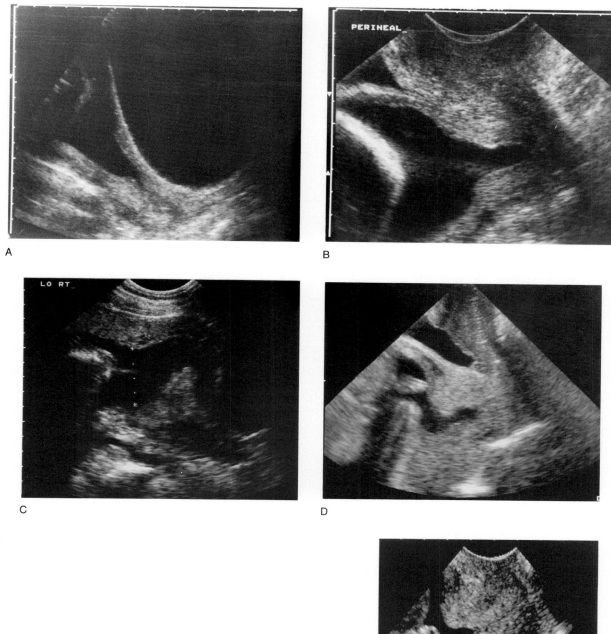

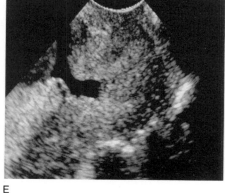

FIGURE 14-4
Incompetent cervix. (**A**) TAS showing a normal-appearing cervix. (**B**) TPS on same patient as shown in **A** showing definite dilation of the endocervical canal. (**C**) TAS showing normal-appearing cervix and lower uterine segment. (**D**) TPS showing slight dilation of the internal cervical os. (**E**) TVS better delineating the cervical length and mild dilation of the internal cervical os. (*continued*)

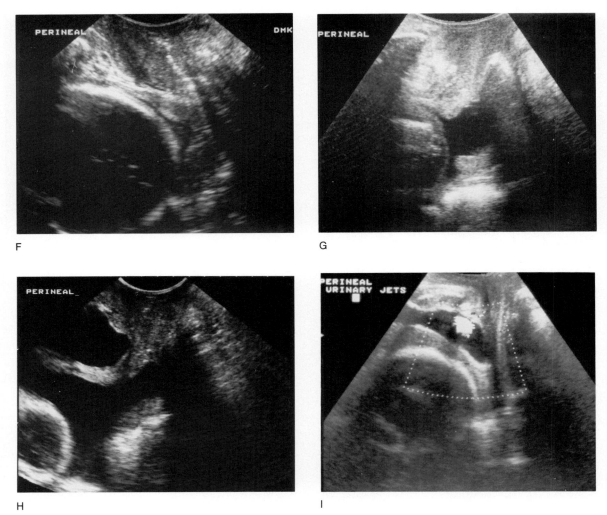

FIGURE 14-4 *(Continued)*
(**F**) TPS showing shortening and effacement of the cervix. (**G**) TPS showing marked cervical dilation.
(**H**) TPS showing marked cervical dilation. (**I**) Color Doppler TPS showing ureteral jet within the
maternal bladder.

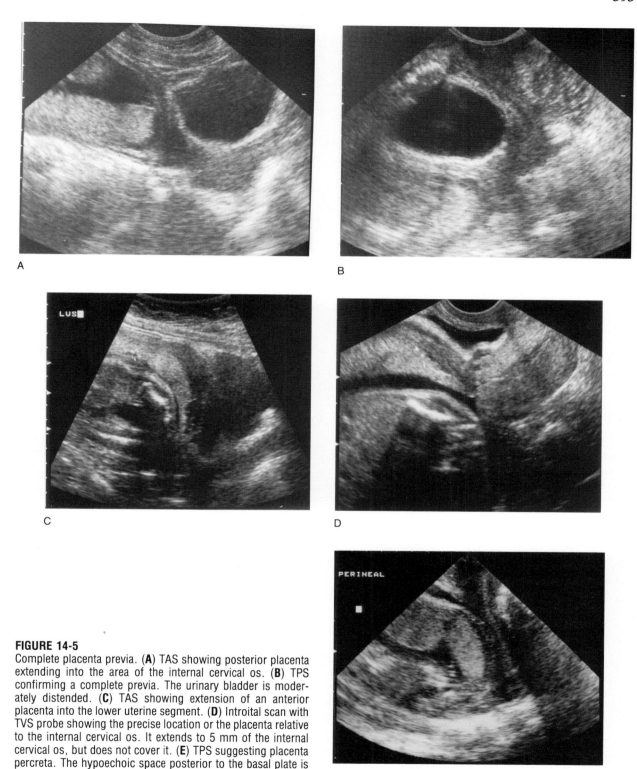

FIGURE 14-5
Complete placenta previa. (**A**) TAS showing posterior placenta extending into the area of the internal cervical os. (**B**) TPS confirming a complete previa. The urinary bladder is moderately distended. (**C**) TAS showing extension of an anterior placenta into the lower uterine segment. (**D**) Introital scan with TVS probe showing the precise location or the placenta relative to the internal cervical os. It extends to 5 mm of the internal cervical os, but does not cover it. (**E**) TPS suggesting placenta percreta. The hypoechoic space posterior to the basal plate is not present. (Courtesy of Thomas Wheeler, M.D.)

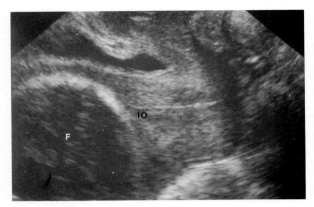

FIGURE 14-6
TPS to rule out placenta previa. The fetal head (*F*) is snug against the internal os (*IO*) with no evidence of placenta previa.

anterior placenta previa with a placenta percreta, which was confirmed by pathologic examination. This diagnosis was made because of a strong suspicion based on clinical history as well as the loss of the retroplacental hypoechoic space on TPS.

An early intrauterine pregnancy in a retroflexed uterus can be difficult to image transabdominally, and documenting fetal heart motion may be impossible because of the attenuation of the sound beam. If a transvaginal transducer is not available, a transperineal scan should be performed. Figure 14-9 is an example of a transperineal scan in a patient with

retroflexed uterus. The gestational sac, fetus, and fetal heart motion are shown.

Urinary stress incontinence has been diagnosed by either the cystourethrogram or a bead-chain cystogram. Genuine urinary stress incontinence in women is associated with a downward and posterior rotational descent of the urethrovesical junction. The increase in intra-abdominal pressure transmitted to the outside of the bladder is then no longer transmitted to the urethra, and urine loss results (Korhorn and coworkers, 1986). Surgery is more beneficial if the anatomic defect can be visualized. TPS to demonstrate the bladder neck and urethra allows all the information previously provided by radiography to be visualized without radiation, catheters, or bead-chains.

Cervical evaluation is difficult in virgins. TAS may not provide the necessary information, and the transvaginal transducer may not be introduced in the virginal vagina. Figure 14-10 is a transperineal scan of a 14-year-old virgin. The patient's transabdominal scan revealed some echoes in her cervix of questionable cause. TPS was performed to better evaluate those echoes. Air bubbles were visualized throughout the vaginal canal. A repeat transperineal scan 1 week later failed to demonstrate any bubbles.

Vaginal atresia has recently been evaluated with TPS. In patients with hydrocolpos/hematocolpos whose obstruction is low lying, TPS can best identify the level of the obstruction and the thickness of the obstructing septum. The study for vaginal atresia is performed with a standoff pad to allow

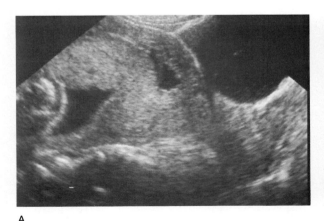

A

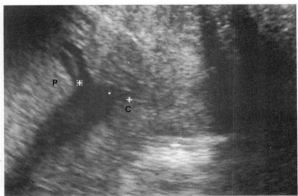

B

FIGURE 14-7
(**A**) Longitudinal midline TAS to rule out placenta previa. The placental edge cannot be delineated from myometrium. (**B**) TPS of the same patient demonstrates a space of 2.4 cm between the placenta (*P*) and internal os of the cervix (*C*), thereby excluding placenta previa.

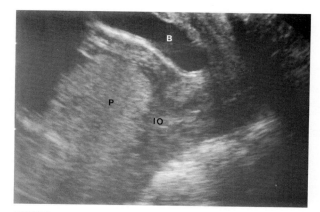

FIGURE 14-8
TPS on a patient with a complete placenta previa. *B*, bladder; *P*, placenta; *IO*, internal os.

TRANSPERINEAL SCANNING IN PEDIATRICS

Pediatric sonography has found TPS to be an excellent adjunct to TAS. Areas in which TPS has proven to be effective include vaginal atresia, anal atresia, vaginal and spinal tumors, and ectopic ureters. TPS is painless, noninvasive and well-accepted by virginal patients. Figure 14-11*A* is a TAS on a 15-month-old child who presented with vaginal bleeding. The scan revealed a pelvic mass, but its origin could not be ascertained. In Figure 14-11*B*, TPS demonstrates the tumor in the vagina. This tumor proved at surgery to be an endodermal sinus tumor. The follow-up TAS 7 months later depicts a normal-appearing vagina, cervix, and uterus (see Fig. 14-11*C*).

SUMMARY

The transperineal scan is a useful supplement to the transabdominal scan (Hertzberg and coworkers, 1991; Mahoney and coworkers, 1990). It is easy to perform, does not require an additional transducer (making the examination cost-efficient), and can be used on young women who are still virgins. Because no transducer is introduced into the vagina, it can be used to assess vaginal bleeding associated with placenta previa. By measuring the urethral angle, information can be obtained for the diagno-

for improved imaging of the superficial structures and a more accurate measurement of the distance from the perineum to the caudal margin of the distended vagina. Once the greatest caudal extension has been ascertained in the sagittal plane, the transducer is rotated to the coronal position. The distance from the perineum to the caudal aspect of the distended vagina is then measured to aid in making decisions concerning surgical reconstruction (Scanlan and coworkers, 1990).

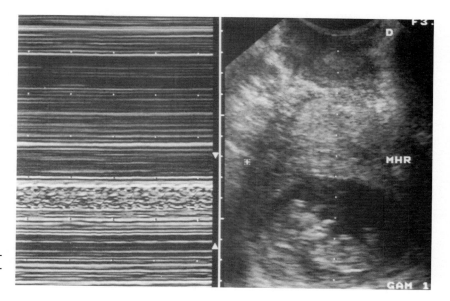

FIGURE 14-9
TPS of a 12-week intrauterine pregnancy with fetal heart motion documented on M-mode.

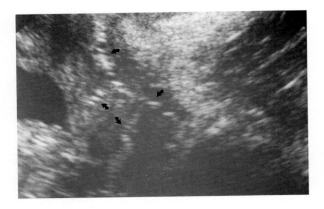

FIGURE 14-10
TPS in a 14-year-old virgin showing echoes within the vagina (*arrows*), probably arising from trapped air after a pelvic examination.

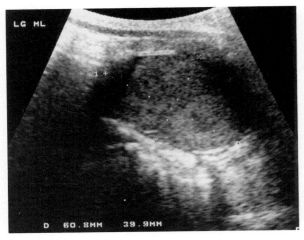

A

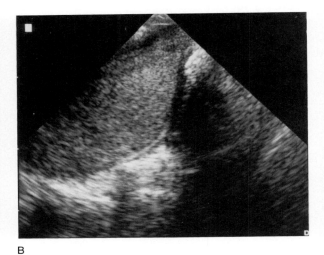

B

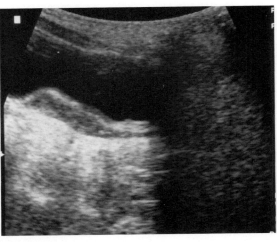

C

FIGURE 14-11
Endodermal sinus tumor in a child. (**A**) TAS showing solid pelvic mass. (**B**) TPS of the same mass in relation to the anteriorly displaced uterus. (**C**) TAS 7 months later showing regression of the mass.

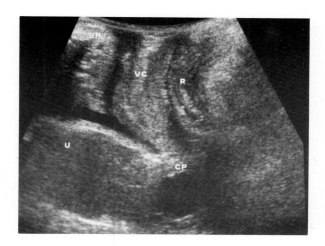

FIGURE 14-12
TPS of a patient with a cervical pregnancy. TVS gave the most information and TAS the least. When TVS is not available, TPS should be the method of choice to evaluate the cervical region. *SP*, symphysis pubis; *VC*, vaginal canal; *R*, rectum; *U*, uterus; *CP*, cervical pregnancy.

sis of urinary stress incontinence. Therefore, when additional information about the cervical area is needed, TPS should be performed (Fig. 14-12).

REFERENCES

Hertzberg BJ, Bowie J, Weber T, et al. Sonography of the cervix during the third trimester pregnancy: Value of the transperineal approach. AJR 1991;157:73.

Jeanty P, d'Altan M, Romero R, Hobbins J. Perineal scanning. Am J Perinatol 1986;3:289.

Korhorn E, Scioscia A, Jeanty P, Hobbins J. Ultrasound cystourethrography by perineal scanning for the assessment of female stress urinary incontinence. Obstet Gynecol 1986;68:269.

Mahoney B, Nyberg D, Luthy D. Translabial ultrasound of the third trimester uterine cervix. J Ultrasound Med 1990;9:717.

Scanlan K, Pozniak M, Fagerholm M, Shapiro S. Value of transperineal sonography in the assessment of vaginal atresia. AJR 1990;154:545.

Transvaginal Sonography: A Clinical Atlas, Second Edition,
edited by Arthur C. Fleischer and Donna M. Kepple.
J.B. Lippincott Company, Philadelphia, © 1995.

CHAPTER **15**

Transrectal Sonography

Arthur C. Fleischer, MD

INTRODUCTION

Transrectal sonography (TRS) can be used in several gynecologic conditions. The same probe used for prostate imaging in men can be applied for visualization of the uterus and adnexal regions and cul-de-sac in women. Although the transrectal approach is not as close to the uterus as transvaginal scanning, it allows the sonographer to have unencumbered access to the vagina for certain intraoperative procedures. Thus, the main applications of this type of scanning are for intraoperative guidance, for difficult dilation and curettage procedures when there is an abnormal cervix, for localization of the cervix for tandem placement for intracavitary radiation when there are cervical abnormalities, for extraction of intrauterine contraceptive devices that may be difficult to retrieve, and for guidance for cerclage in abnormal cervices. Additionally, it may be useful in the evaluation of patients with suspected cystocele or enterocele or lower urinary tract disorder.

INSTRUMENTATION AND SCANNING TECHNIQUES

There are several types of transrectal probes. These include probes that have biplane imaging capabilities (sagittal and axial) and those probes that use a single-element transducer that is rotated in a radial fashion (Fig. 15-1). The biplane probe is preferred for intraoperative guidance of intrauterine procedures. Initially, the cervix is located in its long axis with the longitudinally oriented linear array transducer. The field of view can be confirmed on an image obtained with the axial transducer typically located at the end of the probe.

As opposed to transducer-probe preparation for the transvaginal probe, the transrectal probe has only water placed between the probe and the condom interface. Then fluid within the condom (20 to 33 mL) surrounding the transducer provides adequate transmission through the condom and into the area of interest. Gel is applied to the outer surface of the condom to provide optimal through transmission through the rectal wall.

When the biplane is used intraoperatively, metal objects such as retractors block the ultrasound transmission. Therefore, the smallest retractor possible must be held out of the plane of the incident beam for adequate delineation of the uterus.

NORMAL ANATOMY

As imaged in the long axis on TRS the uterus appears as a pear-shaped structure. Typically, the mucous within the endocervical canal appears as an angled echogenic interface with the remainder of the endometrium being thicker than the endocervi-

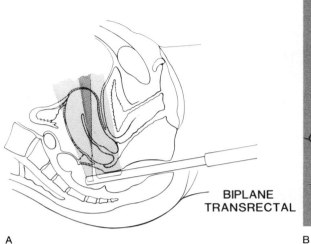

BIPLANE
TRANSRECTAL

A

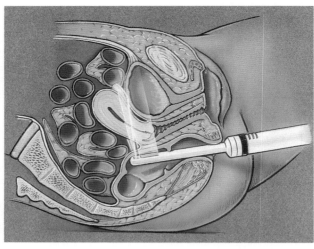

B

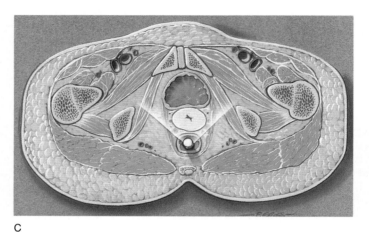

C

FIGURE 15-1
(**A**) Diagram of imaging planes obtained by biplane transrectal transducer-probe. The longitudinally oriented linear array images in the sagittal plane, whereas the axially oriented curvilinear array at the tip of the probe images in the axial plane. (**B**) Field of view of TPS using the sagittally oriented transducer elements. (**C**) Same as B when axially oriented transducer elements are activated.

cal canal (Fig. 15-2). On axial images, the cervix appears as a rounded structure with a central echogenic area representing the endocervical canal. Usually the adnexal regions appear as moderately echogenic areas with no significant soft tissue intervening between bowel and the rectal wall.

Because of the proximity of the transrectal probe to the cervix, it is not uncommon to see small (2 to 3 mm), well-defined hypoechoic structures near the endocervical canal that represent distended endocervical glands. Nabothian cysts can also be demonstrated as cystic structures in this region, but are usually larger than 5 mm. Along the lateral aspects of the upper cervix, punctuate hypoechoic structures can be demonstrated that represent the perforating branches of the uterine artery. These vessels usually enter the myometrium at the level of the internal cervical os and can serve as a landmark for this region of the uterus.

INTRAOPERATIVE GUIDANCE

Transrectal sonography is helpful in difficult cases in which the cervical os may not be apparent to the operator on visual inspection (Fleischer and coworkers, 1990, 1995). Such cases occur when there is cervical stenosis, cervical carcinoma, or a malformed cervix (Figs. 15-3 and 15-4). Scanning through the transrectal approach allows the operator to manipulate instrumentation vaginally.

This approach can be used for initial localization of the cervix before dilation and curettage. It can also be used to locate the cervical lumen when an intrauterine tandem is required before intracavitary radiation (Fig. 15-5). This technique has also been used in localizing the cervical tissue for cerclage, particularly in patients who have had previous conization (Figs. 15-6 and 15-7) (Fleischer and coworkers, 1989).

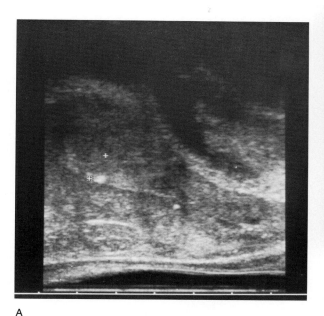
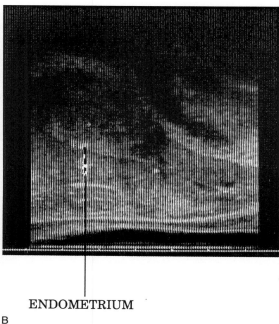

ENDOMETRIUM

A
B

FIGURE 15-2
Normal uterus shown from transrectal approach. Endometrial thickness measured by cursors. (**A**) TRS image. (**B**) Line drawing of **A**.

DIAGNOSIS OF CYSTOCELE AND ENTEROCELE

Transrectal sonography can be used for diagnosis and differentiation of cystocele from rectocele. Cystoceles appear as cystic structures contiguous with the bladder lumen (Fig. 15-8). The structure usually enlarges and protrudes inferiorly when the patient strains. Enteroceles appear as echogenic structures that lie between the bladder and the rectum.

OTHER APPLICATIONS

Transrectal sonography has been used for evaluation of patients with stress urinary incontinence (Bergman and coworkers, 1988). The advantage of this technique over transperineal scanning is that the area is not deformed by the pressure from the transducer itself. Criteria have been established for abnormal displacement of the urethra, as documented by a change in the interface arising from a Q-tip in the urethra. Abnormal angulation and motility of more than 1.5 cm has been defined as abnormal, indicative of stress urinary incontinence (Bergman and coworkers, 1988). Some investigators

have used TRS for diagnosis of recurrence of ovarian and uterine neoplasms (Squillaci and coworkers, 1988). With recurrent tumor, hypoechoic masses in the region of the vaginal cuff have been described.

Using the radially oriented probe, some researchers have evaluated the anus for perianal abscesses and fistula. Using this technique, disruptions in the typical five-layered interface appearance arising from the colon in the area of the internal sphincter can be identified (Law and coworkers, 1989). Intersphincteric abscesses and retained or foreign material, such as sutures and other abnormalities surrounding the anus, can be identified using this technique. TRS can be used to guide needle aspirations of cul-de-sac fluid or pus (Alexander and coworkers, 1994).

SUMMARY

This chapter describes the application of TRS for a variety of gynecologic disorders. It is most useful in intraoperative guidance, but can also be used for diagnosis of enterocele and cystocele (Figs. 15-9 through 15-12).

(text continues on page 415)

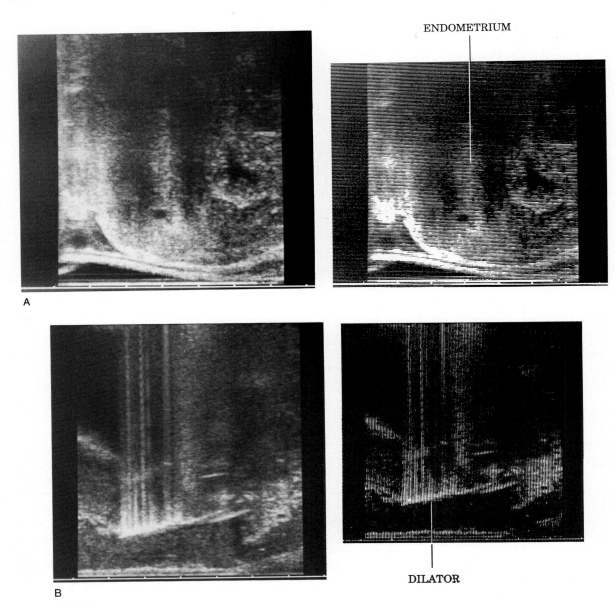

FIGURE 15-3
It was initially difficult to cannulate the cervical os in a patient with thickened endometrium and postmenopausal bleeding. TRS provided guidance for dilatation and curettage. (**A**) Transrectal sagittal scan showing thickened endometrium in an anteflexed uterus. (**B**) Dilator directed posteriorly, causing initial attempts to pass the dilator to be unsuccessful. (*continued*)

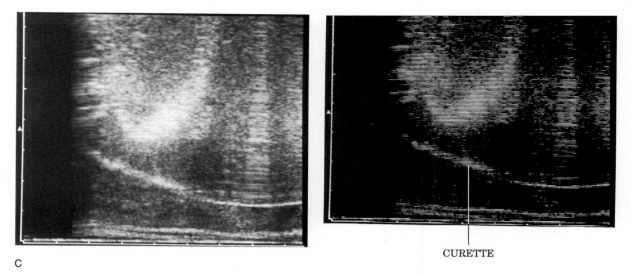

C

CURETTE

FIGURE 15-3 *(Continued)*
(**C**) More anterior direction of the dilator, allowing the cervical canal to be entered and endometrium to be curetted. A mildly distended bladder coupled with posterior pressure on the rectum by the condom-covered probe helped straighten out the uterus to facilitate curettage.

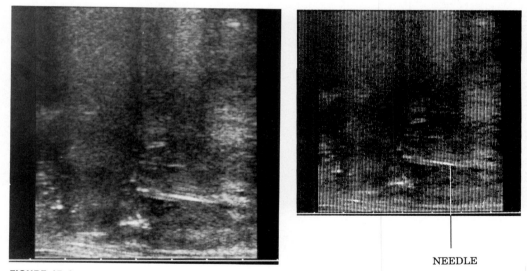

NEEDLE

FIGURE 15-4
Guidance into a blind-ended duplicated cervix in a patient who had purulent discharge.

FIGURE 15-5
Guided Intrauterine Tandem Placement in a Patient With Extensive Cervical Carcinoma

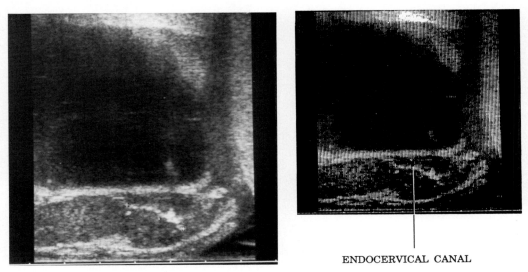

ENDOCERVICAL CANAL

Figure 15-5A. Endocervical canal localized in the long axis.

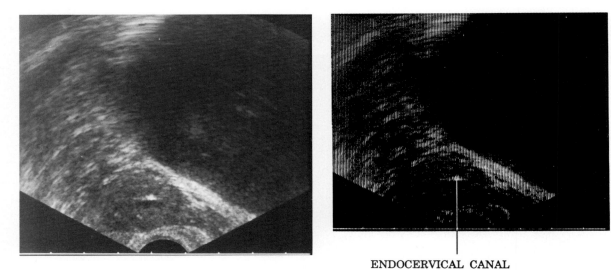

ENDOCERVICAL CANAL

Figure 15-5B. Endocervical canal localized in the short axis.

Guided Intrauterine Tandem Placement in a Patient With Extensive Cervical Carcinoma *(Continued)*

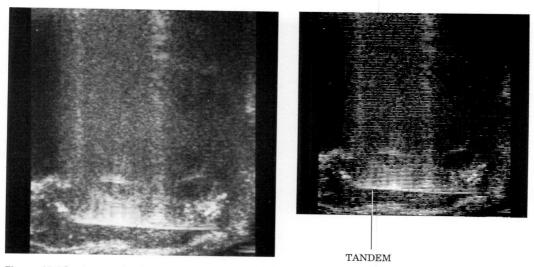

TANDEM

Figure 15-5C. Long axis view confirming that the tandem was in proper position in the uterine lumen.

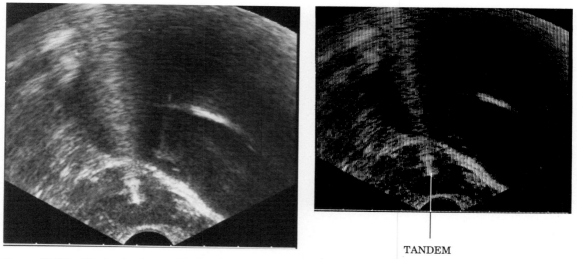

TANDEM

Figure 15-5D. Short axis view confirming that the tandem was in proper position in the uterine lumen.

FIGURE 15-6
Cerclage Placement in a Patient Status Post Three Conizations

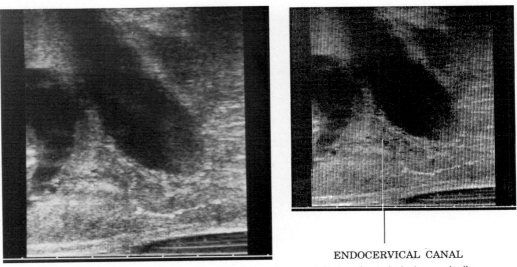

Figure 15-6A. Initial transrectal sonogram showing a shortened (2.1 cm) cervix in long axis (between cursors).

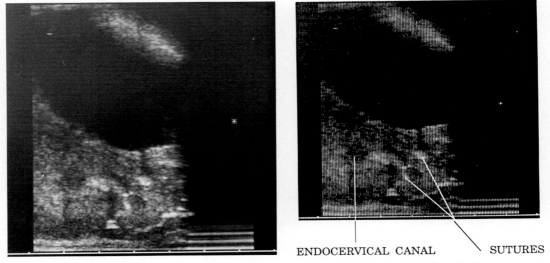

Figure 15-6B. Suture in place around the endocervical canal, approximately 1 cm deep to the external os as seen in the long and short axes. The circular course of the suture could be appreciated on the axial scan.

FIGURE 15-7
Confirmation of Normal Cervix After Cerclage

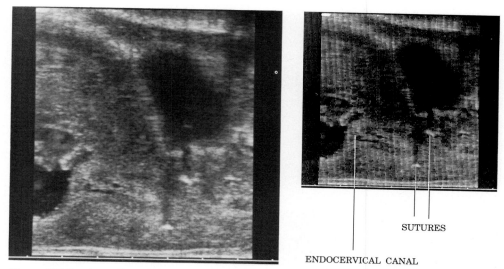

SUTURES

ENDOCERVICAL CANAL

Figure 15-7A. A nondistended endocervical canal as well as the suture within the lower posterior of the cervix.

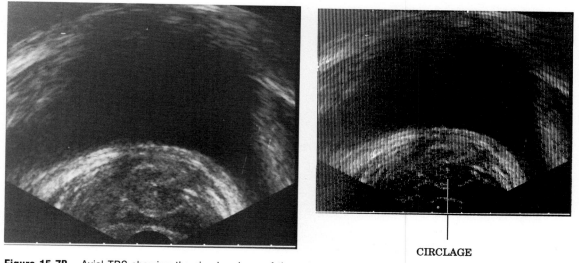

CIRCLAGE

Figure 15-7B. Axial TRS showing the circular shape of the suture.

FIGURE 15-8
Transrectal Sonography of Cystocele

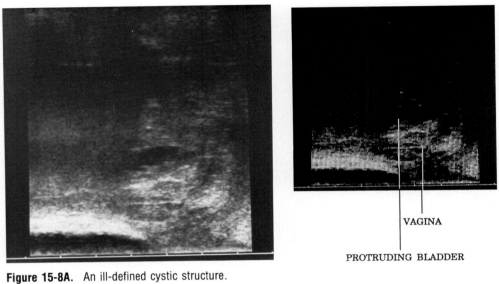

Figure 15-8A. An ill-defined cystic structure.

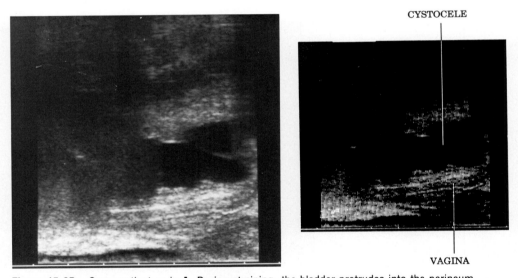

Figure 15-8B. Same patient as in **A.** During straining, the bladder protrudes into the perineum.

FIGURE 15-9
Uterine Perforation

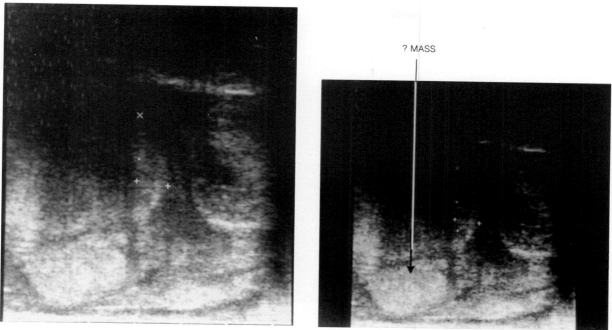

Figure 15-9A. Initial TRS showing anteflexed uterus with thickened endometrium (between cursors). There is an ill-defined ecogenic mass posterior to the uterus.

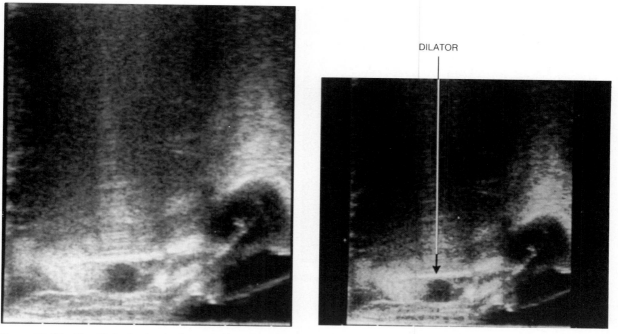

Figure 15-9B. The dilator inadvertently passed into the echogenic structure, which represents colon.

FIGURE 15-10
Transrectally Guided Cul-De-Sac Aspiration of Pus

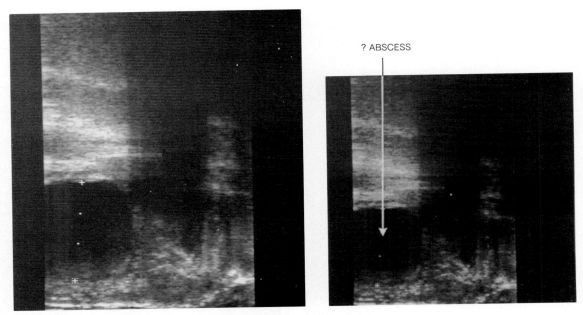

Figure 15-10A. Initial sagittal view showing fluid collection in the cul-de-sac.

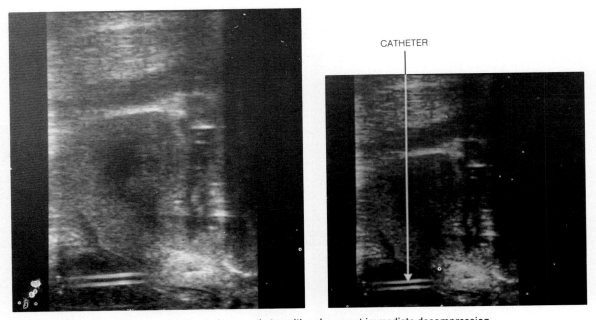

Figure 15-10B. Guided placement of a drainage catheter with subsequent immediate decompression of the pus collection.

FIGURE 15-11
Transperineal Use of Transvaginal Probe in a Patient Who Had a Nonspecific Fluid Collection Status After Pelvic Exoneration

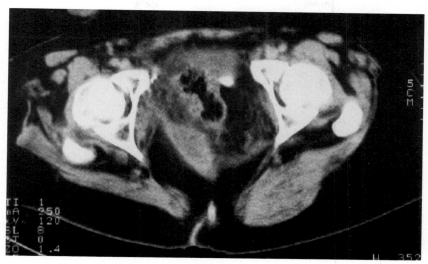

Figure 15-11A. CT scan shows an ill-defined soft tissue density adjacent to bowel loops.

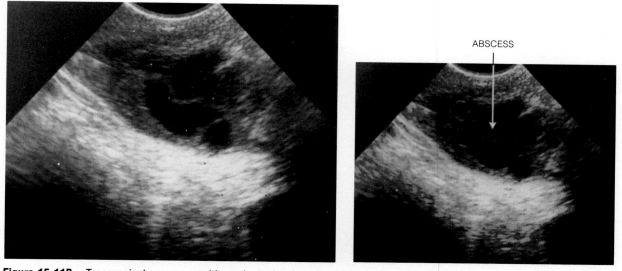

Figure 15-11B. Transvaginal sonogram with markers showing a multiloculated fluid collection.

Transperineal Use of Transvaginal Probe in a Patient Who Had a Nonspecific Fluid Collection Status After Pelvic Exoneration *(Continued)*

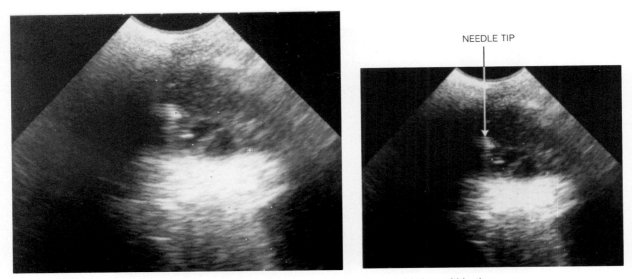

Figure 15-11C. Same as *B*, taken when needle tip (echogenic interfaces) as guided to within the abscess. This patient's fever immediately defervesced and she was discharged the next day.

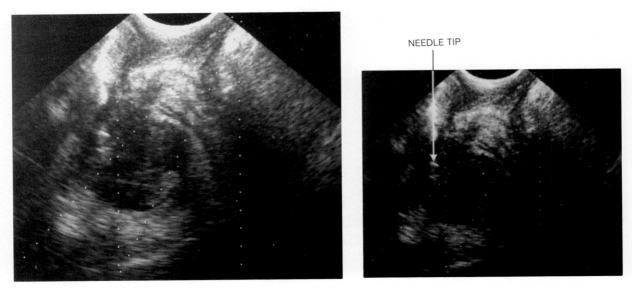

FIGURE 15-12
Transperineal sonographically guided biopsy of a solid lesion. The needle tip is seen within the recurrent tumor.

REFERENCES

Alexander A, Eschelman D, Nazavian L, Bonn J. Transrectal sonographically guided drainage of deep pelvic abscesses. AJR 1994;162:1227.

Bergman A, Vermesh R, Platt I. Ultrasonic evaluation of UVJ in women with stress urinary incontinence. J Clin Ultrasound 1988;16:295.

Fleischer A, Burnett L, Jones H, Murphy M. Transrectal sonography for guidance of intraoperative uterine procedures. Radiology 1990;176:576.

Fleischer A, Jones H, Burnett L. Transrectal and transperineal sonography for guided intrauterine procedures. Ultrasound Med (in press) 1995.

Fleischer A, Lombardi S, Kepple D. Transrectal sonography for guidance during cerclage. J Ultrasound Med 1989;8:589.

Law P, Talbot R, Bartram C. Anal endosonography in the evaluation of perianal sepsis and fistula in ano. Br J Surg 1989;76:752.

Squillaci E, Salzani M, Grandinetti M, Auffermann W. Recurrence of ovarian and uterine neoplasms: Diagnosis with transrectal US. Radiology 1988;169:355.

Index

Page numbers followed by *f* indicate figures; page numbers followed by *t* indicate tabular material.